INTRODUCTION TO NURSING

INTRODUCTION TO NURSING

MAY SPENCER

S.R.N. S.C.M. R.N.T.
Diploma of Nursing (London University)
Senior Tutor
Queen Elizabeth School of Nursing,
United Birmingham Hospitals

AND

KATHERINE M. TAIT

S.R.N. S.C.M. H.V.Cert. Q.I.D.N. O.H.N.
Formerly Education Officer, Education Centre,
Royal College of Nursing, Birmingham

THIRD EDITION

BLACKWELL SCIENTIFIC PUBLICATIONS
OXFORD LONDON EDINBURGH MELBOURNE

ISBN 0 632 09580 6

FIRST PUBLISHED 1965
REVISED REPRINT 1968
SECOND EDITION 1970
THIRD EDITION 1973

Printed in Great Britain by
WESTERN PRINTING SERVICES LTD, BRISTOL
and bound by
THE KEMP HALL BINDERY, OXFORD

This book is dedicated to
PATIENTS, NURSES IN TRAINING
AND THEIR TEACHERS

CONTENTS

Preface ix

Suggestions for the Use of this Book xi

SECTION 1 | PRINCIPLES AND PRACTICE OF NURSING

PART 1 | INTRODUCTION

1 The Development of Nursing 3
2 The National Health Service and the Place of the Nurse in the Service 8
3 The Function of Hospital Departments 19
4 The Nurse and Professional Relationships 21
5 Personal Development of the Individual 25
6 The Promotion of Individual and Communal Health 29
  Further Reading 32

PART 2 | THE ENVIRONMENT OF THE PATIENT (INCLUDING THE CARE OF THE WARD UNIT)

7 Ward Routine 34
8 Ventilation, Heating and Lighting 37
9 Elimination of Noise 44
10 Care and Use of Ward Equipment 47
11 The Ward Kitchen and Ward Meals 51
12 Precautions against Fire 55
  Further Reading 57

PART 3 | NURSING CARE OF THE PATIENT

13 Nursing Care of the Patient 58
14 Progressive Patient Care 77
15 Intensive Nursing Care 79

PART 4 | ROUTINE PROCEDURES

16 Routine Nursing Procedures 85
17 Routine Observations and Reports 120
18 Nursing Care of the Unconscious Patient 130
19 Care of the Dying and Last Offices 134
  Further Reading 136

PART 5 | PAEDIATRICS, GERIATRICS AND
YOUNG CHRONIC SICK

20   Paediatric Nursing   137
21   Nursing Old People and the Young Chronic Sick   145
     Further Reading   147

SECTION 2 | CAUSES OF DISEASE AND
TREATMENT

22   First Aid: Emergencies: Major Disasters   151
23   Medicines and Poisons   160
24   Inflammation and Infection   170
25   Surgery: Bandaging   199
26   Tumours   217
27   Radiotherapy   218
     Further Reading   220

SECTION 3 | STRUCTURE AND FUNCTIONS OF
ORGANS: COMMON SIGNS AND SYMPTOMS:
CLINICAL INVESTIGATIONS: SOME MEDICAL
AND SURGICAL CONDITIONS WITH RELEVANT
NURSING TECHNIQUES

28   Structure of the Human Body   223
29   The Skin   226
30   Movement   240
31   The Cardio-Vascular System   278
32   Respiration and the Respiratory Tract   304
33   Nutrition   326
34   The Alimentary Tract   337
35   Metabolism   367
36   Excretion   372
37   The Nervous System   388
38   Sight   405
39   Ear, Nose and Throat   418
40   The Mouth   438
41   Regulation of Body Temperature   449
42   The Endocrine Glands   455
43   The Reproductive System   464
44   Other Aspects of Nursing Service   490
     Further Reading   496

Index   499

PREFACE

'The unique function of the nurse is to assist the individual, sick or well, in the performance of those activities contributing to health or its recovery (or to peaceful death) that he would perform unaided, if he had the necessary strength, will or knowledge. And to do this in such a way to help him gain independence as rapidly as possible.'*

We recommend the nurse in training to read the above definition carefully and to keep it in mind throughout her career.

This book has been written for the pupil nurse and we have used as a guide to the 1964 syllabus of training for pupil nurses. However, it has been so planned that it will also serve as an introductory text for the student nurse. We have not attempted to cover every illness or aspect of nursing but we have concentrated on Basic Principles of Nursing Care in relation to medical and surgical treatment in hospital.

We hope that through our method of presenting these principles, and by observation and practice in the wards and departments of your hospital, you will be able to lay down such sound foundations in the art and science of nursing that you will be able to build up slowly and carefully a deep understanding of the needs of your patients in all circumstances and develop compassionate nursing skills.

MAY SPENCER
KATHERINE M. TAIT

---

* *Basic Principles of Nursing Care* prepared by Virginia Henderson R.N. M.A., for the Nursing Service Committee of the International Council of Nurses.

A*

SUGGESTIONS FOR THE USE
OF THIS BOOK

This is a book for *reading*. It will be useful to read something from it every day. The practice of nursing will be learned at the bedside of the patients in the hospital wards, but *understanding* the practice of nursing comes from listening, *reading*, discussing and thinking about nursing.

Before becoming a member of a ward team in the hospital it will be helpful to read:

    Introduction
    The environment of the patient
    Basic nursing care
    Routine nursing procedures.

During practical instruction and experience in a particular ward, it will be useful to read the chapter or chapters which are related to the medical and nursing treatments given to the patients on that ward. Several of these chapters are presented in sections as appropriate:

    Structure and function of organs in the system
    Maintenance of health in these organs
    Special care during illness
    Common signs and symptoms in disease
    Observations
    Clinical investigations
    Some common medical and surgical conditions and treatment
    Special nursing care in some cases
    Nursing procedures.

It may then be interesting to read 'Basic Nursing Care' again, bearing in mind the patient being treated and nursed in the ward. Perhaps it will be possible to make one's own notes about nursing care and treatment given to the patient.

After observing a procedure or receiving instruction on the way in which it is carried out in the ward or practical classroom, reading about it helps in remembering the details and understanding the principles involved. At the same time information on the structure and function of the parts of the body concerned with the procedure would make it more meaningful.

The list of chapter headings at the front of the book and the Index at the end of the book are included so that the subject matter may be found easily.

At the end of most sections there is a list of books for reference and further reading. An English Dictionary and a Nurses' Dictionary should always be to hand.

In addition to reading the textbook, a small stiff-covered notebook in the nurse's pocket for very short notes on new or unfamiliar procedures would be useful for future reference. The hospital and training school may have a special procedure book which is consulted regarding procedures the nurse will carry out.

Later on the nurse will find more new books to read. Articles in the nursing press will keep her informed of advances in patient care. Taking an interest in work going on in other wards and departments extends her nursing knowledge. Radio and television and the general press have items of medical and nursing interest.

The main theme throughout every different part of the nurse's training is the bedside care of the patient, and her concern is maintaining its highest possible standard.

SECTION 1 | PRINCIPLES AND PRACTICE OF NURSING

PART 1 | INTRODUCTION

CHAPTER 1 | THE DEVELOPMENT OF NURSING

In this country we have a health service which is available to everybody whatever his age, colour, religion, financial position or disease. It is paid for by the earning members of the community through an Insurance Scheme and through taxation. Doctors and nurses employed in this great service are well trained and highly skilled. You have joined this group and will receive not only training and an allowance but respectful recognition from the community. This has not always been the case and it is exciting to look at the way in which our profession has developed, not only in this country but internationally, over the centuries.

The four main influences on nursing throughout the Ages have been Religion, Politics, the State of Medicine and the Status of Women in the country concerned. These influences have both advanced and retarded nursing as they have every other facet of human progress. It is important to remember that nursing cannot be isolated from current events.

Religion

In earliest times life was hard but simple. The men hunted and the women stayed behind in the family or communal cave and looked after the young, old and sick members of the tribe. The word NURSE comes from the Latin NUTRIRE, meaning to nourish or cherish.

As Man developed, his pattern of life became more complicated and we know that many primitive peoples believed (and still do) that they were surrounded by supernatural powers which could either protect or harm them.

Certain members of their tribe appeared to be given special gifts of magic by which they could protect their fellow tribesmen from harm and drive out evil spirits from diseased bodies. These people were known as witch doctors and medicine men.

Gradually these supernatural powers were given names and the form of men or animals and were called Gods. They had earthly servants known as priests who studied the use of plants in the treatment of disease as well as other ways of appeasing these gods. They became the first physicians. Temples were built so that the gods could be worshipped with greater pomp and ceremony and the sick were often housed in these temples and cared for both by the priests and by temple-women or priestesses.

The Egyptians have left us descriptions of these temples and of the medical and nursing work carried out in them.

In the Book of Leviticus Chapters XI–XV there is a record of the remarkably high standards of personal and communal hygiene practised by the Jewish tribes who had been much influenced by the Egyptians during their years with them as captives. The name of the first nurse ever recorded, *Deborah*, a Jewess, is to be found in the Book of Genesis Chapter XXXVIII v. viii.

Some of the sacred books of India give us the first definition of a nurse. In the surgical book of the Vedas, written about 1600 B.C., a nurse is described as follows:

> 'NURSE. That person alone is fit to nurse or to attend the bedside of a patient who is cool-headed and pleasant in his demeanour, does not speak ill of anybody, is strong and attentive to the requirements of the sick, and strictly and indefatigably follows the instructions of the physician.'

In the medical book we find:

> 'NURSE: Knowledge of the manner in which drugs should be prepared and compounded for administration; cleverness, devotedness to the patient waited upon, and purity (both of mind and body) are the four qualifications of the attending nurse.'

Obviously nurses in India at that time, because of the strong influence of religions, were most carefully selected. We know also that they held sub-priestly rank and were either men or women.

Medicine and nursing received their greatest impetus through the doctrines of Christ and the subsequent decline in the fear of supernatural powers by those people who accepted His teachings that there was only one God and He was a God of Love and that all human life was sacred. In order to follow this teaching, the early Christians set a high standard in caring for their fellow men in health and sickness and it became a Christian duty for dedicated women known as deaconesses to nurse the sick.

As Christianity spread through Asia Minor and Europe, so the sick, the old and the orphans were cared for as never before, either in small hospitals, in private homes known as diakonia, such as that founded by Fabiola, or increasingly in hospitals within a religious community which included hostels as well as churches. One such hospital was built by *Basil the Great, Bishop of Caesarea* (A.D. 329–379) in Asia Minor. It was a small city with streets of houses set aside for every kind of sick or infirm person. There were nurseries for foundlings and schools for children as well as accommodation for physicians and nurses. It is interesting to note that a modified form of this plan is now being acclaimed as a 'new idea' for hospital development in this country.

As the Church developed, various Religious Orders for both men and women were founded. Some had special duties with regard to education and others to nursing. The oldest religious nursing order of nuns is that of the Augustinian Sisters of the Hôtel-Dieu, Paris, founded in A.D. 650. There is a very touching story told of the nuns standing in the River Seine in order to wash the Hospital's linen: the Big Wash on Mondays and the Small Wash on Fridays.

In this country, when Henry VIII dissolved the monasteries, there were no longer any centres for the education of women or for treating the sick, and nursing entered its Darkest Age. Conditions for the sick, the poor and the old became so bad that the king had to refound three London hospitals—St Bartholomew's, St Thomas's and St Mary of Bethlehem (a mental hospital).

St. Bartholomew's is the oldest of London's hospitals and still stands on the site where it was founded by a monk named Rohere in 1123. With its refounding, however, the nursing was performed by women with no particular religious calling and gradually it became harder and harder to maintain the high standards of loving care given by the religious nursing orders. This was the situation in most of the hospitals in this country. As the Church's influence declined so did the community's social conscience, and it was not stirred again to any great extent until men like George Fox, the founder of the Society of Friends (Quakers), John and Charles Wesley the Evangelists, and Charles Dickens the writer, so caught the imagination of the nation that long overdue social and economic reforms were begun. The two women to whom nurses in this country owe so much are *Elizabeth Fry* and *Florence Nightingale*. Both these reformers were inspired by strong religious faith.

It is very difficult today for nursing to maintain its newly found traditions of loving care and selfless service when many sections of the community give increasingly more importance to working shorter hours for higher salaries, and when there are apparently fewer and fewer dedicated men and women to form the backbone and inspiration of the Service. If, however, we believe that our patients should be nursed by skilled hands guided by loving hearts and intelligent heads, we must strive to find a balance between religious and material idealism.

Politics

We have already seen how religion influenced the lives of peoples in many nations. This is also true of politics especially when national pride leads to war. In early times, however, one of the few good things to emerge from the many conflicts that raged between nations was the spread of medical and nursing knowledge from the centres of learning in Greece and Rome.

In this country we have excellent examples of the high standards of sanitation and hygiene enjoyed by the Romans, who built fine camps and towns during their occupation of these islands.

The Crusades or Holy Wars resulted in the formation of the Order of St John of Jerusalem, and the Crimean War gave Miss Nightingale the opportunity she was looking for to put into practice many of her ideas for Army and Nursing reform. Out of the Battle of Solferino came the International Red Cross.

At the beginning of the Second World War nursing in this country received a severe set-back when it was decided by the Government that during the emergency there should no longer be an educational standard of entry into the nursing profession. It took us over twenty years to get that decision reversed for entrants for training for the General Registers.

The extent to which nursing is now influenced by politics will be discussed in the next chapter on the National Health Service.

State of Medicine

We have traced the development of nursing and seen how it has been influenced by religion and politics. Medicine has developed under the same influences. Physicians, because of their religious beginnings, have always been held in high esteem, but Surgeons have had to work extremely hard to break down prejudice. This was caused by the first surgery being performed by barbers, who were considered to be artisans and not professional men.

As scientific knowledge widens and deepens so medicine advances. Nursing must keep abreast but it will only do so if those who wish to nurse are most carefully selected.

Status of Women

Some of the older civilisations such as Greece and Rome gave women equal status to that of men, and so women with ability, education and money were able to travel or make careers for themselves outside the home. The work done by *Fabiola* and her friend *Paula* was possible because of these circumstances. From the end of the 17th century until the beginning of the present century, British women were kept very much in the background and were only expected to excel in home management and the arts of painting and music. It took great courage for intelligent and dedicated women like Elizabeth Fry and Florence Nightingale to break away from that background and pioneer their famous reforms.

The Enrolled Nurse

Whilst British Nursing is subject to a great deal of Governmental control, we are fortunate that most of the responsibility for the training of nurses lies in our own hands through the three General Nursing Councils, the majority of whose members are practising nurses elected by their colleagues. You will take your part in this responsibility when enrolled.

Men and women may train for any of the Registers maintained by these Councils or for the Roll. The Registers were established by an Act of Parliament, the Nurses Act 1919, but the Roll did not come into being until the Nurses Act 1943 was passed. At that time there were a great number of men and women without any formal training nursing in geriatric hospitals. More were needed and it was to meet this need that recognition was given to these nurses and training was based mainly on geriatric experience. Over the intervening years, however, the Enrolled Nurse has been employed in all types of hospitals, in the Public Health Service and in Industry. To meet this wider range of nursing duties a new syllabus of training came into force during 1964.

A further development has been the Nurses' Act 1969 in which the Roll was divided into three parts i.e. General, Psychiatric and Mental-Subnormality nursing. Pupil nurses may train for any one of these parts and when Enrolled may take a shortened course of training for the others. There is also a special training in Orthopaedic Nursing.

As far back as 1962 the Royal College of Nursing advocated the grade of Senior Enrolled Nurse for selected nurses. This grade is now recognised by the Nurses and Midwives Whitley Council with salary and conditions of service to match the promotion.

Following a report in 1971 called 'The State Enrolled Nurse', compiled by the sub-committee of the Standing Nurses Advisory Committee, the Department of Health is being pressed to implement the 36 recommendations. This would result in a national policy regarding the status and duties of the State Enrolled Nurse.

CHAPTER 2 | THE NATIONAL HEALTH SERVICE AND THE PLACE OF THE NURSE IN THE SERVICE

Before the NATIONAL HEALTH SERVICE ACT 1946 came into force in July 1948, the care of the mentally sick, mentally sub-normal and physically sick was undertaken either by voluntary hospitals or by those run by Local Authorities. Patients had to pay according to their means and this often decided the type of hospital to which they were admitted. Many had to pay for attention from their family doctor and also for home nursing either by private nurses or members of the District Nursing Service. Too many people including children and old age pensioners suffered under this system and although there were various ways of obtaining treatment either free or at a reduced rate the public conscience was uneasy about those whose lives were either shortened or spoiled by lack of medical and nursing care at the proper time.

The Act of 1946 which set out to alter this unhappy state of affairs was designed to 'Establish a comprehensive Health Service and to secure improvement in the physical and mental health of the people of England and Wales and the prevention, diagnosis and treatment of illness' (Scotland and Northern Ireland have comparable schemes, although the administrative structures in these countries vary from England and Wales).

Structure of the National Health Service

Ultimate control of the service rests with Parliament. Until 1968 the service was administered by a Minister of Health who was advised by medical, nursing and administrative officers appointed to the Ministry, and by the Central Health Services Council.

In November 1968, in an attempt to improve all our Welfare Services, the Government merged the Ministries of Health and of Social Security into the Department of State for Health and Social Security (DoSHSS), headed by a Secretary of State with a seat in the Cabinet.

Under the Secretary of State there is a Minister of State who has responsibilities in the field previously covered by the Minister of Health. There is a separate Minister of State for the Social Services.

There are variations in the administration of the National Health Service for Wales, Scotland and N. Ireland

The Health Service is one of the largest organisations in the country and is divided into four parts, each of which is responsible at local level to a different committee (Fig.1).

(1) Hospitals and Specialist Services
(2) General Practitioner Services
(3) Local Health Authority Services
(4) National Blood Transfusion Service and Public Health Laboratory Service.

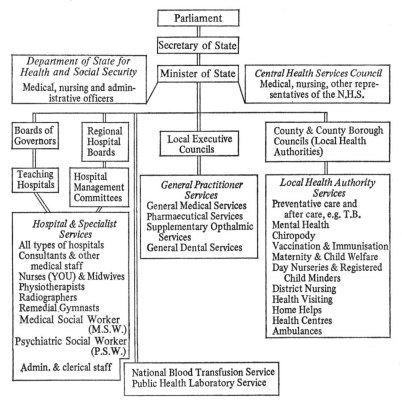

Figure 1. Structure of National Health Service 1968

1 Hospitals and Specialist Services

This is the part of the service you are in at the moment.

The country is divided into *Regions* each with a *Regional Hospital Board*. The Board consists of paid officials including one or more Nursing

Officers and a group of men and women appointed by the Minister who are unpaid. Each Region has an association with a University having a School of Medicine. Hospitals linked with Medical Schools are known as teaching hospitals and have a *Board of Governors* which, like the Regional Hospital Board, is responsible to the Secretary of State for the planning, provision and supervision of the hospitals under its care. Day-to-day administration of hospitals under a Regional Hospital Board is carried out by local *Hospital Management Committees* whose members are also unpaid and who are appointed by the Secretary of State for a specified term of office. There are now nurse members of all Regional Hospital Boards, some Boards of Governors and many Hospital Management Committees.

2   General Practitioner Services

This important part of the Health Service includes:
  (a) General Medical Services
  (b) The Pharmaceutical Services
  (c) The General Dental Services
  (d) The Supplementary Ophthalmic Services.

(a)   General Medical Service
This is based on the general practitioner, sometimes called the G.P. or family doctor. Unless the general practitioner makes full use of the other two parts of the Health Service and unless they use him properly, his patients may not receive the best care which is available for them.

All treatment other than accidents at work or in the street start with a visit to the doctor of your choice. Every citizen has the right to choose the doctor who shall attend him and the doctor has a right to accept or decline a patient. All residents of the United Kingdom who wish to avail themselves of the National Health Service use a medical card on which the name and address of their G.P. is entered when he accepts them as a patient.

Local Executive Councils administer this part of the Service. On this Council, half of the members are professional men and women representing doctors, chemists, dentists and opticians whilst the rest are appointed by the Secretary of State and the County or County Borough Council. There are usually about twenty-five members.

(b)   The Pharmaceutical Services
The local Executive Council which administers the G.P. Service also has to make sure that there is an adequate local supply of drugs and appli-

ances for all persons receiving medical or dental care. Drugs etcetera are only supplied on a prescription from the patient's doctor or dentist.

(c) *The General Dental Services*
Under the National Health Service Act it was hoped that dental treatment would be available for all without additional payment. This has not proved possible mainly because of the scarcity of dentists but also because of the poor level of dental health in this country. Priority and free treatment are given to expectant and nursing mothers and children through the local health authority services and the School Health Service.

The rest of the population can choose their own dentist and pay a small amount (up to £1 or the cost of the treatment, whichever is less) for conservative treatment or extractions. The supply of dentures means an additional charge to the patient. For those unable to afford treatment financial help is available through the Department of Health and Social Security.

(d) *The Supplementary Ophthalmic Services*
It is hoped that eventually a comprehensive service for the care of eyes will be part of the Hospital Service, but until this is possible the Local Executive Councils have the duty to arrange for suitably qualified doctors, ophthalmic opticians and dispensing opticians to undertake this service. Eyes are tested free and if glasses are prescribed for adults they can be supplied for a small charge for each lens and an additional charge for the frames. Glasses for children are supplied free of charge. For an adult to get his eyes tested for the first time he needs to take a letter from his general practitioner to an ophthalmic practitioner or optician.

3. The Local Health Authority Services

Every County and County Borough Council in England and Wales is responsible for administering this part of the Service through paid officials, e.g. Medical Officers of Health, Superintendent Health Visitors and through the Health Committee, i.e. elected and unpaid members of the County or County Borough Council.

The many facets of this part of the Health Service are listed in Figure 1. Whilst looking at these it is as well to remember that these services are mainly preventive, that is, they aim to maintain and improve physical and mental health from before birth to old age.

Many State Registered Nurses are employed in this part of the National Health Service as Health Visitors, School Nurses, District

Nurses and Midwives. An increasing number of enrolled nurses are being recruited into this field of work, particularly into the District Nursing Service.

ANCILLARY SERVICES UNDER THE N.H.S. ACT

Under the National Health Service Act 1946 the Minister of Health was given power to conduct research into the causation, prevention, diagnosis and treatment of illness or mental defectiveness. Boards of Governors and Regional Hospital Boards and Hospital Management Committees have the same powers.

The Minister was also given power to provide a *Bacteriological Service* and a *Blood Transfusion Service*. Both these services have been established on a nation-wide basis.

OTHER IMPORTANT WELFARE SERVICES

At the end of the last war several very important Acts of Parliament came into force to try to improve the health and well-being of people living in the United Kingdom. We have looked at the National Health Service Act in some detail, but this was only one of several. Others, which help to support us through any adversity are:

(*a*) *The National Insurance Act 1946*. Insurance under the Act is compulsory, with a few minor exceptions, for all those over school-leaving age. You pay a fixed weekly contribution to which your employer adds his share (larger than yours). You are covered against loss of income by interruption of earnings.

(*b*) *The National Assistance Act 1948*. This Act makes it possible for persons in financial need to get help either in cash or in goods.

Also under this Act it is the duty of County Councils and County Borough Councils to provide special welfare services for the physically handicapped and for old people.

(*c*) *Family Allowances*. These have been payable since a Special Act was passed in 1946. The first child of the family is not eligible for an allowance; the rest receive it providing they are under the compulsory school-leaving age. This is not an insurance scheme as no direct contribution is made by the parents.

(*d*) *The Disabled Persons (Employment) Acts 1944 and 1958*. The aim of these Acts is not to give financial help but to assist men and women who are handicapped by a disability to find and hold a suitable job or to work on their own account. Special rehabilitation and training schemes have been set up under this Act.

(*e*) *The School Health Service* was established under the *Education Act 1944* and as with the other branches of our Health Services it is of the utmost importance that there should be close co-operation between it and the hospital and general practitioner services.

The main aim of this service is to prevent illness although some curative work is carried out in minor ailment clinics, speech therapy and ear, nose and throat clinics.

Schoolchildren are medically examined periodically so that any abnormalities, whether mental or physical, can be detected and corrected if possible.

(f) *The Occupational Health Service.* Under the *Factories Acts 1937* and *1948* persons working in certain occupations which are known to carry a health risk have to be examined at regular intervals by the Appointed Factory Doctor for the area in which the factory is situated.

The physical conditions of work in Factories, Shops and Offices are controlled by law and in many places of employment First Aid equipment must be provided and be in the care of a person trained in recognised First Aid techniques. Many employers, however, provide much more than the minimum required under the various Acts and you will find, particularly in large organisations, that the employer has set up a comprehensive health service within the organisation. Smaller firms may join together to finance such a service; the pioneer in this field was the Slough Industrial Medical Service. Many nurses are now working in Industry and Commerce all over the country but in doing so they elect to work outside the National Health Service.

Need for Co-operation and Co-ordination

In addition to the statutory services already mentioned there are many voluntary organisations concerned with the welfare of those members of the community who are in need. It is most important, therefore, for nurses to know what help is available for their patients and from what source it can be obtained. In hospital the enrolled nurse is unlikely to have to make the necesssary arrangements as this is the work of the medical social worker, but if she has the knowledge she will be able to give reassurance to her patients.

A simple example will help you to see how the major parts of the statutory services combine to make medical and nursing care possible. A young married woman with two children under five years of age calls in her family doctor because of persistent abdominal pain. The doctor is not sure of the diagnosis so calls on the Hospital Service for consultant advice. This may be given either at home or in the hospital Outpatient Department. If she has to be admitted to hospital her doctor will call on the Local Health Authority Services for several forms of help, e.g. ambulance for the mother, day nursery care for the children. Whilst in hospital, in addition to her medical and nursing care, this patient will have the help of the Chaplain of her choice and the Hospital Library and trolley-shop run by one or more of the women's voluntary organisations. During her stay in the ward, Sister and the Almoner will discuss with her and her husband and the family doctor the various forms of help she will need when she returns home. This may include the District Nursing Service and Home Help Service.

You can see from this example how no one part of the Service is more important than the other and that all contribute to the treatment of the patient.

Finance

The cost of this service is enormous and rises steadily every year. In 1950–51 the Service cost £336 million but in 1968–9 the hospital service for England and Wales alone cost over £750 million.

The money comes from three sources:
   (1) Employers and employees—National Insurance Contributions
   (2) Exchequer funds—Income tax
   (3) Local rates—paid by all householders.
Your hospital receives its money from the Regional Hospital Board or Board of Governors who in turn have applied for the amount they think they need from the Department of Health and Social Services. Every Hospital Management Committee has a Finance Officer who is respon-sible for budgeting for the hospitals in its care. Your training allowance is paid out of these monies, but the cost of the School of Nursing and the salaries of your tutors are paid out of another account administered by the Area Nurse Training Committee. This division was made in order to safeguard the standards of nurse training and to ensure that regardless of the financial state of the hospital, your training should not suffer.

All users of the Health Services and all the people employed within the Service should be as economical as possible. Waste of materials and of time are extremely costly and ultimately mean higher National Insur-ance contributions, income tax and rates for us all.

Future Developments

The second stage in the National Health Service has now been reached. From 1948–62, because Housing and Education were given first priority, the National Health Service had only enough money to improve its facilities, mainly by repairing existing buildings but now a big building programme is forging ahead. This second phase, known as the Ten Year Plan, is seeing the development of large District General Hospitals with facilities for treating acute mental and physical illness and emergencies. These hospitals are supported by a few Regional centres for specialised treatment needing costly apparatus, e.g. cobalt bomb, and by some maternity units and long-stay units for mental and general and geriatric patients mostly in existing cottage hospitals.

General Practitioners will be encouraged more and more to take part-time hospital appointments and they will be supported by the rapid extension of the Health and Welfare Services under the direction of the Local Health Authority.

In the light of the experience of the first twenty years of the National Health Service it is thought that if the three main parts of it were responsible to ONE committee at local level, i.e. an Area Health Board, a better service to the community would evolve. This scheme is now under discussion.

The Nurse's Place

Lines of communication and responsibility are essential in any organisation, and the National Health Service is no exception. Figure 2 will show you to whom you are responsible during and after your training.

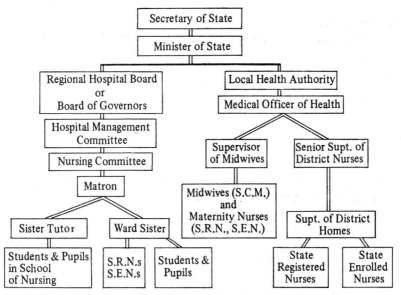

Figure 2. Organisation of Nursing Services (non-Salmon)

You can see from Figure 2 that you are a direct employee of the Secretary of State, who has delegated his responsibilities to Senior Nursing, Medical and lay Administrators at local level (see also page 9).

SALMON REPORT ON SENIOR NURSING STAFF STRUCTURE

In 1966 the above Report was published and has now been accepted as the pattern for the future. All hospitals are being asked to implement most of the recommendations as soon as possible; they are also being adapted to the Public Health Nursing Service.

(a) Objectives

To improve patient care by making Nursing Administration more efficient, attractive and satisfying.

It is especially geared to the District General Hospital concept of patient care.

(b) Structure

(i) a new staffing and grading system will be introduced.

(ii) each grade from staff nurse upwards will have a descriptive name:

Grades 9 & 10 Nursing Officers who decide policy at top management level.

Grades 7 & 8 Nursing Officers who programme policy at middle management level.

Grade 6 Ward Sisters and Charge Nurses who implement policy at first-line management level.

(c) Job Description

Each grade will have clearly defined tasks which should eliminate non-nursing duties.

(d) Management Training

This will be provided throughout the country for first-line, middle and top grades. No promotion until appropriate course completed.

(e) Communications

The Report says 'Where communications are poor, morale in the ward is bad and the efficiency of the hospital low'. Lines of control as suggested in the Salmon Report should improve this vital part of management and make delegation the key to getting quick and authoritative answers to problems.

The General Nursing Councils

Your syllabus of training is drawn up by the General Nursing Council for England and Wales or Scotland, or N. Ireland. S.R.Ns and S.E.Ns are elected by their colleagues to serve on these Councils together with doctors and educationists appointed by the Secretary of State. When

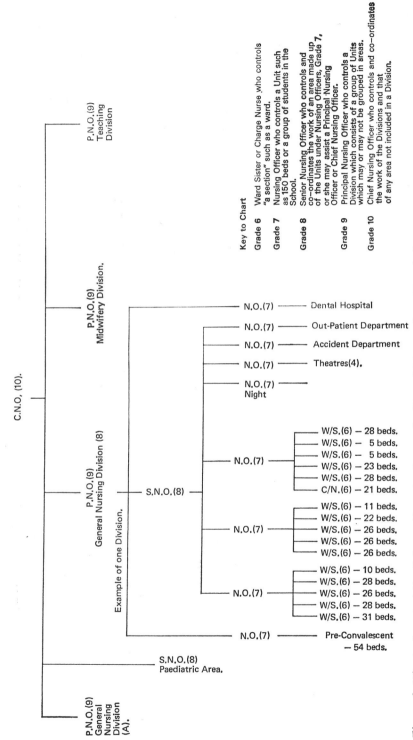

Key to Chart

Grade 6   Ward Sister or Charge Nurse, who controls "a section" such as a ward.

Grade 7   Nursing Officer who controls a Unit such as 150 beds or a group of students in the School.

Grade 8   Senior Nursing Officer who controls and co-ordinates the work of an area made up of the Units under Nursing Officers, Grade 7, or she may assist a Principal Nursing Officer or Chief Nursing Officer.

Grade 9   Principal Nursing Officer who controls a Division which consists of a group of Units which may or may not be grouped in areas.

Grade 10   Chief Nursing Officer who controls and co-ordinates the work of the Divisions and that of any area not included in a Division.

Figure 3. Chart of part of the Salmon Organisation at the United Birmingham Hospitals

you are either Registered or Enrolled you will have the opportunity to vote for those nurses whom you think will serve you best, or you may allow your name to go forward for nomination.

These Councils are assisted in their work by Area Nurse Training Committees whose terms of reference under the Nurses Act of 1949 are 'to advise and assist' the Councils, Boards of Governors, and Regional Hospital Boards, in whose area they work on all matters relating to the training of student and pupil nurses (Fig. 4).

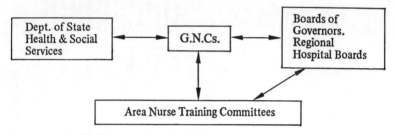

Figure 4. Area Nurse Training Committees

Nurses and Midwives Whitley Council

Training allowances and salaries are negotiated on your behalf by the Staff Side of this Council. Nurses' Professional Organisations, e.g. The Royal College of Nursing, and trade unions with nurse members, e.g. National Union of Public Employees, represent you in this work. The Department of State for Health has recently recommended that ALL hospital employees should join their appropriate organisation.

Pupil and enrolled nurses have their own professional organisation, the National Association of State Enrolled Nurses, but they are free to join a union if they so wish—or not to bother to join anything. The latter, unless it is due to a conscientious objection, is to be deplored, because all nurses benefit from the negotiations between their professional organisations and their employers, and they should therefore support their official representatives both verbally and financially.

Registered and enrolled nurses who belong to their professional organisation have a direct link with the *International Council of Nurses.* This Council, which was the first one for any group of women in the world, was founded by a British nurse, Mrs Bedford Fenwick, in 1899.

The nurse of today has a great deal for which to be grateful to Miss Nightingale and the women who trained under her system, for not only did they raise the standard of bedside nursing care to a level which set the pattern all over the world, but they established nursing education and nursing organisation on really sound foundations. Your title 'Nurse' is protected by law through their efforts. Protect it now by the standard of your work and the use of it *only* by men and women in training or on the Rolls or Registers of the General Nursing Councils.

CHAPTER 3 | THE FUNCTION OF HOSPITAL DEPARTMENTS

The function of a hospital is to provide the best facilities for the reception, diagnosis and treatment of the sick whether as in-patients or out-patients. In addition some hospitals provide facilities for the training of medical, nursing and ancillary service students, e.g. physiotherapists, medical-social workers.

The Secretary of State for Health and Social Security is directly responsible to Parliament for the Hospitals Service, but he delegates his responsibilities for the day-to-day running of hospitals to the Regional Hospital Boards, who in turn pass on some of these responsibilities to local Hospital Management Committees. These committees are composed of persons appointed by the Secretary of State and include doctors, nurses, hospital administrators, and members of the general public. The heads of the four main departments in each hospital report to this Committee either directly or through the Hospital Secretary. Where a Hospital Management Committee (H.M.C.) has several hospitals to look after, it may set up smaller House Committees for the hospitals within the Group.

Four main Services have developed within the Hospitals Service in order that the sick may be cared for in the best possible way.

1 Medical Service

The function of this service is to diagnose, decide on and supervise medical, nursing and ancillary treatment. The medical staff consists of Consultants, Registrars, House Physicians and Surgeons headed in some hospitals by a Medical Superintendent.

2 Nursing Service

The function of this service has been described (*Basic Principles of Nursing Care,* I.C.N. publication) as being 'to assist the individual sick or

well in the performance of those activities contributing to health or its
recovery (or to a peaceful death) which he would prefer to do unaided if
he had the necessary strength, will, or knowledge, and to do this in such
a way as to help him gain independence as rapidly as possible'. This
responsible work must, of course, be carried out under medical supervision, but it implies that nurses have their own special skills to use in the
care of the sick.

3 Ancillary Services

These are also known as the para-medical services and include such
departments as:

Medical Social	Pharmaceutical
Biochemistry	Physiotherapy
Occupational Therapy	Radiotherapy
Pathological Laboratories	X-ray

These important departments assist in the diagnostic, therapeutic or
rehabilitative care of patients and therefore support the work of the
Medical and Nursing Services.

4 Administrative Service

This Service should co-ordinate the other three and help to keep an
adequate and constant supply of skilled hands and equipment to the
patient.

The Hospital Secretary is head of this Service and has the following
departments under his supervision, although each has its own Senior
Officer:

Clerical	Catering	In some hospitals still
Finance	Domestic	the responsibility of
Maintenance	Laundry	the Matron.
Portering		

Once again, you will see that no one department can function properly
by itself and unless all acknowledge the contribution each has to make
to the efficiency and humanity of the hospital, the sick who come to it for
help will not receive the sort of treatment they deserve.

Figure 5 may help you to see how this co-ordination and co-operation
should work.

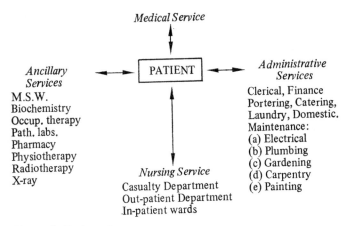

Figure 5. Patient Care

CHAPTER 4 | THE NURSE AND PROFESSIONAL RELATIONSHIPS

All human beings living in groups make rules of behaviour so that living together may be as harmonious as possible. Children learn these rules from their parents by instruction and example and find that if they keep them they gain approval from their relatives and friends. These rules are of two kinds:

(1) ETIQUETTE. These are the simple rules of social behaviour which govern the way we dress, eat, sit, reply to questions, answer letters, etcetera.

(2) ETHICS. These are the difficult rules which govern our behaviour both socially and professionally. They can be difficult because they involve a moral decision, i.e. a personal decision about right and wrong.

Nursing Etiquette

In addition to the normal rules of etiquette governing social behaviour, every school of nursing and hospital have their own special rules which help nurses and other members of the staff to fit into the special com-

B

munity in which they work. Some of these rules refer to the way uniform is worn, others to the way senior members of staff should be addressed and how you address each other.

Nursing Ethics

There are certain moral principles concerned with nursing which help you to do what you OUGHT to do, which may not be what you WANT to do.

You do not have to be a religious person to be a moral one, although those with strong religious convictions should find it easier to make the right decisions.

The International Council of Nurses has drawn up a code of Ethics for the nursing profession and many National Nurses Associations have agreed to accept them on behalf of their members. There are fourteen points in the Code:

1 *The fundamental responsibility of the nurse is threefold: to conserve life: to alleviate suffering and to promote health.* Nothing could be stated more simply and clearly, but it is not always remembered by the hospital nurse that the promotion of health is as much her responsibility as it is for her public health nurse colleague.

2 *The nurse must maintain at all times the highest standards of nursing care and of professional conduct.* Herein lies the safety of your patients and your own peace of mind.

3 *The nurse must not only be well prepared to practice, but must maintain her knowledge and skill at a consistently high level.* Learning should continue after training with the help of professional books and journals, refresher courses, practical experience in other fields of nursing both at home and abroad.

4 *The religious beliefs of a patient must be respected.* To ignore or interfere with another person's faith is the height of impertinence and as well as being hurtful may impede a patient's return to full health. Every effort should be made to enable a patient to maintain his religious observances.

5 *Nurses hold in confidence all personal information entrusted to them.* This includes social background, medical history, diagnosis, treatment and prognosis. Whilst it is perfectly in order to discuss all these with medical and nursing colleagues at a case conference on the ward or in the classroom, it is improper ethical behaviour to have the same discussion with a colleague on the top of a bus or other public place.

6 *A nurse recognises not only the responsibilities but the limitations of her or his professional functions, recommends or gives medical treatment* *without medical orders only in emergencies and reports such action to a physician at the earliest possible moment.* Nurses are frequently asked for *medical* advice by relatives and friends particularly at social functions. You are trained to observe illness, not to diagnose or order treatment, therefore the only advice you can give with safety and ethically is that the questioner should seek MEDICAL advice.

7 *The nurse is under an obligation to carry out the physician's orders intelligently and loyally and to refuse to participate in unethical procedures.* This means that a nurse is the keeper of her own conscience and that she can only obey the physician's orders providing that these do not involve her in the treatment of patients that is professionally wrong, e.g. non-therapeutic abortions, euthanasia.

8 *The nurse sustains confidence in the physician and other members of the health team; incompetence or unethical conduct of associates should be exposed but only to the proper authority.* A nurse should never undermine the confidence of a patient in the people caring for him, either by word, or deed. If, however, she is worried by the professional or ethical standards of her colleagues she should discuss the situation with her matron and, if necessary, her professional organisation.

9 *A nurse is entitled to just remuneration and accepts only such compensation as the contract, actual or implied, provides.* The training allowances of pupils and students and the salaries of trained nurses are uniform throughout this country. They are negotiated on their behalf by the Staff Side of the Nurses and Midwives Whitley Council. Every nurse should know her salary and scale of increases. Patients sometimes offer money to nurses either in the hope of preferential treatment or more often in gratitude for the care they have received. The first offer should always be refused—graciously but firmly—and the reason given. The second offer if refused can cause great distress to the patient, but it should only be accepted in exceptional circumstances and the money handed immediately to your Ward Sister or Matron for amenities for patients or Nursing Staff. Its destination should be made quite clear to the patient.

10 *Nurses do not permit their names to be used in connection with the advertisement of products or with any other forms of self-advertisement.* The reason why this is unethical is that it could lead to bribery and corruption, not only of the nurse but of the National Health Service.

11 *The nurse co-operates with and maintains harmonious relationships with members of other professions and with her or his professional colleagues.* The care of the sick is not confined to one professional group and we can only give our patients the treatment they deserve if we learn to

work with other groups as a team. In this way we can get the support we need in our very difficult profession.

12 *The nurse in private life adheres to standards of personal ethics which reflect credit on the profession.* By our behaviour in the community we either maintain or lower the respect for our profession, therefore our ethical behaviour in private life should be as high as in our professional life. Confidence in and recruitment to our part of the National Health Service is a measure of our personal beliefs and conduct.

13 *In personal conduct, nurses should not knowingly disregard the accepted patterns of behaviour of the community in which they live and* **work.** This applies particularly to nurses who go abroad to work. Only if local behaviour patterns need to be changed in order to improve the health and well-being of the community should the nurse disregard local custom.

14 *A nurse should participate and share responsibility with other citizens and other health professions in promoting efforts to meet the health needs of the public—local, state, national, and international. This* means that because of our training we have a wider contribution to make than at the bedside and that we should take an active interest in community affairs, particularly where problems of health are concerned. We can be effective both as individuals and through our membership of our national and international organisations.

Legal Aspects of Nursing

All nurses are urged to read 'Law Notes for Nurses' by S. R. Speller. In this booklet the requirements under Common Law with regard to Hospitals, Patients and National Health Service employees are clearly laid down. Every nurse should be sure that the procedures she uses come within these requirements e.g.

The Admission and Discharge of Patients.

Care of Patients' property.

Care and Custody of Poisons and Dangerous Drugs.

Consent to Operation etc.

The position of the nurse with regard to litigation is clearly explained and the trained nurse would be wise to be covered by indemnity insurance

Industrial Relations Act 1971

This act will have far reaching effects on all workers including nurses and for the first time all nurses will be required to sign a Contract of

Employment and the National Health Service has to set up a Grievance Procedure which must be explained in the Contract.

Under the Act all workers are encouraged to join a professional organisation or trade union so that advice and help will be available to them if difficulties arise.

CHAPTER 5 | PERSONAL DEVELOPMENT OF THE INDIVIDUAL

'Social psychology deals with the experience and behaviour of the individual in relation to social stimulus situation'.* In other words, it helps us to understand not only how other people may feel and behave, but also why we feel and behave as we do. It is a fascinating subject and a most important one for everyone to study who has to live and work closely with other people.

Nurses must always remember that their patients are people with the same hopes and desires as themselves and that their illness heightens their need for understanding and physical and emotional security.

Basic Drives

We might make an analogy between our behaviour and that of a motor car, for just as machines need power to move them, so do human beings. A motor car gets its power from petrol, oil and electricity and we have several sources of power to drive us, e.g.:

    (a) the instinct of curiosity,
    (b) the instinct of collecting,
    (c) the instinct of self-assertion or self-submission,
    (d) parental instinct,
    (e) gregarious instinct.

It is thought to be one or more of these drives which stimulates us to learn.

Again, just as machines need oiling and servicing to help them to work smoothly and effectively, so also there are certain basic needs to help all human beings to develop and to continue to function smoothly and happily.

* Muzafer Sherif: *An Outline of Social Psychology.*

Basic Physical Needs

 (a) Food
 (b) Periods of rest
 (c) Protection
 (d) Opportunities for reproduction.

If these needs are met, all living organisms can survive, but a human being needs more than the basic physical needs for his development. He has inter-personal relationships with those he comes into contact with and with whom he shares group activities.

Basic Psychological Needs

 (a) He needs to recognise himself as a person in his own right or 'to develop ego structure'
 (b) He needs to have a feeling of belongingness or 'to belong to groups'
 (c) He needs to acquire status and prestige.

These needs if met satisfactorily give a sense of security. They are the hardest to supply because they are not always so apparent as the basic physical needs, and nurses must learn to appreciate their importance.

(a) EGO-STRUCTURE

This begins at a very early age in children (two or three years) and shows itself in various ways, but especially when the word 'I', 'me' and 'mine' are used regularly. Then comes the stage of opposition to parental authority and displays of temper tantrums. All these are natural and healthy but need careful handling if the child is to develop happily. The next stage is picture-building, i.e. when the child sees himself as a person —'I can put on my shoes', 'I can skip', etcetera. This stage should be encouraged and not squashed even though the picture may be slightly distorted! Confidence grows and new situations are tackled with growing assurance, independence and initiative. In the same way you should encourage your patients and junior nursing colleagues. Praise for effort and achievement is essential and blame should be reduced to a minimum, used mainly when carelessness is suspected.

It is useful, at times, to stop and look at oneself and ask: 'What sort of a person do I think I am?' Other people may see us quite differently. This may account for a report on your work from a Ward Sister that seems at first not to be about you at all. Only by discussing one's own development without too much emotion can growth continue in the right way.

(b) BELONGINGNESS

A small child has no desire to belong to any group other than its own family and in the earliest stages is concerned only for the one who provides food and care. Not until a child is seven to eight years old does the urge to push out from the family group occur. Junior youth organisations fulfil this need for some children who revel in being Cubs or Brownies. Some parents resent this stage, but it is essential that children should learn to play with an ever widening group of those of their own age. School groups tend at first to be very unstable, the bosom pal of this week becoming the worst enemy next week, but gradually they become settled and deliberate and lasting friendships are made. As adults we select our friends and the groups to which we belong. For most people five groups provide all we need and at the same time they help us to understand the values and attitudes of other people. These groups usually include: family, religious, work, professional work, leisure interest groups, e.g. tennis club, photography club, etcetera.

Consider the number of groups to which you belong and decide whether you have too wide or too narrow interests. When appropriate, discuss this belongingness with your patients. They often feel intensely lonely in the ward and may need a great deal of help from you to feel at ease in the new group. Introductions by you of new patients to old ones, especially to those in adjacent beds and to ones of similar age and intellect will help a great deal.

It is very important that nursing administrators and teachers should understand the value of the group. The ward team is a group: each member of it is influenced by the group pattern of behaviour and in turn influences the behaviour of the group. To promote and sustain a really good team spirit is vitally important to everyone in the ward—patients, nurses, pupils and to all the ancillary services who from time to time, visit the ward in their respective capacities.

(c) STATUS AND PRESTIGE

Most of us need to feel that we have recognition of our work or achievements in some field. It may not be in our work, but in sport or social activities. The father of a family should have it as the breadwinner, and the mother as the homemaker. They may also get it by achievements outside the family, but unless they have it within as well, conflict may result.

Old people feel this lack of status very much more when they can no longer remain independent. Our attitude towards the elderly chronic sick needs most careful thought. It is not kindness to tie ribbons in an elderly lady's hair and call her 'dear', as this only increases her feeling of resentment at her helplessness and towards those looking after her. Most old people have had a great deal of responsibility in their lives and many have given devoted service to their families and the country. They deserve our respect both in word and deed.

It is however important to stress that there are great individual differences in the basic psychological needs. They are developed in different individuals in very different degrees. Some people do not appear to need a group life, others do not care about status, but the ordinary man in the street has developed them to a normal degree.

Personality

Nurses have to report on their patients and they use words such as 'cheerful', 'co-operative' or 'difficult' when describing the person and not his illness. We think of our colleagues and friends in the same way—and they of us! The words we use to describe a patient or a friend are our opinion of their personality.

We must remember that different qualities are regarded as virtues in different culture patterns: this is certainly true of our manners, habits and general pattern of behaviour. Since we all, staff and patients alike, come from slightly different environmental backgrounds and—in the case of overseas patients and nurses—from very different cultural backgrounds it is kind, before tying a 'personal label' on a person, especially if it is not a very complimentary one, to consider all the factors which may be affecting his behaviour.

In the nursing situation, it may be the nurse who has to adapt her professional habits and social behaviour so that her patients can benefit to the full from their medical and nursing care. On the other hand, it may be the task of the nurse to help a patient to adjust his behaviour to fit into the accepted pattern of behaviour in the ward or department.

In hospital life, where the staff are not expected to show emotion or to display marked personality traits, it is very easy for them to forget that these needs are still very much alive both in their patients and in themselves. Nurses are supposed to know how to handle people—this handling must be both physical and emotional and it will only be truly nursing of the highest order if each patient is handled as an individual who has a right to be understood and comforted according to his own particular needs.

CHAPTER 6 | THE PROMOTION OF INDIVIDUAL AND COMMUNAL HEALTH

This chapter deals with: (1) personal health and good habits, and (2) communal health and the proper use of National and Local Authority Services.

It is old-fashioned nowadays to use the word *hygiene*, but the word means 'principles of health' and comes from the name of the *Greek Goddess of Health—Hygeia*. Safe medicine and nursing as well as ordinary living are only possible if we all understand the basic principles of health.

Let us start with ourselves.

Personal Health

To have the opportunity of enjoying life to the full we need to be able to work and play at careers and games of our own choice, eat and sleep well, dress suitably according to the season, have a weatherproof home to live in, and for the majority of people in this country, to contract a legal marriage and produce a family.

How do we ensure that we can have all these basic physical needs satisfied? We cannot all be guaranteed success, but by observing certain rules, success is more likely!

Good Habits and Health Teaching

We learn many of our habits relating to the care of ourselves from our parents and family. The influence of the mother or mother substitute (this could be a nurse) is extremely important with both boys and girls, for it is she who is responsible for offering food, insisting on rest and sleep, acquiring suitable clothes and providing opportunities for play. It is she who teaches her child to use soap and water on his skin and hair and to use a brush on his nails and teeth. She also is the instigator of regular bladder and bowel movement.

It may be that some of your patients are patients because they formed bad habits in relation to healthy living when they were young and are now suffering from the effects of a badly balanced diet, lack of sleep, unsuitable clothes and housing conditions. Part of the treatment of such patients will be the breaking down of the old habits and replacing them with new ones.

B*

This will be much easier for both staff and patient alike if we practise what we preach both in the cleanliness and quiet efficiency of the ward and its surroundings and in the health standards and practices of the staff attending the patient.

Are you a nice person to be near? Does your hair shine and is it kept from falling over your face or into food by a suitable hair style? Do you wash all the dirt and dust from your skin at very frequent intervals so that it has a chance to do its work properly in helping to keep you healthy? Do you remember to pay special attention with soap and water to those parts of your body where there are two parts rubbing together and do you make sure that you use a deodorant or anti-perspirant daily? Does your face show that you ill-treat your stomach or your feet, or does your body-droop show how little rest and proper food you give it? Do you nibble your nails, or have you grown talons that are a menace to your nylons and your patients' skins?

Having looked yourself over and decided on a reasonably high standard of care, you should now be prepared to give this same attention to your patients. There will be minor differences, of course; for example, you need to bath or shower every day because you do a fairly heavy physical job and your skin will perspire. You are also in constant contact with living and dead organisms and these need to be washed off your skin frequently—that is why you are required to wash your hands so often on the ward. Your patients will probably be happier with a bath every two or three days but daily attention to axilla and groin areas should be taught. In the same way consider the diet, rest requirements and protection of your patients, and try to ensure that they are getting the maximum available under difficult circumstances. This applies particularly to rest and sleep. Noisy nurses and equipment are the best destroyers of sleep and a disgrace to any ward. Check your movements and report noisy equipment so that it can be repaired or serviced as quickly as possible.

One of the main occupations of patients is watching the nurses—how they walk, how they wear their uniform, how they speak and whether they look as though they are enjoying their work. They also like to ask for advice about personal health matters. One of the most controversial subjects at the moment is smoking. To smoke or not to smoke? The medical evidence appears conclusive. There is a definite danger to health and because of this, the Department of Health has asked all hospital personnel to refrain from smoking on duty. The choice off duty remains with the individual but nurses should remember that not only are they health teachers but that the smell of stale smoke in their hair and on their breath can cause nausea in their patients.

Communal Health

In this country there are PUBLIC HEALTH SERVICES which aim to help everyone to live a healthy life. The basic services are those concerned with:

(a) Housing	(d) Sewage and Refuse Disposal
(b) Water Supply	(e) Heating and Lighting
(c) Control of Pests	(f) Prevention of Infection.

If, in spite of these, our health breaks down, we can call on either the Hospital Service or the Public Health Service through the General Practitioner Service for help.

The Public Health Service has nurses on its staff who are either employed as District Nurses or as Health Visitors or as Midwives.

In addition to being nursed at home by trained nurses, we can have a variety of other services, depending on our Local Authority, to speed our recovery or make our chronic illness more bearable, e.g.:

(a) Laundry Service	(c) Home Help Service
(b) Nursing Equipment	(d) Night Attendant Service
Loan Service	(e) Physiotherapy Service.

VOLUNTARY ORGANISATIONS such as the Royal Women's Voluntary Service (R.W.V.S.) the Red Cross and St John Ambulance Brigade help to fill in the gaps in the Local Authority Services by providing such things as:

(a) Meals on Wheels	(c) Home Occupational Therapy
(b) Car Service	(d) Visitors for People Living Alone.

Even if our health has not broken down we may need financial help, especially if we suffer from unexpected unemployment. At this point the great national schemes come into play through their local offices, i.e.:

Ministry of Social Security   Youth Employment Service.
Employment Exchanges

There are also special services for permanently disabled people such as the blind and deaf, for deprived children and the mentally sick.

From time to time life gets too complicated for the parents of large families living in poor conditions and on the edge of ill health. Again there is help available through the Public Health and Welfare Services. Life can get too difficult for elderly people, especially those living alone and they can be supported in many ways either in their own homes or in hospitals or old people's homes. Some hospitals admit old people for one or two weeks a year so that the relatives who nurse them so faithfully can have a holiday.

Although all these services exist it is amazing how many people remain ignorant on how to obtain help either for themselves or others. Nurses working in hospital or on the District can play an important part in the health of the community by bringing to their patients those services which will contribute to their recovery or comfort.

FURTHER READING

Nursing and Medical History

The Story of Nursing. J.Calder. Methuen
The Lamp and the Book. G.Bowman. Queen Anne Press
Florence Nightingale. C.Woodham Smith. Constable.

National Health Service

Law relating to Hospitals. S.R.Speller. Lewis
A Synopsis of Public Health & Social Medicine. A.J.Essex-Cater. J. Wright
Guide to the Social Services. Family Welfare Association

Function of Hospital Departments

Essentials of Out-Patient Nursing. C.Rayner. Arlington Books

Nurse and Professional Relationships

Law Notes for Nurses. S.R.Speller. Royal College of Nursing
Notes on Nursing. Florence Nightingale. Duckworth
Ethics for Nurses. Hilary Way. N. Times Reprint
International Code of Ethics. I.C.N.
Professional Ethic & Hospital. N.Mackenzie. E.U.P.
Industrial Relations Act. 1971. H.M.S.O.

Personal Development of the Individual

People in Hospitals. E.Barnes. Macmillan
Aids to Psychology for Nurses. A.Altschull. Ballière, Tindall & Cox
Psychology as applied to Nursing. A.McGuie. Livingstone

Promotion of Individual & Communal Health

Health. Personal & Communal. J.Gibson. Faber
Health Visiting. M.McEwan. Faber & Faber

PART 2 | THE ENVIRONMENT OF THE PATIENT (INCLUDING THE CARE OF THE WARD UNIT)

CHAPTER 7 | WARD ROUTINE

WARD ROUTINE is the time and work schedule in a hospital ward twenty-four hours in a day.

Purpose of a Ward Routine

1. Planning of the patient's day is necessary so that no item of domestic, nursing or medical care is omitted from his hospital treatment.

2. The rhythm of a daily routine is advantageous to the sick person whose basic needs become more important during illness. When he is ill, he understands that he will receive attention at definite times during the day. As he recovers he will begin to look forward to the *times* when he will have his meals or be made comfortable in bed-making.

3. The regularity and familiarity of a routine produce an atmosphere of relaxation.

4. When a number of the staff are temporary on a ward, or there is a complicated shift system, or several of the staff are part-time workers, the ward routine is a means by which all the staff know which duties are expected of them at the various times during the day.

5. A planned daily routine leaves more time for those in charge of the ward to arrange special emergency measures when these occur such as admissions, urgent treatments or sudden changes in a patient's condition.

In arranging the ward routine, the people to be considered are the *patients*. Their needs may be summarised as follows:

Sleep and rest
Meals
Toilet including bed-baths, bed-making
Sanitary attention
Sitting out of bed and ambulation
Nursing treatments
Medical examinations and treatments

Physiotherapy, Occupational and Diversional therapy
Visitors.
Ward routine may vary according to the type of work carried out in the ward or hospital.

In children's wards the periods of sleep and rest may be lengthened, and geriatric patients will need less medical treatments but more time spent on bathing and ambulation. Where there are operating lists in surgical wards, a special routine may be introduced on operations days.

Patients who are extremely ill are not aware of the day-to-day business in the ward; they require continual or very frequent attention day and night, so arrangements independent of the general ward routine may be necessary. It follows then that the time and work schedule is compiled in the interests of the ward patients, but should not be so rigid that a patient whose care and treatment is dissimilar from that of the other patients is subjected to the routine suitable to the majority. This minority of patients includes the very ill patient, the dying patient, the new admission, the patient for operative surgery or urgent treatment and the mentally confused patient. A degree of adaptability and versatility is required on this account from the ward sister and her nursing team.

Basic Ward Routine

SLEEP AND REST. The wards should be quiet and darkened at night for at least eight hours. Rest periods are usually in the afternoon, after the midday meal. All general activity ceases.

MEALS. Three main meals, avoiding too long or too short gaps between any two of them, e.g.

Breakfast   8.15 am
Dinner   12.30 pm
Supper   6 pm

Drinks of fruit juice, tea, milk either alone or with added foods like chocolate, or soups, e.g. 6 am, 10 am, 3 pm, 9 pm. Some ill patients and small children may need drinks or feeds during the night for 9 pm to 6 am is too long for them to be without food.

THE PATIENT'S TOILET includes a bath once a day either in bed or in the bath. Face, hands and pressure areas are washed and dried once or twice a day, i.e. morning and evening, depending on the time of the bath, and the hands are washed after using a bed-pan or visiting the toilet. The hair receives attention at least three times a day and the mouth is cleaned and teeth brushed early morning and after supper. Regular bowel and bladder action is encouraged in the recovering patient as part of his rehabilitation, and it is found convenient in the day's routine to give bed-pans and urinals to patients immediately after meals, on waking and before lights out at night. These times are approximately every four hours. Patients who are very ill, confused, very young, elderly, have diseases of the gastrointestinal and urinary tracts, or have been given aperients (for constipation) and diuretics (these drugs encourage passing of urine) will require this attention more frequently, and without delay. Some patients need assistance from the nurse when they wish to visit the toilet.

SITTING OUT OF BED AND AMBULATION. A short period of time out of bed is usually arranged in the afternoon, but as this increases, it may be convenient during morning and afternoon with dinner at a table, or the morning and evening with the afternoon spent resting in bed and supper at a table. Patients' ambulation is best at a time when there are few people moving about in the ward to avoid some apprehension on the part of the patient and the possibility of accidents.

FURTHER NURSING TREATMENTS include changing a patient's position, special treatment of pressure areas, oesophageal tube-feeding, administration of medicines, injections of drugs, dressings of wounds, management of drainage tubes. The ward routine is arranged so that nurses carrying out the techniques are not disturbed more than absolutely necessary. There are also duties not at the bed-side such as checking ward equipment, testing urine specimens, keeping records and reporting observations.

MEDICAL EXAMINATIONS take place on the doctors' rounds, which are usually in the mornings, but sometimes also in the early evenings. As the doctor frequently needs answers from the patient, and may listen to heart and chest sounds, it is necessary for the ward to be quiet at this time. This assists in providing for less effort from the patient, and also concentration by the staff concerned in the examination. Medical treatments are arranged in the same way and at the same time (unless emergency measures) as nursing treatments.

PHYSIOTHERAPY, OCCUPATIONAL AND DIVERSIONAL THERAPY. These treatments are carried out either with individual patients or as a group or class in the morning or afternoon. Patients who can walk or be transported in a wheel chair have treatment within the special departments.

VISITORS. There are many points to be considered in the arrangement and supervision of visiting hours. The hospital forms its own rules regarding these. For instance, in Children's Hospitals it is possible for parents to visit at most times of the day. They take part in bathing and feeding their infant and playing with the child. In general hospitals, one or two hours each day are set aside for visitors. This occurs in orthopaedic hospitals. A very ill patient of course is allowed visitors at any time providing no treatment is being carried out at the time. It is generally considered that visitors can be in a main ward outside main meal times, sanitary rounds, rest times and doctors' rounds. The patients' medical and nursing treatment must not be interfered with, neither should he or she be deprived of privacy and quiet. At the same time, the patient needs the comfort and presence of someone familiar and dear to him during the long days of serious illness, and then frequent contact with his own environment outside hospital as he is recovering, particularly during rehabilitation.

In wards such as those in Intensive Care Units and Psychiatric Rehabilitation Units the ward routine will differ from that in the general wards. In the latter unit the in-patient's day is arranged in a more informal pattern and in the former the programme is geared to the immediate needs of the very ill patient.

It would be a useful exercise for the pupil nurse to write in her study notebook the day's routine in the ward to which she has been allocated for practical experience. An alternative exercise would be 'The In-patient's Day', an account of 24 hours in the particular ward.

CHAPTER 8 | VENTILATION, HEATING AND LIGHTING

These are factors in an individual's *environment* which, when satisfactory, contribute to his health. During illness, attention to them is doubly important because they may in small ways hasten or slow down the patient's recovery. An ill person is more aware of discomfort than someone who is fit and well, so a nurse needs to consider these factors in the interests of the patient's comfort.

VENTILATION is important in the maintenance of health for three reasons:

It is necessary for foul air, i.e. air which contains impurities and unpleasant smells, to be replaced by fresh pure air.

Air which contains a large amount of evaporated water prevents a person from sweating and this causes him to be very uncomfortable, hot, listless, thirsty and to complain of headache. Eventually his body temperature rises and he feels unwell. It is necessary for this moisture-laden air to be replaced by air containing less moisture, and then sweat will evaporate from the patient's skin and he will be more comfortable.

Movement of air on the skin, particularly if it is of varying temperature, will stimulate nerve endings in the skin and consequently produce stimulation in the central nervous system. (Notice how people feel less drowsy in a room where there is a coal fire than in central heating where the temperature is level. The heat from the coal fire varies all the time.)

The nurse bears in mind however that ventilation can be excessive for a patient. Then his body will be cooled very quickly, and if he be extremely ill or feverish, or he is restless and the bed-clothes move and leave him exposed, then the fast movement of air (especially if cool) can produce some degree of collapse. Very young babies and elderly people cannot tolerate loss of heat from the body, and should be protected from excessive ventilation. The patient may find the movement of air so irritating in its stimulation of the skin's nerve endings that he complains of the 'draughts'.

When dangerous or toxic substances, smoke or unpleasant smells are produced then it is necessary to have suitable efficient ventilation provided as a safety measure. This can be the case in an operating theatre where general anaesthetics are used.

Methods of Ventilation

1 By Natural Means from a Wind or Breeze
In a building fresh air is admitted through the windows. When these cannot remain opened for any length of time, a ventilation aid may be used, e.g. louvred small panes or a 'Cooper's Disc'.

2 By Artificial Means
That is, by fans which create a movement of air. The simplest form of fan is a piece of stiffened paper either fixed in a handle or held in the hand, moved rapidly by a wrist movement. These fans are seen in hot climates and were used in this country by people who sat in hot rooms where the windows were not opened.

At the present time, fans with metal or plastic blades can be operated electrically and are suspended from the ceiling or stand on a base for table, desk or locker use. The noise is a disadvantage for some people, and they should be placed where they are safe, at least four feet away from a patient. This is necessary if he has poor vision or if it is used during the night, when he may put out a hand and be hurt or frightened.

Artificial ventilation on a large scale may be required in a hospital situated in a dirty and noisy area where windows are unsuitable for ventilation, as well as in a factory where harmful fumes or dust are produced, and in a coal-mine. Artificial ventilation is needed in underground railways, cinemas, theatres, conference rooms and large departmental stores.

The necessary movement of air is accomplished by large fans either drawing air *into* the building (propulsion fans) or drawing it out of the building (extraction fans) or occasionally both. The air is usually filtered as it enters the buildings through grids and this removes dust and dirt. The entry grids are near the floor and the exits are in the ceilings because warmer air in a room rises, but in operating theatres this is in reverse so that any anaesthetic gases in the atmosphere are extracted without passing over the operation field and any personnel in the theatre.

Small extractor fans can be fitted into windows of a domestic dwelling, or in a shop, and are useful when the rooms are small and natural ventilation is inadequate, also in banks where confidential matters may be discussed. Similar small fans have been installed in single dressing stations to reduce incidence of air-borne hospital infection.

It may be useful to consider the application of methods of ventilation.

Ventilation in a City
This is a problem when the buildings are high and close together, the streets are narrow and winding. Wide roads and streets, particularly straight major roads and open spaces such as parks, playing fields and gardens, encourage efficient city ventilation.

Ventilation in a House
Fresh air is introduced through WINDOWS and NOT by room doors, otherwise impure air may be replaced by even more impure air. Aids, e.g. Cooper's disc or small extractor fans are suitable. Air leaves the rooms by the chimney or flue, otherwise a ventilating grille or opening into a flue or outside wall is necessary. Draughts can be a nuisance and are usually due to doors and windows being opposite to each other or because they do not fit the frames correctly. Some fireplaces encourage a floor draught. Electric fan heaters can be used to improve the movement of air in a room; the heating switch is turned off but the fan switched on.

It is useful to know that a sash window opened one inch will admit sufficient air for one person in an average-sized room.

Ventilation in Hospital
Fresh air enters through windows, or there is a system of artificial ventilation. The latter is uncommon in a building as a whole, but is employed in operating theatres, Burns Units, kitchens, also committee and lecture rooms where there is excessive outside noise. In a Burns Unit the air entering will be filtered to prevent wound infection. It is essential to close doors after entering and leaving this department, otherwise the artificial ventilation becomes inefficient.

It is best to open windows on one side of the ward only and then away from the wind, otherwise there will be draughts and also much heat will be lost and artificial heating is expensive.

Small electric wall or table fans may be used in side wards or when a patient is accustomed to spending much time out of doors when he is well and he finds the hospital ward 'stuffy'.

Oxygen and steam tents have an air outlet to assist in some air movement so that the temperature inside the tent does not rise above 24°C. This is especially important when the patient is feverish.

Heating

Requirements for heating vary much from person to person, and from situation to situation. Some people find a well-heated room too warm, others dislike to be cool, and these differences are found amongst patients in hospital. For this reason it is advisable to maintain a fairly constant average temperature in a ward, e.g. 18°C (65°F), but be prepared to add or remove bed-clothes, arrange for a patient who sits up in bed to have a jacket, and open a window if he finds the ward too warm.

Methods of Heating
The sun produces heat by natural means. Rooms facing south do not require as much artificial heating as those facing north. Although pleasant for people who are fit and well, the nurse should understand that patients who are ill find direct sunlight extremely trying and in the evening the patients will have pyrexia, headache, thirst, possibly sunburn, and they will be restless during the night. So it is essential to have sun-blinds in wards facing south, and sun-umbrellas for the patients on balconies. Ambulant patients can move to a shaded place, and it is the person in bed who needs this special consideration.

Coal fires are cheerful and stimulating, but cause smoke pollution and make much work in cleaning and carrying coal. They are unsafe for children, old people and some ill people, e.g. those who may have convulsions or attacks of unconsciousness. In these cases, fire guards are necessary.

Slow combustion stoves will burn smokeless fuel, are cleaner than a coal fire and require less attention but can give continuous heat. They are not as cheerful as a coal fire.

Oil stoves are convenient, clean and efficient. They require special care to avoid the possible danger of fire.

Gas fires are convenient and clean though the air in the room becomes very dry. A flue is necessary to get rid of fumes. Care is required in using the gas tap, which must be kept turned off when the gas fire is not lit, as coal gas contains carbon monoxide, which is a poisonous gas. North sea gas is not poisonous but an accumulation reduces the oxygen content of the atmosphere.

Electric fires are convenient and clean and do not dry the air. They can be moved from place to place providing there is a suitable power plug available, but need to be well protected by a fire-guard.

Convector heaters. These are a variation of the former methods in which the air is warmed and rises in the room. Do not dry clothes or towels etc. on these heaters as they become very hot and may cause a fire.

A fan heater operates electrically. The air is warmed, then driven out into the room by a fan. As with all motor-driven fans, there is some noise.

Electric storage heaters. These consist of blocks of fireclay in a metal casing which are heated by electric elements during the night when fewer people are using electricity and it is cheaper. As the heat is given out slowly and steadily the storage heater is suitable for background heating particularly in an older house where it can easily be installed. Clothing, towels, etc. should not be dried by hanging them over the heater as fire may be caused.

Central heating has been used in large buildings for several years, but is now being introduced into small domestic dwellings. Either steam is produced (only in large buildings), or water is heated by coke, gas, oil or electricity and then passes through pipes in the rooms and corridors. It returns to the heating plant and is reheated and continues on its circuit. The pipes may be in the walls or floors beneath panels. This method is convenient, clean, gives a constant temperature when correctly controlled, and is safe.

Heating Wards in a Hospital

The main method of heating is central heating and the temperature in the hospital wards is maintained at 15°C to 18°C. Additional forms of heating are sometimes used in day rooms where patients sit and have their meals. For this purpose, electric air convectors (movable) or electric fires (fixed to the wall) are convenient, as a nurse is not present most of the time and these forms of heating require little supervision. The fires must be well guarded. Bathrooms have heated towel-rails and no other extra heating is necessary.

In Nurses' Hostels there is central heating as background heating to give a temperature of 15°C (60°F), with extra coal, gas or electric fires in sitting-rooms. Coal fires are disappearing as smokeless zones are introduced in the town or city, and the extra labour for their maintenance is no longer available.

Central heating is also used in the lecture rooms of the School of Nursing to 20°C (68°F).

The hospital maintenance staff supervises the general heating arrangements in the ward etc. and provides supply and service for additional forms of heating. The nurses report any faults as soon as they are noticed and are responsible for observing rules for prevention of fire and protecting ambulant patients from danger. For economy, switch off electric current as soon as the fire or heater is no longer required.

Loss of heat from the building can be reduced in cold weather by closing outer doors, using plastic swing doors in corridors, and by opening windows only on one side of the ward to prevent strong cross ventilation. Young infants and old people do not tolerate low temperatures well (see chapter on ventilation) and their rooms or wards require steady, moderate heating in cold weather. In hospitals where there are premature or ill babies, the ward temperature is maintained at a higher level than in general wards, and some premature infants are nursed in incubators in which the temperature is maintained at 24°C to 27°C. Anaesthetised patients and those suffering from traumatic shock are not exposed to low or varying temperatures, and the air in operating theatres and intensive care units is controlled at 21°C.

In a temperate climate, nurses rarely need to concern themselves with too high a temperature in the hospital wards, but in places where temperatures are high and particularly when the air is humid (moist), keeping a patient cool and comfortable can be as exacting as the provisions of heating in cold weather. Sun-blinds and fans may be essential. Even in moderately warm temperatures the nurse will find that very few patients in bed or in chairs can tolerate direct strong sunlight. Polarised glass can be used in windows facing south but is expensive.

Lighting

The main source of light is the sun and this form of illumination is pleasant, efficient and economical, but available only during day-time. It is admitted to buildings by windows, glass roofs, glass doors and sky-lights, and most of these methods allow for ventilating and cooling a room. Windows allow us to see into or out of the room. When a nurse has several babies in cubicles to care for, the cubicle and corridor walls have glass partitions above two and a half feet, so that she may observe the infants at all times. Curtains or venetian blinds are used to ensure some privacy in houses which are close together and in hospital departments where there are open thoroughfares adjacent to the building.

When daylight (natural lighting) is not available or is obstructed, artificial lighting is necessary. For domestic use this is provided by candles, electric or oil lamps, gas or electric main lighting. In hospitals, electric light is used as it is clean, safer than gas and convenient. However, there is a possibility of breakdown in supply, and this may be serious in operating theatres and by the bed-side of very ill patients. An emergency supply is usually arranged, but a nurse will check the provision in the household stores of a supply of electric battery lamps, in an emergency cupboard.

In hospital wards and corridors there is diffuse lighting from overhead lights, which should be sufficient for general activity and to prevent accident but with 'no glare and no gloom'. Patients lying in bed can be irritated by bright lights in the centre of the ward. This is avoided by the use of shallow opaque bowls by which the light falls on to the white or cream painted ceiling and is reflected downwards into the ward, or by translucent glass bowls surrounding the bulbs.

Patients need reading lamps, and these are fixed on to the wall behind the beds. Illumination for individual work by medical or nursing staff is provided by movable electric lamps of the anglepoise or bull's eye type. Small electric lights may be incorporated in cupboards for dangerous drugs, medicines and instruments. These automatically light the cupboard while the door is open. A night nurse includes an electric torch in her equipment as this has many uses, enabling her to check the drip chamber in blood transfusion, to see the patient's prescription sheet and observation chart, to inspect a pressure area or a wound dressing. The patient is disturbed as little as possible. Any naked light, as from a match, is dangerous when oxygen therapy is in progress. In intensive care units where there are a small number of patients who are all extremely ill, full lighting may be in use all the time, as these patients require constant treatment, attention and observation. It is an advantage when such patients are not in a main general ward, as the lights used (in addition to noise and general activity) prevent other patients from sleeping.

CHAPTER 9 | ELIMINATION OF NOISE

Noise is sound with potential nuisance value. It can be a signal of warning in danger and is a sensory stimulus to motor response in reflex action. The producing of noise can be a source of satisfaction and pleasure, as when a child beats a drum.

Toleration of noise varies among individuals and it is possible to accustom oneself to a great deal of unavoidable noise like that from trains, road traffic, striking clocks and machinery. Intense irregular increases of sound, especially if associated with possible danger, disturb most people, e.g. vehicles changing gears on a hill or at a busy crossroads.

It is unusual, however, to be in a situation without some sounds of background activity and complete silence can cause dread, and even panic. People accustomed to some noise find quiet disturbing, and most people who are ill are comforted by the slight noise of someone near to them.

Noise with nuisance value can be detrimental to health; it interferes with rest, relaxation and sleep, aggravates nervous tension, hinders concentration in mental and creative work, is irritating to those who are near by and cannot escape from it. In industry some machinery produces noise of great intensity and the works managements continue research in an effort to reduce this. The men who work with these machines may become deaf after some years, and are provided with earplugs to prevent this.

People who are ill, or anxious, or have responsibilities towards other people, seem more aware of noise. In the latter instance, the sounds heard may be very slight, e.g. a mother will hear the whimper of her baby but be oblivious to the roar of a heavy vehicle outside the house, and a nurse will notice and learn to interpret small sounds in the ward at night. Many people in activities producing noise usually enjoy the activity and the noise. For this reason it is difficult to control it, and also to maintain some standard of quiet. Discipline is involved, either from an outside source in rules or regulations, such as the 'No talking' signs in a reference library, or the enforced wearing of rubber-heeled shoes by hospital staffs, or by self-discipline in speaking quietly, care in using equipment, reducing noise in the late evening as consideration for others who need rest.

Sources of Noise in Hospital

1. *People:* hospital staffs, of which nurses make up the largest number of those working in the wards, and visitors. Activities producing noise are talking, whispering at night, walking in shoes without rubber heels, slamming the doors.

2. *Equipment:* e.g. the older type of lift, machinery used in the ward like respirators, telephones. The handling of equipment can produce noise—kitchen utensils, crockery and cutlery, bed-pans, stainless steel bowls and dishes, trolleys.

3. *Other patients* who cough or groan, or are irrational at night, and those being admitted or receiving urgent treatment.

PREVENTION OF NOISE IN HOSPITAL

Thoughtfulness and consideration for others are requisites of each person working in, or visiting, the hospital. Some discipline on the part of the individual or by the rules of the hospital is necessary. The investigation of complaints of noise from patients are followed up by the ward sister, and discussion in a ward sisters' meeting will often disclose some solution.

Proper maintenance of equipment will reduce certain noise. This includes cleaning and oiling of trolley wheels, replacement of old washers on taps, rubber shields on wheel chairs and walls where moving space is small, wedges for rattling windows. The preparation and clearing of trolleys in dressing-stations not immediately adjacent to the ward and the installation of telephones in offices instead of corridors assist in preventing unnecessary noise.

It may be an asset if a ward is available, e.g. attached to Accident/ Emergency department into which patients can be admitted during the night, and side wards attached to a main ward for those who need night treatments. Where there are intensive care units, the other patients requiring intermediate nursing care or who are more independent are not disturbed at night by continuous activity.

Television sets are suitable only in day rooms or single side wards, and pillow radio-sets or headphones are used for radio programmes. An individual ear-piece can be fixed to a transistor set.

Visitors consider all the patients in the ward, talk and move quietly, wear rubber-heeled shoes and *not* steel-tipped heels, especially at night. Young children cannot be expected to behave in this way, and this is one reason why it is necessary for the ward sister to be consulted before

they enter a ward. The hospital staff work quietly and with special consideration on some occasions, one of which is in the care of a patient
with tetanus being nursed in a side ward and whose recovery will be
interrupted by noise. Carrying out duties quietly becomes a habit and
one which nurses need to cultivate as they are nearest in their work to
the bed-side, and therefore are most responsible for the patients' basic
comforts. This means taking particular care to prevent noise in rooms
adjacent to the ward, e.g. kitchens, sluices and corridors. Patients find this
noise most distracting, but appreciate a reasonable amount of activity
within the ward as this indicates nurses are at hand when they are needed.
A silent approach to the bed-side can be disturbing to a patient, especially
at night, if he is unfamiliar with hospital surroundings and routine, or
if he is blind. It is then useful to approach him and say 'Good morning,
Mr . . .' or 'I have come to attend to you, Mr . . .' as the occasion dictates.

Ear-plugs may be suggested for a patient who complains of not being
able to sleep in the general wards. These are discs of pink wax which can
be softened in the hand and then moulded into the ears when the time
arrives to settle down to sleep. They are bought at the chemists and need
to be renewed after a few nights. The nurse should know when a patient
has these or she may be anxious when he does not hear her speak even
though he appears to be awake.

In the Nurses' Hostel also, consideration for others is important. If this
be not spontaneous, then some rules may be instituted, and these have
been formed by the residents themselves at some time. It is usual for the
building to be quiet for seven or eight hours at night, e.g. 11 pm to 6 am.
Nurses who enter late, come in quietly and do not use the lifts if these
are near bedrooms. Where there is an internal night duty system, quiet is
essential in the Nurses' Hostel all day and night, as nurses retain their
own rooms during their short period of night duty and night nurses are
sleeping in all parts of the Nurses' Hostel.

It follows that the natural desire for physical activity amongst the
younger nurses needs opportunity for expression. Hours of duty are
shorter, and more convenient in most instances, and allow for more
recreation outside the hospital buildings. For those who remain in the
Nurses' Hostel, recreation rooms for dancing, indoor games or music are
best in a building separate from, though adjacent to, the Nurses' Hostel.
In most nurse training schools the bedrooms are also fitted up for study,
so these, together with the library and classrooms, are part of the nurses'
accommodation which should be quiet.

CHAPTER 10 | CARE AND USE OF WARD EQUIPMENT

Linen

Patients' garments, towels, etc., are transported from the laundry or central linen store in clean boxes or baskets. In the ward they are stored in dry clean cupboards or on shelves in a linen room. Speed and ease in selecting the articles required depend on the methodical and tidy manner in which the linen is placed on the shelves. Clear labelling is useful but it is more important to keep the different articles in the same place permanently. Torn linen or garments without buttons, etc., are withdrawn from the supply either in the central linen store or in the ward. These are repaired in the linen store.

When a patient is receiving treatment in the form of medications which stain the bed-clothes the nurse endeavours to use linen reserved for this purpose or disposable sheets and towels may be available. Removable stains can be dealt with by immediate soaking in cold water.

Mattresses

SPRING MATTRESSES are protected by plastic covers which encase the mattress completely and fasten with a lightning fastener and are mopped with soap and water, rinsed and dried. If heavily contaminated they are disinfected with a liquid disinfectant, e.g. white fluid (Izal) 1 in 300 or Savlon 1 in 40. This removes the need for the mattress to leave the ward to be autoclaved.

DUNLOPILLO MATTRESSES have a rubber surface which can be cleaned or disinfected as plastic-covered mattresses. The surface is damaged by heat and oil or grease. No attempt is made to fold or bend a mattress as this can damage springs or cause sponge rubber to crack.

FEATHER AND FLOCK PILLOWS are stored in the linen room where it is clean and dry. These are protected when necessary by plastic covers beneath cotton covers. After use by a patient they are either disinfected by autoclave, or the plastic covers are disinfected as plastic-covered mattresses.

As an economy measure, the nurse should form a habit of making sure that mattresses and pillows are properly protected from blood, vomit, wound discharges, urine, etc. before possible accidents can occur. Recovering or replacing these articles involves the hospital in expense. If stained mattresses and pillows were kept in use they could be a source of infection to the patient, and most people, including patients, find stained equipment unpleasant.

Cotton cellular blankets are laundered in the same way as sheets. Woollen blankets are difficult to disinfect and need to be treated by special washing and drying processes. They are rarely used in hospitals.

Ward Furniture

BEDS are usually made of iron painted white, cream or aluminium. They are movable but have a brake mechanism to prevent unwanted movement. Beds are available now which are more elaborate and have mechanical means for changing the position of parts of the bed, e.g. raising the foot or head of the bed.

Disinfection is by a liquid disinfectant such as white fluid 1 in 300 or Savlon 1 in 40.

The bedstead wheels require regular attention by the maintenance staff so that bed-fluff does not collect on them and they can be oiled correctly.

LOCKERS vary in size and shape according to the needs of the patients. Washable surfaces are necessary so that they can be cleaned easily twice a day. When some supervision of the contents of patients' lockers is necessary, the cleaning of the lockers is a responsible job. For example, visitors may bring sweets and biscuits which are not allowed in a patient's special diet, the patient may have medicines prescribed before admission to hospital and does not realise he must not now have these, or there may be money or valuables. The Ward Sister will advise in these situations. Articles are not removed from the lockers without the knowledge of the patient or his relatives.

CHAIRS should be of a type which can be cleaned easily and it is usual for two chairs or seats to be provided for each bed.

ARM-CHAIRS are covered in material which can be sponged regularly.

FOOT STOOLS are sometimes supplied with these chairs so that the patients' feet can be raised.

Any chair which appears damaged is removed from the ward immediately to be repaired. This will prevent possible accident.

SCREENS OR CURTAINS provide the patient with privacy. They are laundered each week to prevent infection. Screen wheels and curtain rails require attention by the maintenance staff so that they remain quiet in movement.

WARD FLOORS are cleaned by the domestic staff but any fluid spilled on the floor during a procedure must be mopped up at once. A patient or member of staff may skid on the wet patch and be injured. Any excreta or discharges from the patient are cleaned from the floor using disposable paper towels which are placed in a paper bag for burning. The floor area

involved is then disinfected using a floor mop wrung out in liquid
disinfectant such as white fluid 1 in 10. It may be necessary to leave a
barrier round the area temporarily.

Toilet Equipment

WASHBOWLS, MOUTHWASH BEAKERS AND BOWLS are washed thoroughly
after each usage. Stainless steel equipment can be boiled or autoclaved,
but some plastic materials will not tolerate these methods of sterilisation.
The Supplies Officer will advise on this.

Disposable beakers of compressed paper are available but expensive.

BED-PANS AND URINALS are stored in racks in the sanitary annexe.
Preferably the racks are heated. They are cleaned and sterilised in a bed-
pan steriliser, or cleaned in a bed-pan washer and sterilised in a water
steriliser which is accommodated in the utility room where the toilet
equipment is kept. Disposable bedpans and urinals are available. These
are made of compressed paper and after use are placed in a machine
which disintegrates them. The results together with the excreta are discharged into the sewage system. The bedpan bases are plastic and
permanent. They are cleaned thoroughly using a suitable disinfectant,
rinsed and dried.

BINS to collect waste have tightly fitting lids. If possible a large paper
bag is placed inside. When the bag is filled, it can be easily removed by
the portering staff, otherwise the bins are cleaned every day.

WARD INCINERATORS are usually powered by gas. Any smell of coal-
gas should be investigated at once; the gas from the jet may not have
ignited or there is a leak. The gas taps are turned off before making
investigations and a naked light, e.g. matches, must *not* be used.

Only limited amounts of material can be burned at one time. Metal
parts such as disposable injection needles, plastics, e.g. disposable
syringes, and metal foil will not burn completely in these incinerators and
should be collected in a special box for collection and disposal by the
appropriate hospital department. Incinerators are useful and efficient in
dealing with soiled dressings, sanitary towels and babies' disposable
napkins, and assist in prevention of infection.

Rooms, cupboards or alcoves for urine and faeces specimens and for
urine-testing are well ventilated and have efficient lighting to identify
specimens and observe urine test reactions.

Testing reagents are renewed when out of date. Stoppers are replaced
immediately after use and the bottles are not exposed to strong sunlight.
These are poisons and the cupboard in which they are stored is preferably
kept locked.

BATHROOMS AND TOILETS are cleaned by the domestic staff. The bath is

brushed down after each patient's use. Mops and brushes are stored in a
disinfectant which is changed daily. Sufficient toilet paper is always
available.

Dressing-Station

DRESSING TROLLEYS are washed with soap and water each day. Between
dressings they are cleaned with a suitable antiseptic. The wheels require
regular attention to ensure quiet movement.

INSTRUMENTS are stored in clean cupboards where they can be seen
easily. They are sterilised before use in an aseptic procedure. After use
they are immersed at once in disinfectant. Cleaning of serrated edges,
joints and hinges is very important—a small brush is useful for this purpose. Then they are sterilised by autoclaving or boiling for five minutes.
Instruments and other surgical equipment are very expensive and every
care is taken to prevent damage or loss. Proper inspection and maintenance of equipment are included in the duties of the ward staff. These
include minor frequent attentions such as checking efficiency of equipment or lubricating moving parts. Major repairs or routine maintenance
like sharpening knives and scissors are carried out by technicians in the
instrument stores on request from the Ward Sister.

WATER STERILISERS are cleaned each day using a soap abrasive.

In most hospitals instruments and dressings are sterilised in packets or
containers by the staff of the Central Sterile Supply Department. They
are responsible for routine maintenance and arranging for repairs.

PRE-STERILISED ARTICLES are stored in clean cupboards so that they
are quickly and easily available.

DRESSINGS AND BANDAGES. Stocks of these are checked regularly to
ensure an adequate supply. Use them as economically as possible in
every way, for they are more expensive than may be readily recognised.

DISPOSABLE EQUIPMENT is expensive and should be used without waste.
Methods of disposal are important and details are circulated in the Ward
Procedure Manual.

STORE-ROOM ACCOMMODATION may be necesary for:

(i) *Patients' clothes*. Those awaiting collection by relatives are stored in
bags which are clearly labelled. Damp clothing must be dried thoroughly
before storing in polythene bags, otherwise mould will form on them.
Clothing worn by the mobile patients hangs in a wardrobe cupboard or is
kept in the patients' lockers.

(ii) *Bed accessories* such as cradles, bed elevators, back-rests, intravenous bottle stands.

(iii) *Medical and surgical equipment*, e.g. splints, sometimes respirators.

(iv) *Wheel chairs*, not in use.

(v) *Flower vases*.

General cleaning of the ward may be carried out by the domestic staff under the supervision of the domestic supervisor, but the cleaning of cupboards, etc., is usually the work of the ward orderly.

DUTY OFFICE. In this room will usually be found all records and reports, case-notes, and X-rays concerned with the patient on the ward. The Dangerous Drug cupboard may also be in this room. Special instructions and notices for admissions, operations and procedures are displayed on a board. In some instances equipment required in emergency or for medical examination of the patient is available here.

The Sister or Charge Nurse arranges for private interviews with patients' relatives or members of staff in this office. Nursing staff time-sheets, records of practical experience, ward text-books and procedure notes may be accommodated in this room, as is also the ward telephone.

FIRE EXTINGUISHERS and necessary fire-fighting apparatus are found on brackets or in niches in ward corridors where they are easily available in emergency.

Instructions on the DISPOSAL OF RUBBISH will be issued by the hospital according to the facilities available. For example, the rubbish may be collected in the ward as follows:

(a) burnable rubbish (but NO aerosol containers)

(b) non-burnable rubbish

(c) broken glass, scalpel blades and needles which are disposable.

(a) and (b) are collected in strong paper bags or bins. (c) need to be collected into a container which is readily recognised by the portering staff so that it may be handled with care to prevent accidents.

CHAPTER 11 | THE WARD KITCHEN AND WARD MEALS

Some of the functions of the ward kitchen have changed over the years because very little cooking is now done on the wards. Nevertheless, it is an important part of the ward and needs very careful management, if it is not to become a source of infection.

Kitchen Hygiene

Unfortunately, many ward kitchens are out of date in construction and design, but every effort should be made to keep the ceiling and walls clean. These should be treated with washable material. All other surfaces in the kitchen should be smooth and easily washed, i.e. stainless steel sinks and draining boards and formica working areas. Wooden draining boards and table tops are dangerous and should be replaced. There should be adequate lighting and ventilation, especially over the cooker and sinks. Dish cloths and mops, roller towels and tea towels should be forbidden and disposables used instead. There should be adequate soap and hot water for handwashing and reminder notices on the use of these after the use of the toilet or nose blowing. The ideal is to forbid the use of handkerchiefs and pockets in overalls and to supply paper tissues above a special hand-washing sink with a pedal bin underneath it for their immediate disposal.

The floor should be covered with easily washed, hard-wearing material which is also quiet to walk on and the whole layout of the kitchen should reduce movement to a minimum.

Patients often like to help with the preparation of drinks and the hygiene of the kitchen should set them a good example. Nurses must never forget that they are teachers of healthy living as well as comforters of the sick.

The siting of the ward kitchen is often a cause of difficulty as it is a noisy annexe to the ward and can cause a great deal of irritation to patients during the day and even more so at night. It is important therefore to work as quietly as possible and to keep the door shut when unavoidably noisy work is taking place.

Storage of Foods

All ward kitchens should have a refrigerator for the storage of milk, meat and fats etc. Food left over from main meals should be returned to the central kitchen. Dry goods such as tea, sugar, jam, Ovaltine, etc., should be kept in air-tight tins or jars in lockable cupboards. Bread should be kept in a bin to reduce the risk of mice, and food which attracts flies and can be contaminated by them, such as milk, fish, meat, butter and jam, should never be left uncovered when not being used.

All food put into the refrigerator should be contained in polythene bags, plastic boxes or covered with a plate to prevent either drying or flavouring of other foods. Milk is best kept in its covered bottle. Food belonging to patients should be clearly labelled. Ice trays should be replenished daily and the refrigerator defrosted at regular intervals.

Food scraps should be discarded into a bin with a close-fitting lid and removed after every meal to a central point for collection by contractors. Crumbs should be swept up regularly as they encourage mice.

The presence of pests in the kitchen should be reported to senior nursing staff so that they may be dealt with immediately by a member of the hospital or by the Public Health Department.

Preparation of Food

When food is being prepared the nurses' hands must be spotlessly clean, as must be all the utensils. The ingredients must be both fresh and appetising to look at.

Cleaning and Sterilising Crockery and Cutlery

Every kitchen should have an adequate and constant supply of really hot water and a soap solution or detergent suitable for the type of water in the district. The normal rules of washing-up apply:

1. Rinse all greasy plates and cutlery under running hot water.
2. Wash in very hot water plus detergent, rinse in hot clear water in second sink or bowl.
3. Wash in following order: glass, cutlery, small plates, large plates, saucepans and tins.
4. Drain well in special racks, or dry either by hot air method or with fresh dry paper towels.
5. Store in clean cupboards and drawers.

It may be necessary from time to time or a rule of your hospital to sterilise crockery and cutlery. This is usually done after following the routine washing-up method by (a) moist heat, i.e. boiling, (b) dry heat, i.e. hot-air ovens, or (c) chemical substances diluted with water in which the utensils soak for a prescribed period of time. Increasingly disposable utensils are used where there is a risk of infection.

Some hospitals have installed wash-up machines or central washing-up areas. See that the makers' instructions are followed exactly and know how to wash-up manually in case of a breakdown.

Invalid Cookery

All young people can be expected to know how to cook and be able to use a simple cookery book intelligently. The feeding of the sick is one of the most important parts of a nurse's work and it can be one of the most interesting too. It needs the following:

(a) A knowledge of food values.
(b) A knowledge of cooking methods.
(c) An understanding of the patient.
(d) Imagination and planning.

C

The doctor's orders must, of course, be followed concerning the diet but skill in preparing and presenting the food will ensure that the patient eats it.

In addition to the basic knowledge needed by a nurse in planning her patients' meals the following principles should be remembered:

(a) All food should be of the best possible quality and absolutely fresh.

(b) The most suitable method of cooking should be used. Usually boiling, poaching, steaming or grilling are preferable to frying and roasting.

(c) Patients must be prepared in advance for the meal by emptying the bladder, sponging the hands and being made comfortable in bed or on a chair.

(d) Trays and tables should be set with spotless linen and gleaming cutlery and glass. Small bowls of flowers add enjoyment—as do full cruets.

(e) Meals should be served punctually and a rest period provided afterwards.

(f) Observation of a patient's religious food taboos is essential, and special orders sent to the Catering Officer.

(g) Hot food should arrive at the patient's bedside hot, and cold food cold.

(h) Helpings should be small and well arranged on the plate. Colours and variety are important and second helpings should be available.

A great deal of effort has been made recently to offer a choice of main dish at each meal and menus are circulated to the patients in advance. Choice there should be, whenever possible, but it is not always wise to burden patients with having to make a choice, so menus should be used with discretion.

In the past ten years there has been a great effort made to improve hospital catering. Ward Sisters, Dieticians and Catering Officers work closely together to maintain this service to the patients. New systems of mass feeding are being introduced e.g. Ganymede; but the role of the nurse in observing and reporting on the feeding habits of her patients is as important as ever.

The management of the ward kitchen still belongs to the Sister or Charge Nurse, although the domestic staff may be supervised by a Domestic Supervisor. It is important that both nurses and domestic staff understand the principles of kitchen hygiene and use the same methods for the storage of food and maintenance of cleanliness.

CHAPTER 12 | PRECAUTIONS AGAINST FIRE

These are the responsibility of the hospital management personnel and each member of the hospital staff. Fire officers in the hospital make regular inspections of fire appliances, and members of the Fire Service give advice when problems arise.

These are some of the points which the nursing staff may observe in a hospital ward.

Fire-guards are firmly fixed to the wall on either side of coal fires and cannot be moved, and are attached to gas or electric fires. No tapers or spills are allowed and no articles like handkerchiefs are put on the guards for drying. Whenever possible electric leads are disconnected from wall fittings as soon as the apparatus is no longer required. Any faulty plugs and electric equipment are reported immediately and repaired before further use. Electrical apparatus requires regular servicing.

In the kitchen, gas taps and electric switches are turned off completely. Towels are not hung to dry over a kitchen stove. Care is taken when heating fat in a pan; a large saucepan lid is kept at hand so that if the fat catches fire the pan can be covered by the saucepan lid and the flame extinguished. Do not carry the pan away from the stove; the burning contents may be spilt. Switch off gas or electricity.

Care is also taken in the disposal of cigarette ends. They are placed by the patient into a metal ash-tray on his locker and at the end of smoking hours are collected and burned in the ward incinerator or emptied into a rubbish bin which has a tightly fitting lid. Placing them in waste-paper bins or baskets is dangerous as they may not have been completely extinguished and the waste paper will ignite, perhaps at a time when no one is near. It is inadvisable for bed patients who have a hand tremor or partial paralysis or who are mentally confused to smoke in bed. In many hospitals smoking by staff and visitors is not permitted within the hospital.

Inflammable substances, e.g. ether, are used in small amounts and kept in cool dark cupboards. If a bottle is broken, the room is well ventilated and no naked lights are allowed until the vapour has disappeared.

Precautions are necessary with oxygen and lighted candles, tapers or matches are avoided as a means of illumination at any time. Electric torches are safe and easy to use.

Accumulations of equipment are not allowed in corridors which may be a way of exit. Regulations concerned with the closing of doors and corridors and stairs are observed strictly; in this way spread of fire will be confined to as small a space as possible. Patients' ash-trays must be emptied into a safe place where a fire cannot begin unnoticed. Non-inflammable waste-paper bins, e.g. metal should have replaced baskets. There should be no accumulation of rubbish or inflammable material in out of the way places e.g. ends of corridors or at the bottom of a lift-shaft.

Nurses and other staff familiarise themselves with the *Instructions in case of Fire* as stated by the Hospital Authorities. These are displayed in wards, departments and the Nurses' Hostels. There is a telephone number in each hospital which gives direct access through the hospital switch-board to the Fire Service. Fire alarms are of the press-button type covered by glass which can easily be broken by pressure from a pen, pencil or the blade ends of scissors. There is immediate contact with the hospital telephone room and Fire Service.

Fire extinguishers are operated by removing the valve cover then making a sharp blow with the hand over the valve which is at the top of the extinguisher. Water will spurt from the nozzle and the direction needs control from the operator. Buckets of sand are also available for fires originating in electrical equipment. There may be fire hydrants and hoses at various points in a hospital.

Each ward has an exit in addition to the normal entry and exit. This should always be open or the key kept in a locked glass-covered case by the side of the door, the glass of which is easily broken. When removal of patients may be a complicated procedure, Fire Drill is organised at regular times so that the staff are familiar with the methods of moving patients quickly.

Arrangements may have been made for the Fire Officer to give talks on Fire Prevention and Instructions in Case of Fire, e.g. every 3 months. It may be obligatory for all members of hospital staffs to attend one of these talks annually. Films are shown and equipment demonstrated. A nurse arriving in a new hospital should familiarise herself immediately with the procedures for fire prevention as laid down in that hospital.

Instructions in Case of Fire

Break the glass and press alarm bell or telephone . . . (number as reserved for fire alarm in the particular hospital). In this way the Hospital Fire Officer and the local Fire Station are notified immediately. The person in charge of the ward is alerted quietly. Nurses who are in the vicinity of a fire deal with it by the use of extinguishers, sand, or blankets in an emergency. The remaining staff prepare to remove patients from the ward. Patients near the source of the fire are moved first. Those who are ambulant are taken down the fire escape or out by the ward door. Patients in bed are wheeled into the main corridor or carried down the fire escape in blankets or on mattresses. Do not allow beds or wheelchairs with patients to block exits from the ward.

It is important for people to move quickly and quietly, and to act with confidence and efficiency, thus maintaining the patients' reassurance.

The person in charge of the ward checks all patients and members of staff and reports to the officer in charge of the Fire Service team, which arrives within a few minutes of receiving the fire alarm and takes charge of the situation.

FURTHER READING

Hospital Planning

Noise Control in Hospitals. King Edward Hospital Fund

Nutrition

Nutrition and Dietetics for Nurses. M.E.Beck. Livingstone
Food with Thought. Dilys Wells. Harrap

PART 3 | NURSING CARE OF
THE PATIENT

CHAPTER 13 | NURSING CARE OF THE
PATIENT

'The unique function of the nurse is to assist the individual, sick or well, in the performance of those activities contributing to health or its recovery (or to a peaceful death) that he would perform unaided if he had the necessary strength, will or knowledge. It is her function to help the individual gain independence as rapidly as possible,
1. To breathe.
2. To eat and drink adequately.
3. To eliminate by all means of elimination.
4. To move and maintain desirable posture.
5. To sleep and rest.
6. To choose suitable clothes, to dress and undress.
7. To maintain body temperature within normal range.
8. To keep the body clean and well groomed.
9. To avoid dangers in surroundings and injuring others.
10. To communicate with others in expressing emotions.
11. To worship according to his faith.
12. To play and take part in recreation.
13. To learn, or satisfy the curiosity that leads to normal health.
14. To work at something that provides a sense of accomplishment.'
(From *Basic Principles of Nursing Care* by Virginia Henderson, International Council of Nurses.)

This criterion of nursing care can be applied to a patient in any situation, and during her training the pupil nurse learns the methods by which she may apply the principles of basic nursing care.

BASIC NURSING CARE OF THE PATIENT CONFINED TO BED

Breathing

The atmosphere in which the patient is nursed should contain adequate oxygen and be of average temperature, 18°C. His clothing fits loosely, particularly round the neck and chest, and the bed-clothes do not restrict breathing. If he cannot breathe lying flat in bed he is propped upright supported by a bed-rest and pillows. He may find breathing easier if he leans on a bed-table. His nose is cleaned if necessary with wool swabs on applicators. When breathing is difficult, oxygen may be necessary, and if breathing suddenly stops, artificial respiration by mouth-to-mouth breathing is carried out immediately. Mechanical air-ways, e.g. a tracheostomy or endotracheal tube, may be placed in position by the doctor, and it is the nurse's duty to keep the tube free from respiratory secretions.

Nutrition

The diet of the patient is sufficient for his needs, well balanced and varied so that no dietary deficiencies occur.

The food is served in an attractive manner, and everything is done to encourage him to eat his meal and enjoy it. If the patient cannot sit up in bed, the food is cut up, a diet cloth is placed beneath his chin and he uses a spoon to feed himself. The right-handed person with paralysis or injury to the right hand may require feeding but is also encouraged to use the left hand and, as he recovers, to resume the activity in his right hand. When both hands are incapacitated, the nurse will feed him. A blind patient or one with both eyes bandaged needs special consideration such as an extra large diet cloth, and a deep plate placed immediately in front of him.

The nurse observes how much food a patient has eaten, and if this be insufficient, a milk drink may be needed to complete his food intake.

Diet for the individual who cannot take solid food is calculated in liquid forms and given in small amounts frequently. When the diet cannot be swallowed, it is given to the patient through a tube which passes through the nose into the stomach. This is the procedure when the patient is unconscious. Records are required of the food and fluid intake of very ill patients, and special diets are prescribed by the doctor as part of the patient's treatment.

Elimination of Waste

The patient confined to bed cannot visit the toilet, and his elimination needs are met by the nurse taking bed-pan and urinal to him as required. Constipation is common and is relieved by:
  (a) increasing the fluid and roughage in the diet;
  (b) administration of a simple laxative, e.g. a senna preparation;
  (c) establishment of a habit routine.

Should the constipation become severe or prolonged, then a purgative enema may be necessary though this is only a temporary relief. *Very* occasionally, in patients suffering from:

(i) severe paralysis involving the rectum and abdominal muscles,
(ii) some mental disorders, or
(iii) neglect when they are elderly

the constipation may be so severe it cannot be relieved by ordinary means and the faeces are removed from the rectum manually but this is an extremely skilled operation. This situation is avoided if possible by the following:

(i) adjustment of the diet,
(ii) administration of a mild laxative daily which decreases in dose as soon as it becomes effective,
(iii) taking the patient to the toilet at regular times or giving an arachis oil, glycerine or soap and water enema each day until the situation is relieved. Disposable enemas are available.

It is important that there should be no delay in giving a patient a bedpan when he has a 'call to stool', and the habit of bowel action at regular intervals should be encouraged in the bed patient. A commode is provided as soon as the patient can be lifted or assisted out of bed.

There may be difficulty in passing urine due to:

(a) fear of pain or discomfort.
(b) embarrassment when ordinary toilet facilities are not possible.
(c) in unconsciousness or delirium.
(d) in paralysis of the bladder and abdominal muscles.

The nurse assists the patient by reassuring him and ensuring privacy. Adequate fluid intake is maintained and movement in bed encouraged. Patience is necessary and anxiety must be avoided as the patient becomes tense and then cannot pass urine. Standing by the bed supported by a male nurse or attendant will help a male patient if his condition allows this. Retention of urine is extremely uncomfortable and when it cannot be relieved by ordinary means, the doctor may order catheterisation to be carried out by aseptic technique.

Movement and Posture

The most harmful effects of prolonged rest in bed are:

(i) bed-sores.
(ii) broncho-pneumonia.
(iii) loss of muscle tone.
(iv) absorption of calcium from the bones causing the bones to become less rigid.

(v) formation of stones in the kidneys.

(vi) mental apathy.

It is essential for the patient to move in bed, or to be moved by the nurse until such time as he can be lifted out of bed and use a chair, and later walk.

To enable him to move in bed the bed-clothes are *not* tucked in too tightly, and a bed cradle can support the covers about his feet so that he can exercise his feet and ankles. A pole with chain and hand-grip at the top of the bed provides a means by which he can lift himself up the bed and change his position. Bed-making and bed-bathing are opportunities for exercises, and the patient is encouraged to do as much for himself as he can within the limits of his capacity and treatment. The nurse may find she is needed to put out hairbrush and comb from the locker but the patient will brush his hair himself.

The patient increases his bed-activity as his condition improves and throughout he is encouraged by the nurse's interest and praise in his prowess.

Occupational therapy may be considered. This means he makes something and in so doing exercises his muscles and joints, especially the small movement of fingers, wrists and forearms. The purpose of this activity gives him an aim or object to strive for and a sense of well-being develops. Suitable occupations for a patient in bed include card games, solitaire, leatherwork, making models of motor cars, ships and aeroplanes, knitting, marquetry, embroidery, also lino cuts, setting up printing type, some clerical work, e.g. typing.

The helpless patient is moved in bed by the nurse at regular intervals, e.g. every two hours and at the same time other treatment may be carried out. At bed-bathing or bed-making the nurse flexes and extends as many joints as possible such as wrists and ankles. This prevents stiffness in the joints and difficulty in movement when the patient begins to sit out of bed and walk, but stiff joints must never be forced to move by the nurse.

Sleep and Rest

Sleep and wakefulness form a rhythm which is broken in illness and needs to be re-established in convalescence. Depth of sleep varies, and sound sleep of a short duration is more refreshing than several hours of light, easily disturbed slumber.

In *serious illness* the patient sleeps for short periods at any time of the day or night. His condition may be critical and his treatment more important than sleep but in a few days the medical and nursing care becomes less intensive and his need for sleep apparent. Then the treatment

C*

is arranged at intervals such as two-hourly so that he is able to rest and sleep between these sessions. Later the times become more like those in his normal working day and the ward is quiet and dark from 10 pm to 6 am but rest periods are arranged during the day, e.g. 10.30 am to 11.30 am, 1.30 pm to 2.30 pm and 6 pm to 7 pm. It is useful if a routine of events occurs before sleeping. This is of course difficult when the patient is confined to bed but a routine can be devised. It takes place about 8 pm. The patient is made comfortable in every possible way and it is assumed he will sleep well. The nurse needs to remember that not only are there physical discomforts such as pain, noise, hunger, thirst and cold to prevent sleep, but also mental anxieties, fears and frustrations. As she makes the patient comfortable she will reassure a nervous patient or listen to an anxious one, comfort the distressed and think of means of relieving a sense of frustration when this is within her power.

Some people have developed a habit of reading before going to sleep and this should be allowed if possible by the use of a shaded overhead lamp, though the time will be limited if there are other patients to be considered. Children may be accustomed to saying prayers in the presence of an adult before going to sleep, or having a story read to them, or having a 'cuddle', and this can be done when the child is made comfortable for the night.

When insomnia is interfering with the patient's progress and cannot be relieved by ordinary methods of making the patient comfortable and reassuring him the doctor may order a drug with a sedative or hypnotic effect. This will be administered after he is made comfortable, and the ward is made quiet and dark immediately afterwards otherwise the effect of the drug is lessened. The nurse makes sure that he will be able to have six to eight hours' sleep during which time he will not be disturbed. As soon as the rhythm of sleep is re-established the drug is discontinued as continued use of these medicines can be harmful to the patient.

During the night the bed-bound patient may require the attention of the nurse so she should be available by means of a bell or light, but preferably is near at hand and walks quietly by the beds of the ill patients from time to time.

Waking a patient from sleep is best done by turning on the lights and then speaking to the patient. As in health some rouse quickly and others need half an hour to adjust themselves to the rigour of waking life. Delirious or mentally confused patients should be roused in a very gentle manner and *not* by touching them which they may find most disturbing and to which they may react with increased confusion or resistance.

Rest

Periods of rest are arranged after meals, exercise and occupational activity. Rest means relaxation; the patient is comfortable in bed and his posture maintained without effort.

Fatigue and effort in excess can prevent rest, and the nurse must be quick to notice signs of weariness in her patient and reduce the amount and time of activity temporarily; the patient may be overoptimistic regarding his progress immediately following a serious illness. It is not only physical activity which can produce fatigue in the bed-patient but mental and emotional activity also. Activities like writing letters, making intricate models with measurements can be exhausting, and some visitors may prove too stimulating and exciting. The ward atmosphere needs to be calm with a background of familiar routine and co-operative efficiency.

Prolonged bed-rest is avoided as this may produce complications. Obviously the patient's day is a balance between sleep and activity, rest and exercise.

Suitable Clothes. To Dress and Undress

While he is confined to bed the patient's clothing is loose and easy to put on him and remove. For this reason night-shirts are very suitable for some elderly male patients who cannot be moved easily, for the creases in pyjama trousers cause pressure marks on the skin. When examination of the chest is frequently carried out or there are wound dressings of the upper limbs or trunk, pyjama jackets can be easily removed, and on these occasions are useful for men or women. Gowns which open down the back, fastening with tapes can be changed frequently without disturbing a patient who is extremely ill.

The material is non-inflammable cotton, or wool, or silk or brushed nylon. Cotton is inexpensive and easily laundered, wool is warm but expensive and difficult to launder, silk is warm, expensive, light in weight, and smooth to the skin whereas wool is irritating to some people. Brushed nylon is used for women's nightwear. It is warm and soft, moderately inexpensive, wears well but needs gentle washing. Children's nightdresses and pyjamas are made from non-inflammable cotton, brushed nylon or cellular cotton. This latter is hard-wearing, can be boiled and is comfortable.

Cotton in the form of lawn, batiste, and cellular cotton is suitable for cool bed-wear. Nylon is easily laundered and does not need to be ironed. Not everyone finds it comfortable to wear. Also nylon may make sparks and could be dangerous where oxygen is in use.

Women and girls like to look attractive even though they are ill in bed and appreciate pretty bed-wear decorated with lace or embroidery and in flattering pastel shades, though yellows and creams are best avoided. The same interest is not so obvious in men and boys but their sense of well-being always improves with fresh, clean pyjamas, a shave and their hair brushed.

As vests are difficult to put on and take off, and the hospital wards are reasonably warm, 20°C (68°F), it is not usual for these to be worn by patients in bed. If the patient's shoulders are cold as in the upright position in bed, a cardigan or bed-jacket in dressing-gown cloth is useful. Women, particularly when they wear thin nightdresses, need wool, silk or nylon bed-jackets. Socks are not often required by bed-patients unless they are nursed on balconies or in open wards, but in many ways they are more sensible than hot-water bottles. It is essential they should be large enough but not so loose they slip off the feet. Old people and patients with bed-cradles suffer from cold feet. Such people should be allowed to have a flannelette sheet next to them for warmth and comfort.

Methods of dressing and undressing a patient in bed
The important points are:
(i) the joints are flexed into normal positions *not* into abnormal positions;
(ii) the patient makes as little effort as possible;
(iii) if one limb is injured or disabled this limb is manipulated into the garment first;
(iv) clothing is kept from covering the patient's face during the procedure.

Dressing the patient in a nightdress
The patient leans forward slightly. The nightdress is drawn up to the neck and sleeves. She slips her hands and arms into the sleeves and then raises her arms. The nurse slips the gown over her bent head. As the patient raises her head the gown falls into position and can be arranged comfortably. This method can be used for jacket and dressing-gown also, and in reverse for removing the garment.

To put on a sock, the nurse turns it inside out as far as the mid-foot, places it over the patient's toes, then rolls back the remainder of the sock over the heel and calf.

To maintain the temperature within the normal range 30°C to 40°C

The body temperature rises above normal in fever and in disturbances of the heat-regulating centre in the centre of the brain such as heat-stroke and severe head injury. When the temperature rises to 39°C (hyperpyrexia) there is danger to the patient and it is necessary to reduce the temperature. In fever the patient cannot tolerate a sudden fall in temperature and the methods used are not so drastic, the aim being to reduce the temperature no more than 1·4°C at a time. Treatment for hyperpyrexia in heat-stroke and head injury is urgent and therefore more drastic.

METHODS OF REDUCING THE BODY TEMPERATURE

(i) The room is made cool and well ventilated by opening windows or using fans.

(ii) Bed-clothes are removed as necessary.

(iii) Night-clothes are cool and loose. In severe cases they are removed.

(iv) Simple sponging of the body is carried out with warm water. The skin is mopped dry with a towel.

(v) Tepid sponging in which the body is sponged with tepid water at 27°C using long strokes towards the extremities. The water is allowed to remain on the skin, where it evaporates, thus cooling the body. Bath sponges or disposable flannels are placed in the axillae and groins. The temperature is reduced by not more than 1·4°C. This is a useful procedure in fever and head injuries when the temperature rises to between 39°C and 40°C.

(vi) The bed is made with a sheet covering the patient who is undressed, and over the sheets are two bed-cradles covered by a thin counterpane. Air is allowed to pass through the bed-cradles over the patient. A fan at the bottom of the bed accelerates the flow of air, and ice-bags hung from the cradles will cool the moving air.

(vii) Cold wet pack is ordered when the temperature is between 40·5°C and 42°C. The patient is undressed and lies on a well-protected mattress. He lies between two sheets wrung out in cold water and his limbs are abducted slightly from mid-line, so that the upper sheet is in contact with as much skin as possible. The sheets are kept moist with a water spray and changed daily and as necessary. A more intensive effect can be obtained by placing ice on the sheet by the side of the trunk and limbs but not touching them. The patient may remain in this bed until his temperature is lowered to the normal level.

Cool fluids by mouth and a cold compress on the forehead give comfort to the patient with pyrexia.

Sub-normal temperature below 36°C
This occurs in infants, especially premature babies, and old people who are exposed to cold. The anaesthetised patient cannot regulate his body temperature easily and reacts unfavourably to surroundings of high or low temperature. In shock the body temperature becomes sub-normal.

Methods of relieving sub-normal temperature are gentle and slow so that circulatory difficulties do not arise:

(i) Room heating at a constant level of 21°C to 27°C where patients in the above groups are being cared for.

(ii) No draughts in the ward or operating theatre.

(iii) Adequate clothing where artificial heating is not easily available. The patient's skin is not exposed to cool air.

(iv) Premature infants are placed in incubators for the first few days or weeks of life.

N.B. In shock the blood pressure falls. To maintain a satisfactory flow of blood to vital organs like the brain, heart and kidneys the blood vessels in the skin close down and the circulation on the surface of the body is reduced. Because of this, local heat as from hot-water bottles and electric pads is quite ineffective and may in fact be dangerous by causing a burn.

Keeping the body clean and well groomed

Care of the skin, hair and nails is explained in Chapter 27.

To appear well groomed the patient in bed requires some attention to details:

(i) His clothing is changed when it becomes damp and creased. The collar is turned down neatly. Buttons are replaced when lost and repairs carried out when needed, by relatives or staff responsible for patient's clothing.

(ii) His hair is cut regularly and shampooed each week by the hospital barber. It is brushed and combed as often as necessary. Attention is paid to a woman's coiffure, allowing facilities for styling. Children need hair trimming frequently and small girls may like fresh ribbons in their hair.

(iii) Men patients need to be shaved each day and a woman's appearance may be smartened by some use of cosmetics.

(iv) The bed is made neatly and the linen clean and uncreased. The bed-side locker is kept clear of all unwanted articles and the contents are in their proper places. Not only does the groomed appearance of the patient enhance his own morale but it gives comfort to his relatives when they visit.

To avoid dangers in the surroundings and injuring others

Dangers in the surroundings include articles in the bed which can damage the skin and predispose bed-sores, hot-water bottles placed near to the body and inefficiently protected, beds without sides when the patient is delirious or confused, naked lights where oxygen therapy is in progress, fire, and steam from a steam kettle.

These dangers are removed by:

(i) correct bed-making and supervision of the patient's basic care;

(ii) not using hot-water bottles when the patient is paralysed, unconscious or irrational;

(iii) making use of bed-sides or cot-beds, particularly during the night;

(iv) instructing members of staff and visitors regarding dangers of naked lights near oxygen;

(v) following the precautions against fire and carrying out instructions should fire occur.

Shank buttons on a nurse's uniform, a watch worn on the wrist, a ring with stones and claw settings, and long finger-nails can be sources of injury to a patient. The buttons are covered by an apron and extra sleeves or cuffs. The watch is fastened in a special pocket of the dress, rings are not worn (except plain wedding-rings) and finger-nails kept clean and short. These are customary regulations in the wearing of uniform.

Injury to others is a possible result of irrational behaviour in a mentally disturbed patient, e.g. an alcoholic. The nurse informs the doctor and he will advise treatment. An infectious patient is a potential source of injury to others. He is isolated from other patients and precautions are taken to prevent the nurse from becoming infected.

In a less definite manner a patient can injure another patient by undermining his confidence in himself and the hospital staff, by causing dissatisfaction when there is no cause, and in some cases by making him afraid of his illness or treatment. Sister or the doctor is best able to deal with this situation should it occur.

Communication with others

Patients in hospital and confined to bed who find difficulty in communicating with others cannot make the nurse aware of their physical needs and are also unable to express their feelings. This leads to greater intensity of emotion which is frustrating and exhausting and interferes with the patient's general comfort and peace of mind.

The patient who cannot speak may have had an operation or treatment on his mouth such as fixation of jaw following injury, or radium applied to the tongue, or the larynx may have been removed. Writing pads and pencils are placed near to him and a bell is within reach to summon the nurse. After laryngectomy the patient is taught by the speech therapist how to speak using air from the stomach.

The speech is impaired when a patient suffers from a 'stroke', one side of the body being paralysed including the face. This may be complicated even further by disturbance of the speech centre of the brain and he cannot produce the words he wishes to say. The nurse anticipates the wishes of her patient for he may become distressed in his efforts to explain, and she is patient in listening to him.

The nurse may have a natural aptitude for understanding *a patient who does not speak English* and whose language she does not recognise but she needs assistance from relatives, or the services of an interpreter are sought from other members of the hospital staff, teachers of languages, or students from other countries. Patients who are delirious or mentally confused may lapse into the language of their childhood and this may be unfamiliar to the nurse.

A patient in a single side ward or on a balcony may be unable to communicate with others because of his *geographical isolation*. He should be visited frequently by nurses, relatives and also other members of the hospital team such as a librarian when his condition allows this. Should he be very ill, a special nurse to care for him is an asset when the patient is isolated, in addition to frequent or intensive technical nursing care.

Other groups of patients who have difficulty in communicating with others are infants and young toddlers, very shy or reticent people, and sometimes those who are depressed or apathetic. The nurse needs to spend time with these patients, to listen to them and talk with them or to learn other ways of communication such as encouraging them to paint pictures. When possible, patients should be placed in the ward next to others with interest similar to their own.

To worship according to his faith

The nurse learns the patient's religion when details of information are collected on his admission, and the hospital chaplain or priest in his denomination is informed by Sister that he is in the hospital. If there is no minister of his religion attached to the hospital, relatives then notify his own minister who will be able to visit the patient in hospital.

Ministers of religion are allowed to visit the patient at any time other than when nursing care and treatment are in progress. Services of worship are held in the hospital chapel but the patient confined to bed cannot attend these. Frequently the service is broadcast to the wards. Special services including Communion and Mass can be said at the bed-side and the patient has opportunity for this each week or as arranged by the minister or priest. In some wards morning prayers are said by the nursing staff, and a short service with hymns is held on Sunday.

Patients in hospital may be of religions and creeds other than Christian, and their wishes and those of the relatives are given the same consideration and respect.

The patient who practises his religion needs times for prayer and, on these occasions, the curtains or screens are drawn round the bed to give privacy. Small children who say their prayers at night expect the nurse (mother substitute) to stay with them while these are said. She may be able to comfort the patient who is very ill by repeating a short prayer at the bed-side. The provision of a Bible in the ward is helpful to a man or woman who has not brought his own religious books into hospital or who has been admitted as an emergency. The Roman Catholic priest is informed of a Roman Catholic patient who is extremely ill and who may not recover, so that he may administer the Last Sacrament to the patient.

Christian Scientists may not agree readily to medical and surgical treatment. Jehovah's Witnesses do not agree to transfusion of blood.

When a Jewish patient is very ill and may not recover, the Rabbi (Jewish minister of religion) is consulted about the wishes of the patient regarding last offices. Certain Jews should not be touched after death by Gentiles, and the laying-out is performed by persons of their own faith.

Relatives of patients of other religions are consulted when there is doubt concerning last offices. It may be customary for several relatives to to be with the patient while he is seriously ill.

Diet and Food

Some Roman Catholics do not eat meat on Fridays. Jews do not eat the meat or fat of pigs or rabbit. They prefer that meat is from animals killed in a special manner (Kosher meat). During the Passover they eat no leavened bread, but have special biscuits. Some Jewish patients prefer their food to be prepared in dishes and pans reserved for their type of food. This may mean their cooked meals are brought into hospital providing there is no disturbance of the diet prescribed by the doctor.

Hindus are often vegetarian, eating no food from killed animals or

poultry. Beef is always avoided. Buddhists eat a vegetarian diet. Mohammedans do not eat pork, neither do they drink alcohol.

To Play and Take Part in Recreation

During acute and severe illness this aspect of basic nursing care requires
little attention but, as the patient recovers, his basic physical needs are
more easily supplied and he has time and inclination for the satisfaction
and pleasure which play and recreation provide. It is desirable that
patients should become ambulant and mobile as soon as their condition
allows, but occasionally the treatment necessary for their ultimate recovery is possible only when the patient is in bed. This type of treatment
in an otherwise fit and healthy person is a severe test for an active,
energetic and perhaps impatient person and particularly for him in whose
everyday life there is little time for play or recreation. Creative occupation is usually best for this patient, such as leatherwork and painting.

Some patients enjoy card games, either solo like Patience, or in com-
petition with an ambulant colleague. Chess can also be considered and it
is possible for men completely immobilised but mentally alert to have
mirrors fixed above and in front of them (like a driving or demonstration
mirror) so that they can see a central chess-board. A nurse or visitor
moves the chess-men at the instruction of the patient. To avoid fatigue,
the game may be continued from day to day. Games which can be held
in the hand, such as word-making squares, puzzle bricks (fitting shapes
together to make a cube or object), intertwined bent nails which can be
separated, are inexpensive and sold in many stores. These can be acceptable gifts for visitors to bring but the patient should be given time to
solve one puzzle before another is brought for him, otherwise he becomes
exhausted and his power to concentrate is not allowed to redevelop.
Simple models to assemble and perhaps rearrange on a later date provide
some activity for mind and muscle, and a snow-storm paperweight can
give pleasure to a person regaining strength in the hands after a severe
illness.

Men who when well play field games are interested in following and
assessing the prowess of football and cricket teams. Children need some
playthings either from home or provided for them. They choose those
they want and the remainder should be removed. The nurse or parents
take an interest in the child's play and make time to take part in it if the
child wishes this. It is useful for the nurse to understand which forms of
play are popular in the different age-groups.

Following *recreation* there is a sense of freshness and vitality, the
individual is eager and enthusiastic, he experiences a feeling of well-

being. This is an asset during recovery from illness, and important as treatment in some medical diseases. During recreation the person participates in some form of *activity* either physical or mental or both. A woman can knit a bed-jacket, read a book or solve a crossword puzzle, or paint an original picture—the last demands physical and mental activity. Radio and television, in addition to books, can be a means of recreation, but sometimes the individual can become completely passive in listening and looking, and the recreational benefits are lost. For this reason they should be in use only when being listened to or viewed. Social and festive occasions also provide recreation, and even if the ward patients are confined to bed, it is possible to celebrate the birthday of one of them with perhaps a special cake for tea and some of his birthday cards on the centre table. When play and recreation are part of the patient's day, the nurse will find it difficult to maintain complete tidiness in the ward throughout the day, but the games are put away for mealtimes and at night. The patients need larger lockers, and the ward staff and visitors take a personal interest in the patients' activities.

To Learn, or Satisfy the Curiosity that Leads to Normal Health

As the result of learning, there is a change of behaviour. While the patient is extremely ill, the process of learning is slowed or halted. As he recovers the previous activity of learning returns, but this part of return to independence can be interrupted temporarily or perhaps even permanently by depriving him of the tools with which to learn. These are:

(i) The opportunity of using his senses of vision, hearing and touch, and his muscles.

(ii) Sources of information and stimulation: people, letters, books, newspapers, radio, television. An incentive to learn combined with the affection and personal interest of those surrounding the individual provides the best background for progress. Without the tools and this background and encouragement he becomes apathetic, not only unable to eat and walk and work but also incapable of responsibility for himself and others. In avoiding this situation the nurse assists in providing the tools and the background. She makes sure the patient has his spectacles or hearing aids if he is accustomed to these. He is encouraged to hold articles such as feeding utensils and medicine glasses, later to carry out simple exercises and eventually to sit in a chair, walk in the ward, take part in occupational therapy and become more knowledgable and independent.

Curiosity disappears in acute and severe illness when maintaining life is the prime issue, but as the patient recovers or when he is not very ill (and even more so when he feels well but some investigations are required) he becomes interested in the nature of his illness, the possible treatments, the ward staff, the other patients, the hospital routine and the world outside hospital including details of his own domestic and working life. The doctor will explain his medical condition and treatment. Relatives and friends are allowed to visit as often as is convenient, and should visit regularly, particularly when the patient is in hospital for a long period of time Letters are delivered twice a day, a bedside telephone is sometimes possible, and a voluntary organisation and the hospitals provide library services for patients in bed. Curiosity regarding other patients and their illnesses is discouraged and the nurse gives no information of a personal or professional nature. Conversation in the ward is stimulating but some subjects are avoided when they are likely to cause disagreement, such as religion or politics. Arrangements are made for the children and young people in hospital for lengthy treatment to have school lessons from qualified teachers, and correspondence courses can be arranged for those who need to train for a new kind of occupation on leaving hospital. When neither of these is possible the nurse can encourage the patient to read useful books and magazines, and to make a small collection, e.g. postage stamps, or newspaper cuttings on a special topic such as animals, birds, motor cars or some matter of interest in current affairs.

To Work at Something that Provides a Sense of Accomplishment

For this the patient needs a clearly defined aim, and he should have the ability to carry out the work involved otherwise he will become fatigued, frustrated and discouraged (the doctor or sister confirms the tasks to be selected). He is allowed sufficient time to complete the work as he will be slower than when he is well, and the time of completion is not so distant that his interest will not be maintained.

The tasks may appear very small indeed to the person who is healthy and active but producing even a smile can be an effort for an exhausted and weak patient. The tasks include feeding himself, exercising his hands and feet, changing his position in bed, getting out of bed, dressing and undressing, and walking in the ward. Several patients have a disability which complicates the task—a bandaged hand or an arthritic joint, chronic bronchitis when effort leaves him breathless, the fear of injury on falling. Frequently the nurse finds it necessary to take the initiative in the beginning and persuade the patient, possibly with gentle firmness, to attempt the task. As he gains in confidence, the initiative will change from the nurse to the patient and soon he is ready for the next task. On completion of the present work, and perhaps at each step of the venture, the patient will be encouraged by the nurse's praise and interest. It is necessary at times to remind him of his progress when he is impatient or depressed, and occasionally to explain again the task and the reason for it. When the operation, however small, is completed the patient has all the pleasure of achievement, and indeed the nurse shares in this also. Each of them experiences satisfaction and happiness in the work done.

'Doing something' is another means of gaining similar satisfaction in accomplishment. The 'something' depends on the patient, his condition, and material available. The occupational therapist can provide tools and materials for activities, and teaches the patient how to carry out the task. If the patient is elderly and her hands a little stiff for fine work, knitting squares for dish cloths or blankets is satisfactory for her and useful to other people. In these tasks as with those mentioned above the patient needs praise, interest and encouragement from the nurse.

The Care of the Patient Sitting Out of Bed

A chair gives more support for the upright position than the bed-rest and pillows in bed, there is less likelihood of chest complications and most patients prefer sitting in a chair to being in bed. Sitting out of bed is more beneficial for an elderly patient than continued bed-rest and there is increased opportunity for companionship as the chairs can be grouped together for conversation and meals.

When the patient is expected to walk in the ward at intervals, an ordinary chair is suitable as there can be considerable effort involved in getting up out of a low chair. Otherwise, when he is unable to walk but can sit out of bed for a few hours, an arm-chair is chosen. This has a padded seat and back and preferably padded arms. If the seat is *too long* pillows are placed behind his back and shoulders; if it is *too short* a low stool is placed under his feet. There should be no pressure from the edge of the chair seat on the lower surface of the limbs above or below the knee, as this may cause blood clotting in a vein.

When the feet do not rest comfortably on the ground a foot-stool is essential. Sometimes a padded foot rest is available which can be attached to the seat of the chair. This can prove very comfortable especially when the feet tend to swell but the knee joints should be lightly bent to allow for complete relaxation and comfort (Fig. 6).

If the room is cold, a blanket is wrapped round the patient and covers his legs and ankles and the chair is placed away from draughts. At home a winged chair is warmer for the elderly person.

He is assisted or lifted out of bed into the chair, and made comfortable and secure. There is a tendency for the weak or paralysed patient to slip forward in the chair.

The patient is moved in his chair so that he can see other patients and talk with them. If he is alone in a ward his chair is placed so that he can see the door, and if possible out of the window. A small table (those

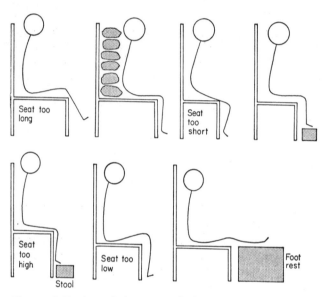

Figure 6. Patient sitting on a chair.

which fit across his knees are particularly convenient) is placed near to him so that drinks, sputum pot, magazines and occupational therapy are near at hand.

Most treatments such as dressings, intra-muscular injection in the gluteus maximus (buttock) are carried out before he is lifted out of bed, but medicines, some injections and exercises are continued as ordered. If the patient is unable to move himself, the nurse changes his position slightly every hour and moves the hands and feet through some degree of flexion and extension and at the same time speaks to him for a moment or two. Some patients sitting out of bed can be more ill than some patients receiving bed-rest treatment and the same principles of treatment and observation apply to their care as to that of the very ill patient in bed.

The problems of nursing the chair-bound patient are:

1. Pressure sores
2. Venous thrombosis (a blood clot in a vein)

3. Postural dizziness (dizziness on moving or in one particular position)
4. Maintenance of suitable position
5. Not being able to reach drinks results in lack of fluid intake.

Additional Points in the Basic Nursing Care of the Ambulant Patient

This patient is able to walk about in the ward. He needs a warm dressing-gown and slippers or light-weight shoes, the latter with non-slip soles, firm uppers and of the correct size. The bed-clothes are removed, the dressing-gown put on and the patient sits for a few moments on the side of the bed to accustom himself to the change in position. His slippers are put on, he presses his feet on to the floor and raises his body from the bed with his hands. A short person needs a firm stool or box at the side of the bed to lessen the distance from bed to floor.

The patient may require the nurse's assistance when he first walks in the ward. Correct posture is important to maintain balance and prevent fatigue so he is persuaded to look straight ahead and not down at the floor, which he is likely to do when he lacks confidence (Fig. 7). Drainage

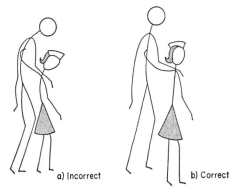

a) Incorrect   b) Correct

Figure 7. Assisting the patient to walk.

tubes and bottles can complicate ambulation following operation. Usually the tubes are clamped off temporarily, or the bottle is carried in a metal basket.

The floors in wards where the patients are ambulant should not be highly polished and slippery, neither should furniture and trolleys remain in places where a patient can collide with them. Articles dropped on to the floor are retrieved immediately and spilled fluids mopped up at once to prevent accidents.

Walking-aids may be used, such as a walking-tripod. Following treatment for fracture in the lower limbs the patient may wear a caliper, a thin metal splint which fits in to the shoe heel. Elbow crutches are another method which assist in bearing the patient's weight during walking.

The Patient During Convalescence

Convalescence is the period of time between completion of the patient's medical treatment and the return to normal daily routine and activities. It is prescribed by the doctor and the length of time varies with the patient's illness and condition. Frequently it is spent as a holiday by the sea or with relatives. The patient who has been very ill needs supervision from a nurse, either the district nurse when he is at home or the nurse in charge of a convalescent home. Several firms and employing authorities arrange the services of a convalescent home through a contributory scheme, so that their employees may return to work fit and well. These convalescent homes may be used by the employee's family also after illness.

During convalescence the patient needs a nutritious, well-balanced diet with protein and vitamins (meat, fish, eggs, milk, fresh fruit and vegetabls) in each day's menu. The amount is controlled by his appetite, which may be greater than usual. If the appetite be poor, it is stimulated by giving him food he particularly likes, increasing his exercises in the fresh air and providing some active interest. He becomes fatigued more quickly than when he is well, and this is avoided by adequate regular sleep, eight hours each night when seven hours is the normal habit and an hour's rest after dinner and after supper either reading or listening to the radio. Exercise increases each day, and walking is easily the most convenient form of exercise, suitable for taking the patient into the fresh air with a change of surroundings to stimulate his interest in activities outside the hospital or home. He becomes more independent, more willing to make decisions, small though these may be at first and regains confidence. Habits are re-established except those which may interfere with continued health and prevention of complications, and these are replaced by new habits which are instituted during convalescence.

If the time before return to work is likely to be extended, the patient, his relatives and the social worker may arrange some productive organised education, including study for an examination, or lessons in painting, or learning to play golf when he is retuning to a very active occupation.

CHAPTER 14 | PROGRESSIVE PATIENT CARE

Nurses who read this book will realise that patients vary in their nursing care needs. The nurse's experience in the ward situations will reveal many instances of the differences between patients both in the nature of their diseases and also in the treatments and in the modes of their recovery.

In progressive patient care an attempt is made by those who have the patients in their charge to assess the patient's dependency on the nursing service. (As the hospital service is composed of several staffs such an assessment could be expanded to consider his dependency on the hospital as a whole but here only the demands on the nursing service are discussed.)

An example of groups in an assessment:

    (a) The patient who needs a minimum of skilled nursing attention.

    (b) The patient who requires expert basic nursing care, but no advanced nursing treatments.

    (c) The patient who requires skilled nursing attention at intervals during the day and night.

    (d) The patient who requires 24 hours' continuous skilled nursing attention each day.

It may be considered an advantage for the patients in the above groups to be accommodated in separate wards or units although the various buildings may be in the grounds and served by the united hospital services.

Patients who need a minimum of skilled nursing attention are accommodated in small units or wards. Single cubicles may be available. Equipment is according to the requirements of the patients and the facilities available.

Here are some of the amenities which have been thought suitable:

Beds (divan type).

Carpets on the floor (non-skid type).

Bedside lamps.

Locker wardrobes. The patient will wear his own clothes. He will need outdoor clothes when walking in the grounds or outside the hospital area when this is arranged in his treatment programme.

Dining-rooms are shared by men and women patients. They collect their own cutlery, etc., and sometimes their meals, from the serving table or trolley.

The sitting-room is also shared. Tables are useful for writing letters and playing games like cards or chess. The television room is shared and has comfortable chairs. The patients have use of the kitchen at stated times for making hot drinks and/or snacks.

Toilet facilities include a small laundry so that patients can wash small personal linen.

They are encouraged to arrange their own flowers, have access to the hospital shop and library, and are able to attend services in the hospital chapel when they wish.

The patient's schedule is arranged and supervised by the sister or charge nurse in consultation with the medical staff. The nurses are trained to listen to the patient, give him instructions on ways by which he may regain his health quickly and preserve it, and provide him with the emotional support he needs during his return to a normal active personal and working life or the adjustments to a modification of this.

REHABILITATION PROGRAMME

The patient attends the physiotherapy and/or occupational therapy departments on the instruction of the doctor and sister.

Treatment, e.g. care of ileostomy, is carried out in a treatment room, not in the ward. The diabetic would be taught how to give his own injections of insulin.

It is helpful if the patient can have access to the doctor and sister, and to facilitate this a small discussion room may be provided. Here he can be given explanations regarding his illness, treatment, etc. and he has an opportunity to talk to the staff about these or any other matters relating to his rehabilitation.

PREPARATION FOR DISCHARGE

The patient should be renewing contacts with his previous environment. Visitors' times may be extended, e.g. 11 am to 8.30 pm. He may need advice from the medical-social worker. A welfare officer from his place of employment may be able to make suggestions concerning any assistance which is necessary. If the services of a domiciliary nurse are to be arranged by the general practitioner it may be possible for her to visit him before he is discharged from the hospital.

The maximum time in such a unit would be about two weeks.

Patients who require continual expert basic nursing care but no advanced nursing treatment. These are the bed-fast patients, the chronic sick, those with long-term illness and the elderly who are incapacitated. The most important concern here is the retaining of each patient's individuality with the maintenance of a high standard of care.

These patients need bright, cheerful surroundings with a rather informal atmosphere. They can wear their own clothes or choice of clothes and have round them some personal possessions, e.g. a photograph of loved ones or a cherished ornament. Visitors are encouraged and it may be possible for arrangements to be made for some of these patients to go on occasional outings. Voluntary organisations often play a great part in contributing to the patients' well-being by arranging social activities.

Physiotherapy and occupational therapy are important in the maintenance of the patient's activity and improve his mental alertness.

In the nursing care of these patients the nurse should be gentle, quiet and slow. Absence of hurry is particularly necessary in feeding and dressing them and it takes time also to communicate with some of these people.

There are problems such as incontinence, and the nurse should familiarise herself with all the methods of dealing with these matters as they can be the cause of much distress.

Well-balanced meals, carefully served, are important. Assistance with feeding may be necessary. The patient's visitors may like to feed the patient and perhaps provide some small variation from the general menu.

The patient who requires skilled nursing care at intervals during the day and night. The care of this patient is described in the following chapters.

The patient who requires continuous skilled nursing attention is often accommodated in an Intensive Care Unit. (See the next chapter.)

CHAPTER 15 | INTENSIVE NURSING CARE

Patients in Intensive Therapy (or Care) Units are those who need skilled medical and nursing care 24 hours a day with continuous observation and assessment of their condition.

They may be accommodated in a unit attached to a group of wards or in a large Intensive Care Unit which serves a hospital area.

Situations in which patients require intensive care:
  A. following major surgery, e.g. repair of heart defects or seriously complicated surgery.
  B. coronary thrombosis with severe myocardial infarction.
  C. poisonings and overdose of drugs.
  D. severe toxaemia.
  E. relief or prevention of severe shock associated with severe or multiple injuries.
Also where maintenance of an adequate air-way is required and/or the use of mechanical or electronic aids.

The patient's stay in the unit varies between 48 hours and 4 days. He is admitted from:
  (a) Accident/Emergency Department; or (b) Operating Theatre; or (c) a main general ward.

The nursing staff usually comprises a sister on duty during each shift and one S.R.N. for each patient with other nurses as required. Medical staff are either in the ward or easily available. The cleaning of the unit is important. Maintenance of structure, appliances, furniture, etc. is essential.

The patients are extremely ill and many are unconscious as the result of illness or injury. A patient may appear unconscious as he cannot move or speak *but he can hear*. The staff must understand this and continue to communicate with the patient and comfort him. Some of the patients will not recover from a severe phase of their illness or injury and the new nurse may find the work distressing. She would do well to consider the increased number of recoveries due to this highly skilled service and bear in mind the contribution she can make in her technical duties and in her consideration for and vigilance over her patient.

ADVANCED TECHNICAL EQUIPMENT is used. It is expensive, easily damaged, and is maintained by expert technicians who are part of the I.T.U. team. A nurse will be told which parts of the equipment she is concerned with in her nursing duties, how to carry out techniques which depend on the equipment, how to recognise faults in the apparatus, and how she may preserve its working life.

Although many highly technical procedures are being performed at the bedside the patient continues to need the same degree of BASIC NURSING CARE given to all very ill patients, e.g.:
  mouth toilet
  care of pressure areas
  careful lifting—special devices may be necessary
  maintaining correct position, e.g. in an unconscious patient
  changing his position, e.g. every 2 hours
  care of paralysed limbs.

Adequate nutrition is maintained by:
    (a) oral feeding;
or (b) oesophageal tube, sometimes gastrostomy tube;
or (c) intravenous infusion.
He requires a well-balanced diet up to 4,000 calories a day. The diet in (a) and (b) may be an egg-and-milk mixture or Complan or an ordinary diet liquidised by a machine in the kitchen. Strict cleanliness of food and utensils is essential.
    (c) the doctor prescribes nutrients, e.g. Aminosol-digested protein, Intralipid—a vegetable-fat emulsion.
All food and fluid is measured carefully and given in accurate amounts as prescribed.

DRUGS are administered accurately as prescribed. Those required in emergency are made easily accessible.

The pupil nurse will assist the trained nurse in the SPECIAL NURSING PROCEDURES. There may be in the unit an Intensive Care Manual to which the nursing staff can refer for accepted procedures.
Examples of special procedures:
    Oxygen administration.
    Suction through tracheal or endotracheal tubes.
    Underwater seal drainage of the chest.
    Management of wound drainage tubes.
    Management of retention of urine, urinary incontinence, bladder drainage.
    Management of mechanical respirators.
    Reduction of temperature—use of fans, tepid sponging.
    Sterilisation of special equipment, e.g. by miniature autoclave.
    Isolation of infectious patient or patient who is susceptible to infection.

General Environment in the Intensive Care Unit

HEATING AND VENTILATION. Temperature 20°C to 22°C. Artificial ventilation, e.g. by extractor fans, is necessary if the room is small and several people work on it.

LIGHTING. Efficient general lighting with a dimmer mechanism is desirable. Do not allow overhead lights to shine in the patient's eyes. Portable and/or anglepoise lamps are useful when performing treatments.

BEDS may be of the trolley type with accessories built into them, e.g. intravenous stands, cot sides, oxygen cylinder racks, and resuscitation apparatus. This removes the necessity of lifting the patient from the admission trolley to the bed. The bed head can be removed, and the bedstead can be raised or lowered at either end as required. The wheels are large for easy movement.

SHELVING is of the open type so that equipment is easily accessible. All equipment of course has its own particular place on the shelves and supplies are made up each day to the required amount.

ELECTRIC SOCKETS. Several of these are necessary. There is usually an alternative supply of electricity in case of failure in the general supply.

SUCTION OXYGEN and sometimes COMPRESSED AIR are laid on, i.e. 'piped' to each bed.

DOMESTIC CLEANING is by vacuum appliances and damp disposable cloths to prevent accumulation of dust.

REFRIGERATOR accommodation is provided:
    (i) for food and beverages
    (ii) for specimens
    (iii) for certain drugs.

The nurse will see SPECIALISED EQUIPMENT by the bedside, e.g. monitoring devices. The special machine is attached to a patient by thin cables called 'leads'. A moving line is seen on a small screen and this is produced electrically from the patient's heartbeat. It is therefore a useful early indication of any change in the condition of a patient who has heart failure or some heart disease.

At each bedside there is some means of calling a nurse, e.g. an electric bell or Cass/Com equipment.

CLINICAL INVESTIGATIONS will be requested by the medical staff. These are often of vital importance and the nurse's role in them is an important duty. It may include, e.g. collecting the patient's urine and testing it, making sure that specimens such as cerebro-spinal fluid are delivered to the laboratory without delay, assisting the radiographer in taking X-ray films by supporting the ill patient in the correct position, ensuring sufficient and suitable equipment for carrying out clinical procedures.

OBSERVATIONS AND METHODS. In Intensive Care units there is usually a more detailed method of reporting than in general wards. Charts and notebooks may be at the bedside and the nurse is requested to write briefly on all observations and treatments. The reporting may be made on Kardex and/or in a Nursing Report and signed.

These notes can be of extreme importance to the medical staff at some future date.

Reports of course should be brief, clear as to meaning, accurate and *legible*.

EMERGENCIES. Nurses who are allocated to the units will be instructed in certain procedures on their arrival and included in these will be procedures to be followed when an emergency arises. The situation varies according to the type of unit.

cardiac arrest
respiratory failure
severe haemorrhage.

There is always an experienced sister in the unit. The nurse learns what to do first, how to contact a doctor or resuscitation team, which equipment may be required, and how to assist the senior members in the unit team.

PATIENTS of both sexes are nursed in the same ward. These patients are too ill to have any interest in their neighbours and numbers of available beds are small. Proper use is made of curtains or screens when these are necessary. The ceiling lights are switched on most of the night to aid observation of the patient and performance of procedures. Often the patient is undressed and covered only with a sheet. The room temperature is higher than in a general ward, e.g. 20°C to 22°C. Members of the unit team are working in the unit throughout the 24 hours of the day —physicians, surgeons, anaesthetists, nurses, physiotherapists, radiographers, technicians.

If a patient in such a unit is conscious he needs a window from which he can look outside, a clock and a calendar so that he can be aware of place and time and so avoid the possibility of some disorientation.

The conscious patient being transferred to a general ward or being received from a general ward should have some explanation and reassurance from the doctor and sister before the transfer as there can be a great deal of unrecognised apprehension. It would be advantageous if a nurse whom he knows could take part in his transfer and see him established in the new surroundings. The conscious patient also needs to be reassured frequently and given emotional support. In the midst of the highly technical and often disturbing treatment he needs someone to preserve his identity as an individual and the nurse is the best-equipped person to do this. Do not talk to the patient; he needs just a brief word of comfort.

When the patient is unconscious the nurse must not lose touch with him as a person but maintain his dignity which is the human right of every human being.

The RELATIVES AND FRIENDS of these patients need a great deal of help, reassurance and sympathy from the staff. They visit someone for whom they have great feeling but with whom they cannot at the moment communicate. The deprivation of contact with a loved one can cause the deepest distress. There is in addition to this the discipline of 'living from minute to minute' with self-control, and also continuing their responsibilities at home and at work. The doctors and sister will keep them informed of the patient's progress. The nurses can be considerate and thoughtful in many small ways. Optimistic cheerfulness can be out of place but sincerity never is.

The relatives appreciate some accommodation in or close to the unit with comfortable chairs and perhaps a bed-settee may be available. Meals can be obtained in the hospital cafeteria/restaurant or ordered from the hospital kitchen, depending on the facilities available. Access to a public telephone is useful.

Preferably only one or two near relatives stay in the hospital when it is necessary. They visit the patient one at a time and then only for a very short period but as frequently as the situation allows. It should be explained to them that the patient may be aware of their presence even though he appears unconscious or semiconscious and that he may hear them and recognise their voices. Because of complicated equipment it may be difficult for the relative to touch the patient, e.g. hold the patient's hand, which would have been a comfort for both of them. It is the understanding of situations of this kind which tests the nurse's skill in the nurse-patient-relative relationship.

PART 4 | ROUTINE PROCEDURES

CHAPTER 16 | ROUTINE NURSING PROCEDURES

PRINCIPLES OF ADMISSION, TRANSFER AND DISCHARGE

There are two main aspects concerned with the admission, transfer and discharge of patients.

1. The Humanitarian Aspect

This is very much the concern of the nursing staff, not only to see that they treat all patients with courtesy from the moment they arrive at the hospital gates until they leave, either for another hospital or for home, but to ensure that non-nursing members do the same. This courtesy should be extended to relatives and friends also. Remember that when people are frightened or nervous they often show this by being aggressive and difficult. Hospitals are frightening places unless you work in them, and the first duty of the staff is to put the newcomer at ease—like any good hostess in her own home.

2. The Legal Aspect

To protect both the patient and the staff certain definite rules have been laid down concerning the care of patient's property, his detention in hospital, his case notes and his discharge.

It is important that your hospital rules on these matters be obeyed implicitly, so that the patient, his relatives or the hospital be saved embarrassment or even legal action against the latter.

A. ADMISSION

You receive your patients as a hostess, taking particulars and dealing with property with a minimum of fuss, but completing all the forms and adhering strictly to the hospital rules. Introduce the newcomer to other members of the nursing staff and to her bed neighbours. Be sure that

D

relatives and friends know when to visit and how to make telephone enquiries.

If the patient walks into the ward for admission and looks clean, leave him out of bed as long as possible. Help him to unpack his personal things and store them in his locker. Your hospital will have definite rules about the bathing of new patients, either in bed or in a bathroom and also whether every patient has to have a hair inspection. Mostly, nowadays both these procedures are carried out at the discretion of the ward sister. If they are performed they must be done with as much skill, privacy and warmth as possible.

There are definite procedures with regard to verminous clothing, check your hospital rules on this matter. Legally, you may not destroy a patient's clothing without his signed permission. If this is refused the clothing must be put into a special bag for disinfestation either on the premises or by the Public Health Authority. The patient must be isolated until it is certain that he is free of body and head lice.

Your hospital will also have definite rules about the use of hot-water bottles and electric blankets. Unfortunately, in the past few years some patients have received burns from these normal sources of comfort and because of this, some hospitals have banned their use. This seems a pity, especially for new, conscious patients who would probably sleep better, at any rate on their first night, if they were allowed to cuddle a hot-water bottle.

If the patient is in a side ward or isolated in any way make sure that he understands how to call a nurse and look in to see him at frequent intervals without being called.

The Ministry of Health has made it clear to all hospitals within the National Health Service that they are not responsible for patients' belongings except those handed over to the hospital for safe keeping. It is important to make this point clear to a patient and to list those articles handed over, seal them in an envelope if possible and have the patient sign it as well as the nurse. The patient should also sign the total list. In emergency admissions or accident cases where the patient is unconscious, the envelope and list should be signed either by a relative or friend and the nurse, or by two nurses.

No valuables should be handed to a relative unless the patient signs a form permitting this, and it is also important to describe articles correctly, e.g. unless you are sure the stone in a ring is a diamond, better to describe it as a white stone cut in facets.

The same basic rules apply to the property of mentally disordered patients, but medical guidance is usually sought as to what is therapeutically right to leave with the patient. Where the patient is unable to sign the list himself, two nurses will check and sign as for unconscious patients.

Property that is removed from a patient for safe keeping must be properly stored. A list is made of money and valuables and these are then handed in to the cashier in the hospital administrative office who gives a receipt for them to the patient. Clothing is marked clearly with the patient's name and hung or folded neatly in a cupboard which can be locked. A receipt should be given.

B. TRANSFER

Again, think of the patient as a person and deal with his worries about the move first and the administrative duties second.

Apart from ordering transport on the right day, ward sister will have advised relatives about accompanying the patient to the new hospital or convalescent home and about the visiting arrangements.

Discuss with sister any of the patient's worries concerning the move, as these can often be smoothed out with help from the medical social worker or Public Health Service if they concern the family.

The transfer of medical notes, nursing reports, X-rays, etc., is usually bound by hospital rules. Find out what these are and obey them. In principle it is unwise to allow any of these papers to leave the first hospital unless further treatment is required. A covering letter from the first doctor to the second may be sufficient. If the notes have to go, they are usually sealed in a large envelope with all the reports and handed to the Senior Officer in Charge of the patient during the transfer. These should be signed for on delivery and the receipt returned to the ward sister.

The transfer may well be to another ward in the same hospital. The kindest way to do this is for the new ward sister to come and meet the patient some time before the move and to discuss with her colleague the previous nursing care. On the day of the move make sure that everything is ready at the receiving end and take the patient by the quickest and warmest route, using either a stretcher or chair for the majority of patients. His relatives and friends should have been notified where to find him on their next visit.

C. DISCHARGE

The majority of patients accept that the date of their discharge from hospital will be decided by their doctor. Where a patient is not prepared to wait there are special steps that have to be taken to safeguard both the patient and the hospital. We will deal with these later.

When the approximate date of discharge is made by the doctor in charge of a patient it is usually the job of the ward sister to discuss the arrangements with the patient and, where it is necessary, to help the patient and his relatives in any way. Arrangements should be made as quickly as possible with the local Public Health Services. For example, a home help may be required or the laundry or meals-on-wheels services. If the care of the District Nurse is called for, she should be contacted and invited to visit the patient before discharge so that patient and nurse can become known to one another. This also enables the District Nurse to discuss treatment with the doctor and ward sister. She will then visit the house and with the help of relatives have everything in order for the patient's return.

On the day of discharge the patient will then have returned to him any clothes and valuables he gave into the hospital's keeping on admission and he will sign a receipt for them after checking them. This receipt must be filed with his notes or wherever your hospital orders.

D. SELF DISCHARGE

Unless a patient is mentally disordered, lightheaded or delirious, suffering from a notifiable infectious disease, or a child, he can discharge himself whenever he wishes. When such action is known to be in the patient's mind the ward sister must inform the matron and the doctor in charge. Every argument will be used to detain him, but if he still insists he must be made to understand the risks and to sign a form stating that he does so understand. If he refuses to do this he still cannot be kept in hospital, but the person who gave the warning must record that he did so and have the record signed by a witness to the warning. The patient must be given every assistance in his return home and relatives and his own doctor notified.

A patient who has discharged himself or who has been discharged for non-co-operation must be re-admitted at any time and given the same courteous treatment as any new patient.

PRINCIPLES OF BEDMAKING

The hospital bedstead is of iron and of a height which makes bedmaking less of a physical strain for the nurse. In hospitals where most of the patients get up during the day the beds are conveniently low for the patient. *A spring or Dunlopillo mattress* is the basis for the bed, which is made up with two long sheets, two or three pillows, blankets to keep the patient warm and a counterpane which prevents the blankets from becoming soiled and makes the bed more attractive. The spring mattress is protected from possible soiling by a *sealed plastic cover*. When the patient is confined to bed *a draw sheet* is used. This can be pulled (or drawn) through at any time to provide the patient with a cool part of the sheet on which to lie. It gives added protection to the mattress, and can, if soiled, be removed more easily than the bottom long sheet. Disposable draw sheets are used in some hospitals. *Pillows* are usually soft (feather) but those of flock may be used for support when the patient sits up, and for a patient who is allergic to feathers. Dunlopillo pillows and cushions are soft and comfortable but make some patients feel hot. *Sheets and pillow-cases* are of cotton and easily boiled and laundered after use. Stains are removed as soon as they are found. Soiled sheets are disinfected before laundering as they are contaminated by discharges and for this reason are collected in bags separate from the used dry linen. *Blankets* are of cellular cotton, light in weight, warm in winter, cool in summer, easily boiled and laundered. Wool blankets are difficult to disinfect, and need special laundering methods. *Counterpanes* are of cotton and are easily laundered. The pattern and design form part of the ward colour scheme.

Bed Accessories

Back-rests are placed behind the patient and provide a firm support for the pillows when the patient is nursed in an upright position. They are adjustable.

Bed-cradles, fitting either over the patient or with the end under the mattress at the bottom of the bed, are used to keep the weight of the bed-clothes from the patient, particularly his feet.

Elevators or wooden blocks raise the foot or the head of the bed.

Fracture boards are placed beneath the mattress to ensure a firm, rigid foundation to the bed. They are used when the patient has fractures of the spine or lower limb and in some orthopaedic conditions causing backache. A plaster of paris splint applied to the trunk or lower limbs is very heavy and its weight will damage mattress and springs; the boards are necessary to prevent this. For the same reason they are used beneath the mattress on which a water-bed is placed, and below metal or wooden frames which support plaster beds when no mattress is used.

A pole and chain can be fitted to the top of most hospital beds when the patient's exercise is limited to activity in bed. A hand grip is attached to the chain which hangs over the patient's shoulders and provides a means by which he can lift himself up the bed and use his shoulders and upper limbs, thus making him more independent.

A foot board is fixed across the bed to support the patient's feet in a flexed position when he cannot exercise them, e.g. in paralysis or extreme weakness, and prevent drop foot. It is padded by a thin pillow or thin sponge rubber, and its distance from the foot of the bed is adjustable. If the patient has some active movement at the ankle joints, the board supports the ball of the foot only and he exercises by pressing his heel towards the board.

A sponge rubber (sorbo) cushion relieves the pressure on the buttocks as the patient sits upright in bed. It is placed in a cotton cover which can be laundered.

Water-pillows are useful in preventing bed-sores but their weight is cumbersome.

Bed-sides are necessary to prevent a restless or mentally confused patient from falling out of bed, and one bed-side will give support for a very heavy patient with hemiplegia (paralysis of one side of the body). It may be necessary to pad the bed-sides with pillows.

Bed-tables either as trays with feet, extending shelves from lockers, cantilever tables or on metal supports fitting over the bed, are used for meals, drinks, washing-bowls, book-rests, etc.

Accessories may be part of the bed structure, e.g. fracture boards, cot-sides, bed-rests or elevators. Special beds are available when certain equipment is in constant use; these include cot-beds, cardiac beds.

HOT-WATER BOTTLES can be used to warm the bed before the patient is put into it if the ward is cold and the use of them is permitted by the hospital.

Filling of a rubber hot-water bottle
Water below boiling point is used, and it is poured into the bottle from a jug to avoid spilling. It is practical to rest the bottle on a table while it is being filled so that it does not slip out of the hand. The air is squeezed out of the top of the bottle, which is filled only two-thirds full with hot water. The stopper is replaced firmly and the bottle held upside down to check that there is no leak round the stopper. It is dried with a towel and placed in a wool cover which covers it completely and can be tied securely. The cover should be laundered efficiently after use to prevent infection between patients.

A hot-water bottle is rarely necessary to keep the patient warm in hospital, where the wards are heated, but at home it may be a comfort for the patient in a cold bedroom. The bottle in its cover is placed between two blankets and *not* over or against the patient's body, as his skin may become reddened before he is aware of it. Hot-water bottles are *not* used in the beds of patients who are unconscious, paralysed, mentally confused or restless, in order to avoid accidents.

Bottles are stored in a cool, dark place after they have been emptied completely and allowed to fill with air.

Stone or metal hot-water bottles are very useful for warming a patient's bed before admission, but are unsafe to use when he is in bed, as they are heavy and difficult to move away from the patient's body. They are filled to the top with boiling water.

An ELECTRIC PAD is easy to use, quick and convenient. It can be used to warm a patient's bed before admission.

Plugs and flex are inspected for faults before use, and the nurse makes sure this electric appliance is safe to use. It is not used where there is any moisture as this may cause the electricity in a faulty pad to be transmitted to anyone who touches it. A clean cover is placed on the pad each time it is used.

Electric pads should not be folded or creased as this can damage them.

These appliances are *not* used in an occupied bed without medical permission.

The bed of the patient whose treatment includes bed-rest is made twice a day, and then at other times when necessary. This may be during bed-baths, when the patient's position is changed, and following medical, nursing or physiotherapy treatment. If he is ambulant the bed is made once a day in the morning.

SIMPLE BED-MAKING consists of preparing the equipment which may be required, closing open windows, drawing curtains or placing screens round beds unless all the beds are being made at the same time in a closed ward, and explaining to the patient what is to be done. The bedclothes are loosened from under the mattress and the covers are removed neatly and gently without shaking them, on to two chairs, leaving the patient covered with a blanket or flannelette sheet. It is necessary to know whether the patient is to be rolled from side to side or lifted from top to bottom of the bed and this is determined by his condition or ailment. The former method is more usual, removing the pillows except one under the head. If he cannot lie down he is moved to the foot of the bed. If he is very heavy and cannot lie down, he is lifted to one side of the bed. When possible, the patient is *lifted* wrapped in his blanket, into a chair while the bottom of the bed is made. If he cannot be moved in the bed he is lifted a few inches from the bed while two nurses deal with the under-sheets. This will occur in multiple fractures or total paralysis, and four to six people will be required. A lifting crane may be available and useful. The draw sheet is removed to cool and air it. The long sheet is smoothed, crumbs, etc. removed, and is tightly tucked in. If a long mackintosh is used it is also pulled taut. Clean linen replaces used linen where necessary. The draw sheet is replaced, feather pillows 'puffed up' and replaced, the patient moves or is lifted into his proper position and is made comfortable. The upper bed-covers are replaced up to chin level, but loosely so that there is no pressure on the feet and he can put his arms in or out of the bed-clothing as he pleases and there is no constriction over his chest. Some patients, including babies, the very ill and the elderly, appreciate being well tucked in but active children and adults, restless patients and those who feel hot or feverish find it exasperating.

The patient's hair is brushed or combed. He is given his spectacles, his book or a drink as needed. There is a word of conversation, then the curtains are drawn back and the windows opened. The trolley and linen carrier are removed. Any observations during the procedure are reported to Sister or recorded.

POINTS IN BED-MAKING

Two nurses are required to make a bed occupied by a patient. Further assistance may be necessary in lifting a helpless or unconscious patient. All accessories are removed when possible during bed-making for greater ease of moving the patient and making observations. It is less trying for the patient and more methodical for the nurse to perform other basic nursing care at the same time as bed-making; e.g. bed-bathing, face and hand washing, special two-hourly attention for the helpless patient, hair washing, changing the patient's position, treating pressure areas or sitting the patient out of bed.

Drainage bottles attached to tubes in wounds are moved carefully, and not lifted above the level of the bed. If they are to be detached from the tubing the latter is clamped off first. No tension is placed on the tubing and when the bed is made the nurse checks that there are no kinks in or pressure on the tubing, and the drainage is satisfactory.

If the bottom sheets, mackintosh or plastic covers need to be changed after a long period of time in bed and the patient is heavy and helpless, it may be useful to consider lifting him on to another clean bed, and disinfecting his former bedstead and mattress with cover together with the laundering of the sheets. More pillows and blankets may be needed by the patient for comfort or warmth. If he is too warm some may be removed.

The accomplishment in bed-making may be classified as follows:

1. A contribution towards the patient's *comfort*. Clean sheets and a neatly made bed improve his appearance and morale.

2. The treatment may include a *particular position in bed*; the patient is placed in this position during bed-making using suitable accessories. A patient who is very weak finds it difficult to maintain *correct bed posture* and tends to slip into a cramped position, his chest sinking into the pillows. This can be corrected when the bed is made.

3. The bed-linen is changed when damp, soiled or crumpled, as a *hygienic measure*.

4. Some of the practices in bed-making are directed towards *the prevention of bed-sores*. Pulling bottom sheets taut, removing crumbs and small articles belonging to the patient, hair-grips, combs and coins, and changing the patient's position prevents pressure on certain areas of the body by the bed.

5. Smooth movements in bed-making and careful handling of the bed-clothes, taking care not to shake dust into the air, assists in the *prevention of spread of infection* in the hospital ward.

6. When the bed-clothes are removed the patient has more freedom and this is a suitable time for him to *exercise* for a few moments. He bends his hips, knees and ankles as he lies flat, then bends and straightens his back as he rolls onto his side. If he is weak he is assisted by the nurse. Moving to the bottom of the bed or being assisted out of bed for bed-making each day prevents some slight dizziness which results from lying flat in bed for a long time. He also has a different view of his room or ward (including the other patients) and this provides mental stimulation for someone recovering from a severe or debilitating illness.

7. Bed-making, especially when combined with bathing and washing the patient, gives the nurse a unique opportunity for *observation* of changes in the patient's condition, his progress, behaviour, also any medical and surgical procedure in progress, e.g. blood transfusion, dressings covering wounds, drainage, etc. There may be evidence of pressure on the skin, a rash, incontinence of urine, distension of the bladder. The reticent patient may use this occasion to inform the nurse of fresh symptoms or anxieties rather than call her from another nursing duty.

8. The bed-patient who is unable to talk with the other patients in the ward relies on the nurses and other members of the staff and his visitors for *social contacts*. In bed-making the nurse provides this opportunity twice a day for a few moments' conversation with the patient, to listen to him. In some way difficult to describe, the very ill, helpless and semi-conscious patient will respond to a few kind words and gentle handling from the nurse even though he is unable to express himself in words. This is important also when nursing infants and elderly patients, as well as those who do not speak or understand the nurse's language; then the tone of voice becomes more important than words.

It is obvious that bed-making is not the simplest of the nursing arts. It requires knowledge, patience and skill, and sufficient time and attention should be given to this part of the patient's nursing care.

D*

POSITIONS USED IN NURSING

Recumbent Position. The patient lies flat in bed with one or two pillows.

Semi-Recumbent Position. He has three or four pillows.

Upright Position. A bed-rest and at least four pillows are used to support the patient in this position. The patient needs one pillow in the hollow of his back and one behind his shoulders and head. If two pillows are used to give some support to the arms (known as the 'arm-chair' position) then three others are needed to support the back and head. If he sinks between the two arm pillows, his breathing will become restricted. A bed-table is a useful accessory.

In the *left lateral* position the patient lies on his left side. He may need a pillow to support his back and maintain his position. If his lower limbs are paralysed a protecting pillow may be placed between his knees and ankles. In the *right lateral* position he lies on his right side (Fig. 7).

When the patient lies on his back, both arms and legs outstretched and no head pillow he is in the *supine position.* It is usual to maintain the curves of the spine by placing small, thin pillows or cushions under the neck, the hollow of the back and a very thin one below the knees also. A bed-cradle is essential to protect the feet.

If the patient is placed face downwards, he is in the *prone position.* Then the thin pillows are placed under the upper part of the chest, under the pelvis and beneath the ankles. In all these positions, maximum freedom for breathing is allowed, pressure areas receive special attention and the limbs are placed in the most comfortable and relaxed position.

LIFTING AND MOVING THE PATIENT

These are simple matters when the patient is fairly active, of average weight and not very ill or incapacitated, but even then there are correct and incorrect methods. The main points are that the patient should be lifted competently and decisively, the nurse *and* the patient should be confident that it will be done well, and the procedure carried out in such a way that the nurse is not exposed to muscle and joint stress or fatigue.

The methods of lifting a patient are:

    (a) The forearm lift.

    (b) The shoulder lift

    (c) Using a lifting sheet.

(a) One nurse grasps the wrists or hands of her colleague beneath the patient's buttocks (*not* the thighs; the lifting force needs to be at the *centre* of the lifted weight). The patient rests his hands on the nurses' shoulders.

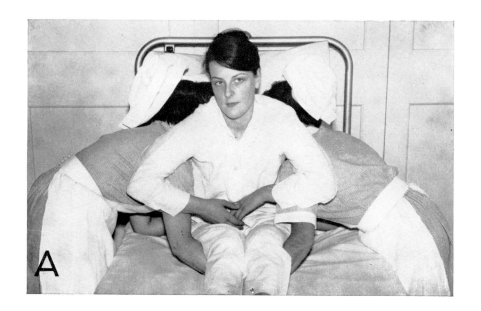

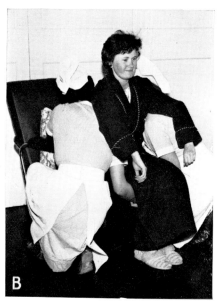
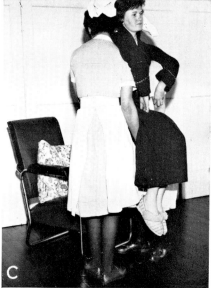

Figure 8. Shoulder lift (by courtesy of the Board of Governors, Charing Cross Hospital, London).

Both nurses lift at the same time, and it is useful if one nurse counts 'One, two, three, lift' then the patient knows when they will lift him and he can be more helpful.

(b) In the shoulder lift two nurses take the weight of the patient on their shoulders instead of the forearms by facing the patient, then placing a shoulder under his arm-pit (Fig. 8). The nurses stand upright supporting his lower limbs by grasped hands under the pelvis. The other hands are placed behind his back. This method is unsuitable for patients with hemiplegia, inflammatory conditions of an axilla, fracture, etc. involving a shoulder, and following amputation of the breast. It is most useful for carrying patients from bed to chair, and causes little fatigue.

(c) When changing sheets, a lifting sheet may be used to move the patient. This is a strong draw sheet folded in four to about 18in. to 24in. width, placed beneath the patient's pelvis. The ends are grasped securely by the two nurses about six inches from the patient and he is lifted to one side or down the bed. By this method he may be moved from one lateral position to another also.

The methods used to move and lift the patient when he is lying flat in bed and covered by a blanket:

(i) the pillows are removed except one which is below his head. When moving him into the left lateral position, his right arm is placed across his waist, the right lower limb is flexed at his knee and turned inwards. The nurse at his left side draws his left upper limb a little towards her. She places her right hand behind his right shoulder and the other behind the pelvis and rolls him towards her. She stands close to the bed to provide resistance should he roll a little too far. It may be necessary to lift him into the centre of the bed.

(ii) to lift him towards the head of the bed, the nurses place their forearms beneath his arm-pits, he bends his knees, presses his heels in the mattress and straightens his knees as the nurse lifts him towards the top of the bed. *If he is helpless*, they grasp hands or wrists below the pelvis and lower chest after folding the patient's hands across his chest, asking him to keep his chin towards his chest. *If he is unconscious*, his head is turned to one side and maintained in position by a third nurse.

When lifting an ill or unconscious patient from stretcher trolley to bed or stretcher to theatre or X-ray table and vice versa, at least three people are necessary and they stand at one side of the patient with the bed and stretcher trolley or table in one long line (Fig. 9). One nurse lifts the head, one lifts the pelvis and the other lifts the feet. They lift together with the patient in the horizontal position, move sideways, and gently lower the patient down. The male attendant responsible for the patient's transport takes the middle position for lifting.

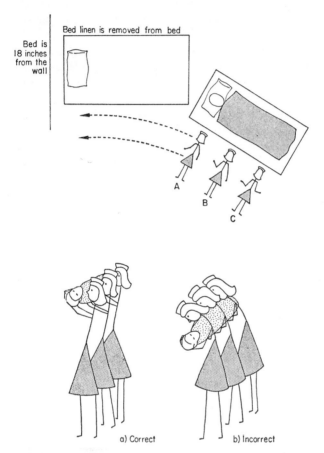

Figure 9. Lifting the patient from stretcher to bed.

The shoulder lift can be used *when lifting patients from bed into a chair*, and back again. If a nurse is lifting a patient alone, it is best to sit the patient on the side of the bed so that the feet touch and can press on the ground. She places her hands behind the nurse's neck, the nurse grasps her at the waist or by a securely fastened belt. The chair is along-side, and in one movement the nurse swings the patient into the chair. Lifting her back into bed is more difficult and in wards where many patients are lifted out of bed it is necessary to have beds of a height so that most patients can sit on the sides of the beds with their feet on the ground, the short patients being provided with stools. Chairs should not be so low that it is difficult to assist or lift patients out of them. *Lifting patients in and out of the bath* sometimes needs some thought. A damp towel on the side of the bath is less slippery than the porcelain, bath boards can be placed across the top of the bath or seats suspended in the bath. Proper hand-grips fixed at the side of the bath can be used by the patient himself. Sometimes lifting devices are available, e.g. an Ambulift. It is important to have not more than 10 inches of water in the bath.

To avoid strain and fatigue the nurse does not bend her back when lifting but flexes her knees and hips and then straightens up. She lifts with her shoulders and *not* her forearms as far as possible. She stands with both feet firmly on the floor about six inches apart with the weight of her body balanced evenly between her feet. The patient's co-operation and confidence are obtained, whilst foreknowledge of the nurse's skill is a great advantage. When actually lifting the nurse breathes through her mouth to avoid a raised intra-abdominal pressure. This would result from contraction of the diaphragm as she takes a deep breath, and contraction of the abdominal muscles when lifting. Skill in using muscles is more important than the actual strength of the muscles.

THE PATIENT'S TOILET

Bathing the Patient in Bed

This procedure is necessary when the patient is unable to go to the bathroom to take a bath and patients confined to bed are bed-bathed once a day.

The reasons for bathing a patient in bed are:

1. To remove dust from the skin, also dead particles of skin, some natural skin oil and sweat, and any urine and faeces which may remain on the skin when toilet after using a bed-pan is difficult.
2. To freshen the patient and make him more comfortable.
3. To increase his sense of well-being and maintain his self-respect.

At the time of bed-bathing, the personal clothing and bed-linen are aired, or replaced if necessary.

Elementary physiology applied to bed-bathing the patient
The upper layers of the skin are formed from cells which are no longer living and have become flat, hard and waterproof. They protect the body from injury and infection. During illness the skin is likely to be unhealthy,

there are more germs on it, or wounds have been made through which infection can take place. For these reasons it is necessary to keep the skin free from dust and dirt by washing it regularly with soap and water. The upper layers of cells are replaced by new cells growing up from the deeper skin.

Washing with soap and water removes some of the natural skin oils in which the dust and skin particles can become clogged, and prevents its collection over the pores of the sweat glands. If a great deal of oil is removed in washing with soap (this would occur very quickly with a soap containing soda) a skin cream or ointment with an oily base is used to protect the skin and keep it waterproof. Silicone applications form a waterproof surface on the skin.

It is essential to dry the skin thoroughly after washing, otherwise it eventually becomes soggy and is likely to break down into a sore. Skin surfaces in contact with each other, or sweat and urine on the skin, hasten the breaking-down process. Then the deeper layers of the skin are exposed to injury and infection.

Massage with the soapy flannel during washing or with a dry powdered hand after washing and drying, and friction with a warm, dry towel during drying encourage the circulation of blood through the skin. This assists in keeping the skin healthy.

Washing the patient who is feverish cools his skin and he is more comfortable. On the other hand, a draught over the patient's body during bed-bathing would cause the water on the skin to evaporate quickly and cool the patient rapidly. This is serious in infants, particularly premature babies, elderly patients, anaesthetised patients or those suffering from fever or shock.

The patient

A fastidious patient who sweats during his illness is relieved to have the sweat washed from his body so that he is more comfortable and does not smell of stale sweat.

To appear before his visitors and fellow patients as a neat, clean and not unattractive person raises his morale. It gives him confidence and security to be 'cared for' during his illness, particularly when his condition includes symptoms which are unpleasant to him. Patients can be embarrassed by the thought of this procedure, particularly children at puberty (10 to 13 years), male patients and people who live alone. Bed-bathing is part of the patient's treatment while he is ill and is carried out by the nurse like any other treatment or as a personal service to someone who is unfortunate enough to be ill or helpless. The nurse's lack of embarrassment causes the new patients to be less nervous. At the same time she must be aware of the need for privacy by using curtains or screens round the bed. She does not expose the patient any more than is absolutely necessary; almost all parts of the body can be washed and dried with some cover from the bath sheet. A male patient is given the opportunity of washing the genital area himself when is able to do this. For some small degree of enjoyment a patient is given a chance of dabbling his hands or placing his feet in the bowl of water for a moment or two during the bed-bath. A towel can protect the bed from a minor splash by the slightly mischievous patient.

Bathing a patient in bed takes up to an hour, especially if the procedure is complicated by the patient's breathlessness, or inability to move easily, or apparatus and equipment. This gives the patient and nurse some time in which to talk and listen to each other. The patient can ask questions and explain difficulties; the nurse begins to understand her patient as a person.

The patient, when clean and comfortable, will relax and may even sleep after his bed-bath. The procedure should not be so lengthy that he becomes cold or fatigued, otherwise his condition will deteriorate.

Equipment for Bathing the Patient in Bed
Large bowl of *hot* water, a jug of *very hot* water, a pail for used water.
Face flannel. Body flannel or sponge.
Face towel. Bath towel.
Soap. Talcum powder. Barrier cream.
Hair brush and comb.
Nail scissors.
Tooth brush and tooth paste, mouth wash and bowl, or tray for cleaning the mouth.
Treatment or bath sheet.
Clean nightdress or pyjamas.
Clean bed-linen.
Used linen carrier.
It is preferable that two nurses bed-bath a patient. Lifting and moving him is more easily performed and with less effort from the patient. A senior nurse can train a junior nurse in this situation.

Preparation of the Patient
He is told of the procedure to be carried out and asked if he wishes to use a bottle or bed-pan first.
Screens and curtains are drawn round the bed. The windows near to the bed are closed. The bed-clothes are removed leaving the patient

covered by the bath-sheet. His night clothes are removed and put in a warm place if they are to be used again.

The face, ears and front of the neck are washed, using the face flannel and towel, rinsed using not too much water to run into his eyes, then dried thoroughly. The arms are washed one at a time, the hands placed in the water for a few moments before drying. The nails are trimmed. Then the chest is washed. Drying the skin beneath the breasts is important in plump women.

The flannel is changed. Using the body flannel the abdomen is washed, paying attention to the cleanliness of the umbilicus. After washing of the genital area (this may be done by the patient) the water is discarded into the pail and replaced by fresh hot water.

The legs are washed one at a time, and the feet placed in the bowl for a few moments. The nails are trimmed. Lastly the patient's back, the back of his neck and thighs are washed while he lies on his side.

Special attention is given to the areas where skin surfaces are in contact or moist, e.g. behind the ears, in the armpits and groins, beneath the breasts in some female patients, the crease between the buttocks. The skin is washed gently but thoroughly, dried well, then powdered very lightly with talc.

Pressure areas are inspected before they are washed, dried and then massaged using deep, firm but not heavy pressure. Clothing is replaced and the bed is made, using clean linen when necessary.

His hair is combed and brushed and he cleans his teeth and rinses his mouth.

His position in bed has been changed if possible and he is made comfortable.

Extra equipment at the bed-side such as drainage bottles are dealt with.

The curtains are drawn back and the windows are opened.

Personal equipment is returned to the patient's locker and towel rails. General articles such as bowls and jugs are cleaned thoroughly before further use.

Nurse reports to Sister that she has completed this procedure, any abnormalities she has noted and the patient's general condition.

Bed-bathing the Patient on Admission

This procedure is similar to that of the daily bed-bath, but the patient will already be between treatment or bath sheets.

The patient's general condition is assessed by the doctor or ward sister before he is bed-bathed. If he is very ill, the procedure is postponed until his condition is improved.

Night clothes will be required and also equipment for inspecting the hair if infestation by pediculi (head lice) is suspected.

When the patient has been admitted as an emergency or has travelled some distance in the ambulance he may wish to pass urine before any procedure is carried out; the specimen is saved to be tested for abnormalities. The temperature, pulse and respiration rate are noted.

His clothing is removed carefully and gently. His skin may be dirty, depending on the situation in which he was taken ill. If this is the case, several replacements of hot water may be required.

Observations are made and these are reported later:

1. Complaints of pain.
2. Deformities, artificial limbs, a wig, etc.
3. Mental state, whether delirious, semi-comatose, unconscious.
4. Position in bed, e.g. with his knees drawn up.
5. Inability to move or raise a limb (paralysis).
6. Skin: cleanliness, scars, any abrasions or wounds, bedsores, unnatural colouring of the skin. Lice on body or in clothes.
7. Head: lice (pediculi), nits, dirt, sores, use of dyes.
8. Ears: deafness, discharge, hearing aid.
9. Eyes: inflammation, squint, artificial eye, spectacles.
10. Mouth. unpleasant smell of breath (halitosis), decayed teeth, furred tongue, cleft palate, peculiar voice, loss of voice, dentures.
11. Nose: discharge.
12. Incontinence of urine and/or faeces. Distended bladder indicating retention of urine.
13. Fear, anxiety, apathy, aggression, nervousness, timidity.

The procedure is carried out with a minimum of effort from the patient and in as short a time as possible. He is addressed by name and made to feel welcome, confident and secure. The nurse encourages him to talk if he wishes to but does not question him when he is obviously ill or tired. A few words of explanation regarding ward personnel and routine are given if possible.

Bathing the Patient in the Bathroom

The Ward Sister decides whether he baths in the bathroom or is bathed in bed.

Preparation of the Bath
The windows in the bathroom are closed, a screen is placed across the door. Clean clothes and towels are hung over the warm towel-rail.

Flannels and soap are in readiness on the bath rack. A clean cork mat is placed on a bath mat or the floor.

Cold water is run into the bath first, then hot water to a depth of not more than 10 inches. The water is well mixed with the hand and the temperature recorded with the bath thermometer. It should be 40°C (105°F). A towel on the bottom of the bath is useful for a heavy or unsteady patient to stand on. The patient visits the toilet.

During the Bath

He is not left unless it is known he is reliable, and then the door is not locked. A female nurse remains with a child or female patient, and a male nurse or orderly with a male patient. A small child may be afraid of a large bath, and if so, is bathed in a large bowl.

The patient is assisted into the bath and remains in no longer than 5 to 8 minutes. Some help may be necessary; a plump person cannot wash the back easily. He is assisted out of the bath and in dressing, the nurse making sure that his skin, nails, etc., are clean, his hair brushed and neat.

After the Bath

His bed has been made, if necessary with clean sheets. If the ward is cold a hot-water bottle or electric pad has been placed between the sheets to warm the bed.

The patient returns from the bathroom either walking or in a wheel-chair. The hot-water bottle or electric pad is removed before he is assisted into bed. He is made comfortable and the nurse observes his general condition.

The bath is mopped with a disinfectant, left for 5 minutes, and then washed thoroughly. The towel bath mat is sent to the laundry. Windows are opened and the bathroom is left tidy.

The ward sister will decide whether the patient who is admitted will bath in the bathroom. Usually his temperature, pulse and res-piration rate are recorded first and any abnormalities of these are reported.

Washing in Bed

This is the procedure carried out in the morning or evening when the patient is not bed-bathed. The patient's pyjama jacket is removed, his face and hands are washed and the pressure areas are treated. His hair and mouth receive attention also. The bed is remade, and linen is changed as required.

Toilet of the Incontinent Patient

This procedure is performed as soon as it is known that the patient has been incontinent.

Equipment is prepared:

Cellulose wadding to remove excreta from the patient's skin. A pail containing a thick paper bag in which to discard used cellulose wadding.

A large bowl of hot water. Replacement if necessary.

Disposable flannel, soap, bath towel.

Barrier cream, either zinc cream and castor oil, anhydrous lanoline or silicone cream.

Clean personal and bed linen, mackintoshes, special waterproof bag for soiled linen.

The procedure is similar to that in bed-bathing or washing the patient but the excess excreta is removed with the cellulose wadding while the patient lies on his side supported by a nurse. The skin is washed well with soap and water, rinsed and dried thoroughly, then massaged and treated by the application of a thin layer of barrier cream. It is important to make sure that all parts of the skin affected have been treated, buttocks, groins, vulva, etc. Soiled linen is removed and replaced by fresh, clean linen, as is also a soiled mackintosh. Sometimes a disposable incontinence pad is placed beneath the patient's buttocks. The soiled section of plastic mattress cover is washed with soap and water and dried.

The nurse protects her hands by wearing disposable rubber gloves and prevents cross infection in this way. An unpleasant odour can be removed by opening the windows after the procedure or using an air deodorant in an inconspicuous place .

The patient who is distressed by this occurrence is comforted by the nurse. Maintaining the cleanliness and comfort of the patient is part of the patient's treatment and care. When the reasons for the incontinence are known, steps can be taken in some cases to prevent it from recurring.

Washing of the patient's hands is performed at least twice a day, and after performing toilet which follows the use of the bed-pan when the bowels are opened. Ambulant patients can wash their hands before meals. The patient requires a bowl of warm water, a piece of soap and his hand towel.

Care of the Patient's Hair

The hair is combed and brushed twice a day and then when necessary for the patient's comfort and general appearance. It is arranged in a simple style without thick hair or hair grips beneath the female patient's head which would cause discomfort. With the patient's agreement it is cut or trimmed at intervals by the hospital barber or hairdresser. In an emergency or before operation it is cut sometimes by the nurse, but with the knowledge of the patient.

Washing the hair is usually necessary about every three weeks but may be delayed when the patient is very ill. The ward sister requests this to be done by the nurses or perhaps by the hairdresser who visits the hospital.

Washing the Hair of the Patient in Bed

Equipment
Large bowl.
Large jug of water 40°C (105°F) (use bath thermometer or test carefully with hand).
Small jug for pouring water.
Liquid shampoo mixed with warm water in small jug, or cream shampoo in tube, or olive oil soft soap mixed with warm water to form a lather.
Dressing comb, hair grips or rollers for setting the hair.
Treatment sheet to protect the patient's shoulders.
Waterproof sheeting to protect the bed.
2 bath towels, (a) under the head, (b) to dry the hair.
Face towel to protect the face and eyes.
Hair dryer.
Pail for used water.
Protective covering for the floor if necessary.

Preparation of the Patient
The procedure is explained to the patient. Her upper garments are removed and her shoulders protected by the treatment sheet. The bedclothes are turned back neatly.

When the patient is sitting up in bed the bowl is placed on the bedtable, which is protected by the waterproof sheeting. She sits forward with her head over the bowl, supported by a nurse.

When the patient lies flat in bed, the mattress is pulled out 1½ feet over the foot of the bed on to the back of a chair. The wire frame is protected by the waterproof sheeting, and the bowl is placed on this.

The patient's head is supported over the bowl by the nurse, her eyes are covered by the face towel so that the soapy water does not flow into them.

The second nurse tests the heat of the water with her hand; it should be warm. If the patient is nervous, a little water may be poured over her head first so that she is assured it will not be too hot or cold. Nurse wets her hair, applies the shampoo and massages the scalp. Then she rinses the hair, using the small jug. When quite clean and free from soap (the hair 'squeaks' when rubbed) the head is wrapped in a dry, warm towel. The bowl is removed, the bed remade and the patient made comfortable. The hair is mopped or rubbed until fairly dry, then arranged in a suitable and attractive style and dried using the hair dryer.

Special care should be taken with the patient who has a tendency to be dizzy. She should avoid bending forward and needs some assistance from a nurse while her hair is washed. It is unwise for this type of patient to wash her hair in the bathroom.

Following the patient's admission to the ward the nurse observes and reports the condition of his hair and scalp. This may include.

(a) cleanliness of hair and scalp,

(b) abrasions, scratches, sores or bald patches,

(c) pediculi (lice).

Head lice are not common but when this infestation is present it should be recognised and treated without delay so that there is no risk of other patients or staff becoming infested. The lice are most easily seen in the hair above and behind the ears. There may be very few; in severe cases the large numbers cause the patients to scratch, when infected abrasions are seen on the scalp. Eggs of lice, called nits, are attached to the hair by a cement which is difficult to remove. They are grey in colour. The lice hatch out in 3 to 5 days.

An examination of the hair is carried out if head lice are suspected or to make sure there are no lice. This is a personal matter and the nurse explains tactfully to the patient that she needs to fine-comb her hair. The procedure may be part of the routine admission.

Curtains or screens are drawn round the bed. A *towel cape* is arranged round the patient's shoulders. The hair is combed with a *large dressing-comb*. If it is tangled it may be necessary to separate the hair gently with the fingers to avoid pain. A brush is unsuitable as the lice would be brushed on to the bed. The hair is combed in sections using a *fine comb*. This may be done more easily if the comb is dipped first in *water*. The combings are collected into *white wool swabs* which can be examined easily. These are discarded into a bowl of *disinfectant* which will destroy lice should there be any present. The combs and towel cape are disinfected afterwards. The hair is arranged as the patient wishes.

Pediculosis (Infestation by Lice)

Treatment of an Infested Head
If the treatment is severe, the nurse may wear a gown with her hair well covered by her cap.

The treatment proceeds on Sister's instructions immediately following the examination of the hair. Lorexane (lethane oil) is usually prescribed. The liquid is applied using a pipette along partings made in the hair. Depending on the size of the head and the amount of hair 10 to 20 millilitres (2 to 4 teaspoons) of liquid are used. It is massaged into the hair so that each hair is covered by a thin film of the solution.

The hair is washed about 12 hours afterwards and the dead lice are combed out. If there are numerous lice it may be necessary to cover the hair after the application with a disposable paper cap or a triangular bandage. Lethane oil applications do not kill the eggs (nits). These hatch out within 5 days, and each day for a week following treatment the hair is fine combed. The treatment is repeated if necessary. Vinegar, dilute acetic acid, can be used for removing old nits from the hair.

It is thought that pediculi are becoming resistant to lethane oil preparations. An alternative treatment being used is a preparation of the insecticide malathion.

Pubic lice are uncommon. The patient admitted with this infestation suffers from neglect in personal hygiene. The lice are large and may be present on any of the hair on the body. Hair is removed by shaving or by cutting it close to the skin. Then the patient is bathed and puts on clean clothes. His former clothing is autoclaved.

Body lice are extremely small and greyish in colour. They exist in the seams of clothing and are not easy to distinguish from wool fluff. Any patient with them has usually worn his clothes continuously for some time before admission. His clothing is removed and placed immediately at the bed-side into a large bag or sack which is sealed and sent to be autoclaved, or sprayed with insecticide powder to destroy the lice. (Clothing cannot be destroyed without the patient's permission as it is his personal property.) He is given a bath, then put into clean clothes.

When the patient attends the Accident-Emergency Department and is mobile, he may be transferred to the Local Authority disinfestation centre for treatment. Should he require medical treatment also he will return to the hospital for this.

Scabies

Treatment of *infestation of the skin*. This, like pediculosis, is not common. It is caused by a mite, the female of which burrows into the skin to lay eggs. The areas affected are between the fingers, the wrists, hands, buttocks and skin folds. The burrows appear like tiny lines and the skin itches. The treatment prescribed is usually benzyl benzoate emulsion and the procedure is as follows:

In the evening the patient has a hot bath and the affected areas are scrubbed. The skin is painted with the emulsion and allowed to dry. The painting is repeated and the emulsion dries on the skin. Clean clothes are worn. Next morning the procedure is repeated.

In the evening the emulsion is washed off the skin and the patient has a bath. All clothes and bedding are changed.

Recently it has been found that one application of benzene hexachloride is sufficient.

Enquiries are made in the patient's family or close associates to discover if others also have scabies; if this is so, they are advised to have treatment.

Care of the Hands

The *patient's hands are washed* twice a day to remove the loose upper layers of dead tissue cells from the skin. They are washed after the patient has used a bed-pan or when his hands have been in contact with any body discharges to prevent infection being carried on his hands to his food, etc. It is important *to dry the hands thoroughly* after washing, particularly between the fingers, as this skin easily becomes unhealthy, soggy and may break down. There are a large number of sweat glands in the skin of the palms and in excessive sweating, as in fever, frequent sponging and drying of the hands is comforting to the patient. In this case the hands should be placed on top of the bed-clothes where they will be cooler, not beneath the blankets.

Dryness of the skin is due to lack of skin oils from the tiny sacs near the hair roots, or its continual removal by washing and rubbing of clothes, dressings, etc. against the skin. Poor general health and blood circulation may be the cause in some illnesses. *A skin cream or ointment* with an oily or grease base is applied to the skin after the hands have been washed and dried.

The nails grow continually from the upper layers of the skin and are made up of dead cells. However, the deep part of the skin to which they are attached (the nail bed) is plentifully supplied with nerve endings of pain. It is necessary to cut the nails regularly to prevent them from becoming long, when they would damage the skin elsewhere or become deformed. Nail clippers are the most suitable equipment, otherwise short-bladed scissors are used. It is difficult to cut neglected nails, and if possible the tips of the fingers are first soaked in warm soapy water. It is usual to trim the finger-nails to a rounded shape, taking care not to damage the skin on either side, as infection can quickly occur here, and is extremely painful. A piece of wool is held under the end of the fingers to catch the tiny cuttings and prevent these from falling into the bed where they may scratch the patient's skin.

Inactivity leads to muscle weakness and wasting. Weakness can be observed in the patient's hands when he tries to grasp objects like a cup, and wasting in the hollow between the bones in his hands where there would normally be thick muscle.

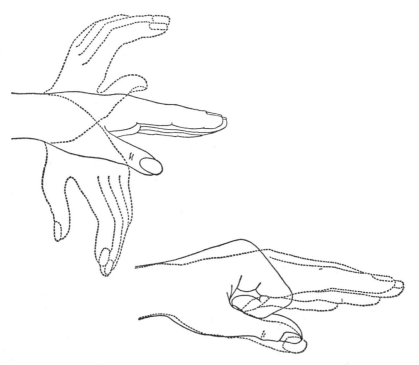

Figure 10. Hand exercises.

As the patient recovers from his illness, his exercise programme includes movements of the joints by the physiotherapist and nurse. Then active movements are made by the patient himself (Fig. 10) such as squeezing a ball or making a fist. Activities like knitting, basket-making, leather work, painting, making models, assist in preventing muscle weakness and joint stiffness in the hands, besides the general exercise afforded by dressing, going to the bathroom and toilet, eating, etc.

While the nurse cares for the patient's hands she makes observations:
Colour of skin and nails.
Warm or cold.
Moist or dry.
Swelling.
Abnormalities of skin or nails.
Redness due to friction or pressure when the patient is restless or completely inactive.
Wasting or weakness of muscles.

Care of the Feet

Much of the care of the patient's feet is similar to that of the hands. They are washed each day during the bed-bath or in the bathroom. Thorough drying is important, especially between the toes. When these are close together and the skin is soggy, light powdering with a little talc and thin pieces of dry wool between the toes help to keep the skin dry.

There are many sweat glands on the soles of the feet, and in excessive sweating the skin becomes unhealthy and soggy. There can be, too, an unpleasant smell. This can be prevented by placing a bed cradle over the feet and washing them as frequently as possible. A little methylated spirit and talc cool the feet and the patient is more comfortable.

When the upper layers of the skin are exposed to friction or pressure they become thickened. These areas are called 'hard skin' and are sometimes found on the feet. When the patient is very ill and is confined to bed, the hard skin softens and frequently flakes off. The skin beneath is tender and rather red: it is easily damaged and should be protected from pressure by the use of a bed cradle and occasionally loose bed-socks. Frequent massage will improve the state of the skin.

Hard skin may be ingrained with dirt caused by the patient's occupation, lack of facilities for washing, etc., or by neglect. Scrubbing with a nailbrush is of little use and may damage the skin. A better method is to spread a thin layer of petroleum jelly over a large piece of old linen (about 12 inches square), wrap it round the foot and bandage lightly. At the bed-bath next day this is removed, the foot is washed if it is clean. If not, the application is repeated.

The nails are cut straight across, taking care to avoid cuts and abrasions. If there is difficulty in dealing with hard, tough nails, or the patient has corns or suspected foot infection, the doctor may request that the services of a chiropodist be obtained.

A bed-cradle prevents friction by bed-clothes on the toes and ankles. A small, thin pillow beneath the ankle prevents a sore heel when the patient lies or sits still in bed. Changing position every two hours helps to prevent this type of pressure sore.

Because the feet are extremities of the body, inefficient blood circulation is apparent here. The skin becomes white and cold. It is unwise to apply heat to the skin at these times as local burns can occur easily, and hot-water bottles must not be used. The doctor may request the foot or feet to be left exposed on special occasions, otherwise moderate warmth is applied by a flannelette sheet close to the body beneath the bed-clothes and the room is kept warm.

In the case of poor blood circulation in the feet, the skin must be kept dry and free from injury and infection. This problem arises in older patients, those with certain diseases of the blood vessels and in diabetes mellitus. Similar care is taken when the feet are very swollen due to water under the skin (oedema). A cradle is useful to prevent pressure from the bed-clothes.

Movement of ankle joint and exercises of the feet prevent muscle weakness and joint stiffness (Fig. 11).

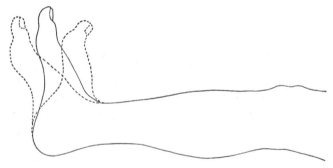

Figure 11. Foot exercises.

'Drop foot' is inability to raise the foot at the ankle and is due to lying in bed for a long period of time and pressure of the bed-clothes on the feet. It is prevented by adequate nutrition, a bed-cradle, foot exercises, changing the patient's position at intervals during the day and perhaps supporting the feet by a board fixed across the bed.

While washing and exercising the patient's feet, the nurse observes:

colour of the skin,
warm or cold,
moist or dry,
swelling,
inability to raise the foot,

corns, hard skin, soggy skin between the toes,
rashes, abrasions,
redness due to friction or pressure,
abnormalities of skin or nails.

Care of the Mouth and Teeth

Reasons for Keeping the Mouth and Teeth in a Healthy Condition
A. The appetite and enjoyment in eating food are improved. Digestion
is aided by adequate production of saliva which is the natural liquid
in the mouth, and the mixing of this with the food during chewing. Discomfort in the mouth discourages the person from chewing food.

B. Certain conditions are less likely to occur in a healthy mouth such
as halitosis (unpleasant breath), gingivitis (inflammation of the gums),
carious (decayed) teeth.

C. The mouth is a cavity which opens into the digestive tract, the lungs,
and the salivary glands. Infection of the mouth can result in infection in
these parts of the body.

General methods ensuring the health of the mouth and teeth include:

1. Sufficient food in a balanced diet to provide healthy tissue in the
mouth.

2. Nose breathing is encouraged to prevent the mouth becoming dry
and lowering resistance to infection.

3. Adequate fluid intake is necessary to make sure there will be a
satisfactory flow of saliva from the salivary glands, i.e. 2 litres a day.
Eating fruits like oranges and drinking the juice of oranges, lemons,
limes or grapefruit stimulates the flow of saliva.

4. Mastication (chewing) stimulates the salivary glands to produce
saliva. For this reason meat and raw fruit and vegetables like apples,
pineapple, celery, carrots and cabbage, also nuts, are an asset in the
diet. Chewing gum has a similar effect on the production of saliva.

5. Cleanliness of the mouth and teeth.

6. Avoidance of the continual eating of foods containing sugar such
as sweets and biscuits. This habit encourages the decay of teeth.

7. Periodic inspection of the mouth by a dental surgeon or dentist,
for example every six months.

THE PATIENT'S MOUTH AND TEETH
In illness, particularly fevers, the mouth becomes dry and unpleasant.
This occurs also when the patient in respiratory distress breathes through
his mouth as in pneumonia or congestive heart failure. Dryness of the
mouth prevents the appreciation of taste. This sense of salt, sour, sweet

and bitter (acid) takes place through the taste buds on the tongue surface, which must be moist to fulfil this function. Loss of the sense of taste removes pleasure in eating food. Speech is altered as the mouth becomes very dry, and a harsh croak will replace intelligible words when the mouth is neglected.

The patient with a sore mouth cannot tolerate food in the mouth.

One complication of an infected mouth is the inhalation by the patient of infectious material. This may result in lung infection. Inflammation of the parotid salivary glands (just in front of the ears and close to the jaw joints) is called paratitis and this may also complicate an infected mouth.

Care of Patient's Mouth and Teeth
The principle of this treatment is to keep the mouth moist and clean.

Whenever possible the patient cleans his own teeth. This is done twice a day at least, i.e. morning and evening, and after all meals if possible.

(a) If he can go to the bathroom he cleans his mouth there, but it is helpful for the nurse to make sure this has been done. Some health education may be necessary if the patient has not been in the habit of caring for his mouth and teeth.

(b) The patient in bed who is able to brush his teeth and gums needs the following articles:

Beaker containing mouth wash.
Tooth brush with medium or soft bristles.
Tooth powder or paste.
Bowl or receiver.
Face towel.

(c) If he is unable to clean his teeth then this is done by the nurse.

Cleaning the Mouth of an Ill Patient who is Conscious
The nurse explains to the patient what she is about to do and places his *face towel* below his chin. His co-operation is essential as he must open his mouth as necessary. With clean hands the nurse attaches *dental squares* dampened with *cleaning lotions* to *swab-holding* or *clip forceps*. Suitable lotions include *soda bicarbonate* 1 teaspoonful to 600 millilitres of water which dissolves mucus, and *glycothymoline*; dilute as directed.

A *torch* is useful when inspecting the mouth and a *tongue depressor* can be employed when cleaning the inside of the cheeks and the back of the tongue.

Some routine in cleaning the mouth is useful.

(a) The tongue is cleaned first with strokes from side to side making

sure the back of the tongue is clean (swabbing the tongue from front
to back may cause the patient to retch or vomit);

(b) then the upper teeth, inner and outer surfaces of the upper jaw;

(c) then the lower teeth, inner and outer surfaces of the lower jaw;

(d) next inside the cheeks—food collects here;

(e) finally the roof of the mouth, and the floor if necessary.

A little glycerine and lemon in the mouth may assist in keeping it moist
but is uncomfortable in a sore throat. White petroleum jelly or lanoline
can be applied thinly to the lips to prevent them from becoming dry, sore
and cracked. The nurse may assist the patient in using a mouthwash
when she has cleaned his mouth with swabs. This is more refreshing for
him and helps towards keeping the mouth moist besides providing him
with a little activity and feeling of independence. It is unwise, however,
for him to use a mouthwash if he has difficulty with breathing or any
paralysis of the throat.

The Cleaning of the Mouth of a Patient who is Unconscious or Mentally Confused

A mouth gag may be required to open the patient's mouth. It is placed
between the molars or back teeth. Dental squares are held firmly in swab-
holding or clip forceps, and the edges are folded in so that no loose threads
are likely to come off the dental square. The mouthwash is not used.

After treating the mouth, equipment is disinfected or placed in a bag
for disposal.

Mouth or oral toilet is carried out every two or four hours, before and
after meals, for these patients:

(a) very ill or unconscious patients;

(b) those with high fever.

(c) those who have fluid diets, are being fed by tube or who cannot
have food by mouth.

(d) those with infections of or injuries of or operations on the
mouth.

Care of Dentures

Dentures are cleaned with the patient's tooth brush or a special denture
brush and are rinsed in cold water. When a patient is not able to wear his
dentures they are kept in a labelled container in his locker.

Patients who are unconscious or about to have a general anaesthetic do
not have dentures in the mouth as the denture may obstruct the throat.
The nurse will find that the patient's lower dentures are removed easily.
The upper denture is attached to the roof of the mouth by suction and to

release it the nurse can press upwards on the back of the plate; this removes the suction and the dentures can be taken out. Plates which support one or two teeth are fragile and require careful handling as indeed do all dentures.

Unless there is a definite reason for the patient not to wear his dentures the nurse should enable him to have them for they are important in his appearance, speech, taking food and general self-respect.

Care of the Patient's Pressure Areas

Pressure areas are the parts of the body which are exposed to pressure (Fig. 12). This pressure on the body may be due to:

(a) weight of the body on the bed;

(b) bed equipment such as cradles;

(c) splints, bandages, clothing, etc.

The effects of pressure are made worse by friction (rubbing) and dampness. A *bed sore* is an ulcer (loss of skin surface) which may occur when the patient lies in bed a long time. The weight of the body causes pressure on blood vessels and nerves resulting in lack of nutrition and loss of 'feeling' in the area of skin exposed to pressure. If this skin breaks down, a bed sore develops.

If the nurse has an opportunity to place the classroom skeleton in a bed using the different positions in which the patients are nursed, she will see the parts of the body where bed sores may form:

back of the head,	the spinal column,
the ears,	the sacrum,
the shoulder blades,	the buttocks,
the elbows,	the hips.
the knees, heels, ankles, toes.	

Then perhaps a colleague nurse can lie in the different positions on the bed, and comparisons can be made between the bony prominences in the skeleton and the pressure areas in the living person.

PREVENTION OF PRESSURE SORES

A. An adequate nourishing diet is necessary to keep the tissues of the body (including the skin) healthy and therefore less easily damaged.

B. Absolute cleanliness of skin, clothing and bed-linen is essential.

C. Relieving parts of the body from pressure by changing the patient's position regularly (i.e. throughout day and night). This may be every two hours for patients who cannot move easily or as often as every half hour when the patient is deeply unconscious. Encouraging a patient to move in bed, sitting him out of bed and early ambulation are all methods of

relieving continuous pressure on certain parts of the body and thus
prevent bed-sores.

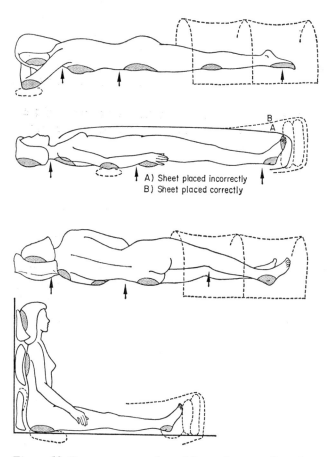

*Figure 12. Pressure areas: dotted lines show small cushions or air rings,
footboards and bed-cradles. Arrows show positions for pillows.*

D. Efficient bed-making. This includes removing crumbs and other
articles from the sheet beneath the patient, also pulling these sheets tight
to prevent creases. Linen on beds of incontinent patients is changed
immediately it has become wet or soiled.

E. In long illness various beds or mattresses may be used, e.g. ripple
beds (these are of rubber in narrow sections through which air flows in
waves or 'ripples'), Dunlopillo (sponge rubber) mattresses, air beds, packs
of pillows or Dunlopillo sections.

Sponge rubber rings or air rings are useful for very fat or very thin patients, particularly those in sitting positions. Bed-cradles prevent pressure of the bed-clothes on the feet. A thin feather pillow under the lower calves and ankles relieves pressures on the heels as the patient lies or sits with legs extended. Pressure sores can form on the heels when the patient sits out of bed with his feet on a stool. A thick sponge-rubber cushion should be fixed to the top of the foot-stool. Small, thin feather pillows are useful to place between the knees and ankles when the patient lies on his side.

They can be made about 16 inches by 10 inches, a size which fits into small spaces for the patient's comfort when the usual pillow is either too large or too thick.

Sheepskin has been found useful in protecting pressure areas. The patient can lie on a sheepskin. Small pieces of sheepskin which fit over the heels are available.

F. Careful lifting of the patient so that he is raised clear from the bed and not dragged along the draw sheet. Giving and removing bedpans also requires attention; the patient may be too ill to raise himself on to and off the bedpan, in which case two nurses lift him.

G. The nurse's finger-nails are trimmed short and round, otherwise when lifting a patient she may damage his skin. Watch wrist bands, and rings, particularly those with stones, can scratch the skin and quickly predispose a bed-sore. For this reason nurses do not wear watches or rings other than wedding rings while they are in uniform.

ROUTINE TREATMENT OF PRESSURE AREAS

This procedure is carried out twice a day when the patient is confined to bed and is included in the bed-bath and evening toilet. It is repeated more often if the patient is unable to move in bed, or is unconscious, incontinent, restless or very thin

After preparing the patient as for a bed-bath the pressure areas are inspected. A satisfactory light is required for this as a tiny crack or abrasion can easily be missed, particularly in places like the crease between the buttocks. (A small electric torch is part of a night nurse's own personal equipment.)

Cleanliness. The skin over the pressure areas is washed and dried thoroughly twice a day and also at other times when the patient is incontinent or has been sweating excessively. Clean personal and bed-linen replace soiled linen. Sheets beneath the patient are drawn tightly to prevent creases.

Massage with the palm of the nurse's hand in firm movements improves the circulation of blood to the skin. This is aided by the use of a little talc.

Local applications include *barrier creams* which contain olive oil, nut oil, castor oil or cod liver oil, or a grease such as lanoline. These and silicone creams form a waterproof surface on the skin and are useful in treating incontinent patients. Sometimes a little methylated spirit is rubbed over the skin to harden it; this is also cooling and refreshing. Only small amounts should be used otherwise the skin dries and may crack.

Changing the patient's position is undertaken at the same time. This relieves the pressure on certain parts of the body as it lies on the bed and allows the blood to circulate through the skin. Pressure due to other causes such as bandages or equipment is removed where possible.

The patient's *comfort* is considered so that he is able to rest and relax in the position best suited for his medical treatment.

If redness or an abrasion occurs, it is reported to Sister at once. Bedsores may develop from these stages to slough formation (death of tissue). The ward sister is always informed of the progress of pressure areas. She directs any treatment required. Forms of treatment vary depending on the patient's condition, area involved, etc.

TREATMENT OF PRESSURE SORES

1. *Redness* due to inflammation. Pressure is removed, e.g. if the reddened area is over the sacrum the patient lies on his side or has a Dunlopillo ring. Routine treatment is carried out more frequently.

2. *Abrasions* are treated by medication such as tincture of benzoin compound or Aristol powder. These are applied to the abrasion only and *not* to the skin round it. This latter is treated as for all pressure areas, but more frequently. Cleanliness is important.

3. *Pressure or bed-sores.* As the skin in this area is damaged, the dressing is applied by aseptic technique, and a dressing trolley is prepared. Medications include eusol and liquid paraffin, red lotion, a petroleum jelly gauze and chlorhexidine cream. The skin surrounding the area is kept clean and dry, and is massaged gently at frequent intervals. Pressure or friction over the area is removed or prevented.

In some cases the doctor requests the physiotherapist to give heat treatments to the bed-sore which stimulate the growth of new tissue.

Pressure sores and bed-sores cause the patient much discomfort and delay his recovery. They are difficult to heal, lower the patient's general condition and can interfere with the treatment of his illness. Prevention is easier than cure. Conscientious inspection and treatment of pressure areas are essential parts of the patient's nursing care.

E

Sanitary Arrangements for the Patient

The male patient who is confined to bed uses a bed-pan when emptying the bowel (defaecation) and a urinal when emptying the bladder (micturition).

The female patient uses a bed-pan on both occasions.

Bed-pans are made of:

(i) *Plastic*. These are light and easy to clean.

(ii) *Stainless steel*. These are non-breakable and easily cleaned, but expensive. They are cold unless stored in heated racks or held under hot water from a tap and dried.

(iii) *Compressed paper pulp*. These are light in weight. After use they are placed in a special destructor machine which disposes of both bed-pan and contents. This is convenient and also a consideration in prevention of cross-infection. The machines are expensive. The disposable bed-pan is used with a plastic base which supports it beneath the patient's weight.

When giving a bed-pan to a male patient in bed, the nurse draws the curtains round the bed for privacy. A urinal and toilet paper are taken at the same time. The female patients' ward is closed to non-nursing personnel when bed-pans are being used or curtains are drawn round the individual beds.

A helpless patient is lifted carefully by two nurses when necessary, and the bed-pan is slipped under his buttocks so that its flat top curve lies beneath the sacrum (lower part of spine). If the patient is extremely thin it may be helpful to pad the top of the bed-pan with wool to prevent discomfort and possible damage to the skin.

When the patient is unable to carry out his own toilet, the nurse assists using disposable paper tissue and water when necessary. The bed-pan is removed and immediately covered with a sheet of paper tissue which can be disposed of with the contents of the bed-pan.

OBSERVATIONS are made of the contents before emptying and sterilising the bed-pan, and any abnormalities are reported. Records on a chart may be necessary.

The patient is given a bowl of warm water, soap and towel to wash his hands, and the nurse washes her hands at a ward sink. The ward is ventilated.

Urinals are made of:

(i) *Glass*. These are easily broken but can be cleaned thoroughly and the contents are easily observed.

(ii) *Metal*. These are expensive but not easily broken. There should be no rough joints in the metal. The contents are not easily observed.

(iii) *Plastic.* These are light in weight and perhaps easily overturned. Most of them can be sterilised in the bed-pan steriliser and some are suitable for autoclaving.

(iv) *Disposable compressed paper pulp* similar to the bed-pans previously mentioned.

In some wards the patient has his own urinal, and it is stored in a rack which is fixed to the side of the bed. Curtains are not usually drawn round the bed when the male patient uses a urinal (he calls it a 'bottle'). Disposable paper tissue covers the urinal as it is removed from the bedside, and the urinals are taken to the sluice in a wire carrier.

Non-disposable bed-pans and urinals are washed and sterilised by steam-heated water in a bed-pan steriliser. The process takes about 2 minutes and the door of the steriliser is tightly closed during this time. The steriliser must be cleaned thoroughly every day.

SANITARY ARRANGEMENTS FOR THE PATIENT WHO CAN
GET OUT OF BED

A *commode* is more comfortable than a bed-pan and in some cases the patient is less precarious than when using a bed-pan. He usually has a better bowel action and is less likely to become constipated. Privacy is essential as when using a bed-pan. It may be necessary to lift the patient out of bed. He must be well wrapped up and not left on the commode too long. Some assistance may be required with toilet. A bowl for washing the hands is given afterwards. The commode, stool or chair and receptacle are kept very clean.

It may be useful to have a chamberpot in the ward utility room, particularly when there are likely to be children or elderly patients admitted to hospital in a delirious or mentally confused state. The patient may have more success and less distress using this article, a commode or the toilet than in trying to use a bed-pan when this is a completely unfamiliar contraption.

Sani-chairs are arm-chairs of the upright type with a bed-pan fitted into the seat of the chair. There are also wheel-chairs in which the patient can be taken to the toilet. The seat of the chair is similar to the top of a bed-pan. The chair enters backwards into the toilet and over the water closet basin. Assistance is required from the nurse as the patient enters and leaves the toilet and perhaps with clothing. An opportunity is made for the patient to wash his hands.

Hand brackets in the walls of the *toilets* are useful for patients who cannot raise themselves easily. Toilet paper should be conveniently placed. It is advisable that the door is not locked in case the patient needs attention. If the doors do lock, the master key should hang in a prominent place in the Duty Office where it can always be found.

CHAPTER 17 | ROUTINE OBSERVATIONS AND REPORTS

Temperature, Pulse and Respiration

THE PATIENT'S TEMPERATURE indicates the degree of heat being produced in his body. A normal response to infection of the body tissues is to produce more heat, and a raised temperature is one sign of infection. The type of thermometer used is a *clinical* thermometer, and the range is 35°C to 43°C. A low-grade thermometer begins at 30°C. Unlike other thermometers (bath, lotion, food and room thermometers, the temperature on the thermometer can be read *after* it has been removed from the patient's body. This is possible because of a small constriction made just above the bulb which prevents mercury passing back into the bulb of its own accord. The thermometer is shaken after using so that the mercury returns to its original level.

The normal body temperature is 37°C but it may vary within a range of 36°C to 38°C. It is usually higher at night than in the morning.

The body temperature is estimated by placing the clinical thermometer in the mouth, axilla (arm-pit), groin or rectum.

When taking the temperature in the mouth the patient is in bed or sitting quietly on a chair. He should not have had hot or cold drinks or mouthwashes or have been smoking immediately before the procedure, neither should he have had a hot bath. His thermometer is taken from its jar, dried on a swab and examined for cracks. Check that the mercury is below 35°C—if not it is shaken down. The bulb of the thermometer is placed beneath his tongue. The patient closes his lips, but not his teeth, and he does not talk with it in position. It is left in position for two minutes, then removed. The bulb is wiped with a moist swab to remove saliva, the temperature reading is taken, the mercury shaken down to 35°C and the thermometer returned to its jar. The temperature is recorded on the chart, using a graph.

This is an unsuitable method of taking the temperature of small children, and of patients who are delirious, unconscious, irrational or who have fits.

The temperature of a patient who has a disease of, or operation on, the mouth, or who cannot breathe through his nose, is taken in the *axilla* (or in the *groin*) after drying the area with a towel, as sweat will cause some lowering in the recorded temperature. The bulb of the dry thermometer is placed in the axilla. The arm is flexed across the chest or the thigh across the pelvis, so that the bulb is in contact with two skin surfaces, otherwise the reading is inaccurate. Inaccurate readings can occur in some very thin patients. The thermometer in the axilla is left in position, but if it is placed in the groin the nurse holds it in position for two minutes, then the reading is taken.

In infants, or when an accurate reading is essential, the temperature is taken in the *rectum*. The patient is in the left lateral position. The thermometer, a special type with a thicker bulb, is lubricated with paraffin molle (petroleum jelly) inserted one inch in the rectum and held carefully in position for one minute. The thermometer bulb is wiped on a swab, then washed in cold water after the reading has been taken.

When a patient has suffered head injuries and his temperature rises above 39°C he may be treated by hypothermia, i.e. cooling the patient. He is usually comatose and temperature readings are important. A subnormal thermometer is required, the lowest temperature indicated being 30°C. This is a rectal thermometer.

Rectal temperatures are 0·5°C higher than those in the axilla or groin, and slightly higher than those in the mouth. The body temperature is slightly lowered in sleep, old age and starvation, and slightly raised after a hot bath and in excitement. In a patient the temperature is raised in infections and heat-stroke, and is lowered in haemorrhage, shock and anaesthesia.

A rise in temperature is called *PYREXIA*.

THE PULSE is the wave of distension felt in an artery when the left ventricle of the heart contracts and forces blood into the aorta. The pulse may be counted at any point where an artery crosses the bone near to the surface of the body, e.g. at the wrist, at the front of the ankle and over the temple.

The method is to make sure the patient has been resting for at least five minutes, and his arm, leg or head is in a relaxed position. The nurse places three fingers over the point where the pulse can be felt and counts the pulse for one minute.

There is no fixed normal figure for the pulse rate as it varies from person to person, in an adult between 60 and 80 beats per minute, though in athletes it may be lower than 60. In infants and children the rate is faster, and the nurse is advised to use a stethoscope to count the heart beat. In physical exercise and emotional states it is raised. The rate slows down in rest and sleep and old age.

The nurse may find the pulse of a patient to be slow in head injuries, some heart diseases and as a result of drugs which are prescribed to slow the heart rate. In infections, haemorrhage and shock and following the administration of some drugs which stimulate the flow of blood to the heart, the pulse rate quickens. Besides the *rate* of pulse beat, the nurse may also observe its *rhythm*, i.e. the regularity of the beats, or its *volume*, i.e. when it is bounding or full, weak or feeble.

The respiration rate is counted for one minute when the patient has been at rest for a few minutes, and the results are often more accurate if he does not know the respirations are being counted. If the breathing is not obvious, the rise and fall of the chest is observed. In adults the rate is 16 to 20 per minute, and quicker in infants and children. The rate rises and the inspirations become quicker in physical exercise and emotion, and also in respiratory infections and some lung and heart diseases. The rate is slowed down in coma. Breathing may be noisy, i.e. stertorous. Difficult breathing is called dyspnoea. Sighing respiration occurs in internal haemorrhage, and shallow breathing is noted in shock.

In practice it is usual to take the temperature, pulse and respiration at the same time, and it is an advantage for the patients to be in bed or sitting by their beds some minutes before the observations are made. When the thermometer can be left in position for two minutes, the pulse and respirations are counted one minute each, then the thermometer is removed and all three recorded. The nurse frequently retains her fingers over the pulse while the respirations are counted, as most people breathe more quickly when their attention is drawn to their breathing.

Fluid Balance

The body requires an adequate amount of water in order to carry out its various functions. This fluid is taken into the body in food and drink. Excess water is excreted by the kidneys, and when the intake is limited, the kidneys produce less urine. In this way a balance is maintained.

During illness the intake of fluid may be interfered with as in vomiting when the swallowed fluid is rejected. There is an increased loss of fluid from the body in diarrhoea or excessive sweating. Kidneys which do not function correctly prevent the normal loss of fluid as urine. Fluids administered by artificial means are not controlled by thirst and appetite and, unless skilled care is used, can be given in excessive or inadequate amounts.

In all these cases it is necessary to observe the intake and output of fluid, and at the end of the day assess the balance.

Fluid Intake is by:
  Mouth.
  Oesophaegeal tube.
  Gastrostomy tube.
  Rectal infusion.
  Intravenous infusion.
  Blood transfusion.

Fluid Output in:
  Urine.
  Vomit.
  Aspirations from body cavities,
    e.g. stomach.
  Drainage from wounds.
  Diarrhoea.
  Excessive sweating.

In measuring *fluid intake*, it is necessary to include small additional amounts such as medicine. If a patient is given a glass or jug of water and this is to be replaced with a clean vessel, any fluid left in the glass or jug is measured and subtracted from the original figure. The result shows the amount the patient actually drank and this is recorded.

In measuring fluid output it may be difficult to assess the amount of drainage from wounds, blood or serum loss, or excessive sweating, but the nurse reports that the loss has occurred, and informs Sister that dressings have been renewed or repacked, or the patient's damp clothes have been replaced by dry garments, or he has been incontinent with urine.

When the output is considerably less than the intake, the amount of fluid given to the patient will be reduced. In kidney failure, the patient passes little or no urine and the nurse may be instructed to give him a small amount of fluid each day, e.g. 500 millilitres, and this will be increased as the urine output increases as shown on his Fluid Balance Chart.

In severe blood or serum loss (in haemorrhage or burns), or diarrhoea or severe sweating, the fluid ouput will be greater than the intake, and the patient's blood pressure will fall if it is a sudden major loss, or he will become increasingly dehydrated. These complications are avoided by the administration of an increased amount of fluids. When the patient is extremely ill or incapacitated it may be difficult to give these by mouth (though a nurse can often show her skill in the management of the patient and his care on these occasions), and the water is given by other routes—through the oesophagus, the rectum, under the skin or into a vein.

From these examples the nurse will understand the *importance of the Fluid Balance Charts*. Not only do they indicate how much fluid has been given and the amount excreted from the body, but the balance indicates the patient's progress and provides the doctor with useful information when he orders further treatment. It is obvious that in the measuring of the fluid intake and output nurses must be careful and accurate. The amounts are written down at the time they are measured, at the bed-side when drinks are given to the patient, and in the sluice when bed-pans and urinals are emptied. The metric system of measurement may be used and the totals are expressed in millilitres. There are thirty millilitres in one fluid ounce.

Electrolyte Balance

In the blood plasma are certain substances in solution, e.g. sodium chloride (salt). The particles which make up these substances are found in the plasma as sodium ions, chloride ions, potassium ions, and alterations in the amounts of these ions (or electrolytes) are a reason for a patient feeling very ill. It is necessary, therefore, on the occasions when this may occur for the doctor to know the amounts or levels in the blood, and this is done in the Biochemical Laboratory by an examination of a blood sample. Then the intake is adjusted to maintain the correct level of electrolytes. Prescribed quantities of sodium chloride can be administered in rectal, subcutaneous and intravenous infusions, and the nurse notes not only the amount of water given but the strength of the solution. Normal saline is 0·9 per cent of sodium chloride in water, 1/5 normal saline is 0·18 per cent sodium chloride in water. Tap water contains no sodium chloride.

Observation of Excreta and Discharges

OBSERVATIONS ON URINE

In a healthy person the urine is pale amber in *colour* and clear without deposits. The *amount* excreted varies with the amount of fluid taken in food and drink and an average quantity is 1,500 millilitres a day (nearly three pints).

Observation of a patient's urine:

The *colour* varies. The urine may be dark green due to the presence of bile, or smoky red when blood is present. There may be *deposits*, white, pinkish white or yellow.

The *amount* excreted is decreased when the intake of fluid is limited, when sweating is excessive in fever and in some kidney and heart diseases. More urine is passed as the fluid intake increases, and following the administration of certain drugs.

Simple tests may be carried out to ascertain whether abnormal substances are present in the urine, such as protein (albumin), glucose or sugar, or acetone. Chemical reagents are used, and the following are supplied ready for use, together with colour charts to indicate presence and amount of abnormal substance.

To test for the protein in urine: the reagent is ALBUSTIX prepared in strips.
1. Dip the test end of Albustix in urine and remove immediately.
2. Compare colour of dipped end with colour scale.
No colour change—negative.
Green or blue-green at once—positive.

To test for the glucose in urine: the reagent is CLINISTIX prepared in strips.
Dip test end of Clinistix in urine and remove.
No colour change—negative.
Blue colour within one minute—positive.

To test for and estimate amount of sugar in urine: the reagent is CLINI-TEST tablets.
1. Place five drops of urine in a test tube. Rinse the Clinitest dropper and add ten drops of water.
2. Drop in one Clinitest tablet and *watch reaction.*
3. Fifteen seconds after boiling stops, shake tube gently, and compare with colour scale.
Blue colour—negative.
Any colour other than blue—positive.
Compare with Clinitest colour scale. Record as indicated on colour chart.

To test for diacetic acid and acetone in urine: the reagent is ACETEST tablets.
1. Place one Acetest tablet on a clean white surface.
2. Put one drop of urine on a tablet.
3. Compare tablet with Acetest colour scale after 30 seconds.

Reagent strips (LABSTIX) are now used for detecting a number of abnormal substances at the same time—raised acidity or alkalinity, protein, glucose, ketones, blood. A colour chart is necessary for comparison with the results.

Urine is examined for other abnormal substances in the laboratory and the nurse collects and prepares the specimen.

OBSERVATION OF FAECES

In the healthy person, normal stools are passed once or twice a day, the amount being approximately 120 grammes. The consistency is soft solid, the colour light brown and the odour characteristic but inoffensive. There are variations which can occur during illness. Stools may be more frequent and more fluid, this is diarrhoea; or less frequent and harder in consistency, this is constipation. The faeces are clay or putty coloured in jaundice, green in some gastro-intestinal infections, tarry (called melaena) when they contain blood altered by digestive processes in the

E*

small intestine. There may be bright red blood from bleeding in the rectum or round the anal canal.

Abnormalities in faeces are blood, pus, mucus, worms and swallowed foreign bodies.

The nurse may be asked to test for blood in faeces by using HEMATEST reagent tablets.

    1. Place a *thin* smear of faeces on test paper provided.

    2. Put one Hematest tablet on centre of smear.

    3. Place two drops of water on the tablet.

No blue colour on test paper at the end of two minutes—negative.

Blue colour appearing on test paper around the tablet within two minutes is positive.

OBSERVATIONS OF SPUTUM

Sputum is a discharge coughed up from the respiratory tract.

When a specimen is required the sputum is expectorated into a glass flask or waxed cardboard container with screw lid. The latter should be marked in millilitres on the inside if a measurement is required. In colour the sputum may be red or pink due to the presence of blood, yellow if pus is present, or frothy if it consists largely of mucus mixed with air as it is coughed up.

The odour is fetid in untreated bronchiectasis or abscess of lung.

The nurse will notice the times at which the patient expectorates sputum. These may be when he awakes in the morning, after moving or being moved in bed, after steam inhalations with tinctures of benzoin compound or menthol crystals, or following breathing exercises by the physiotherapist.

When bleeding occurs in the respiratory tract as a consequence of injury or disease, the blood is coughed up by the patient and, being mixed with mucus, appears red and frothy. This is *haemoptysis*. The amount of blood varies enormously, appearing as a pink or rusty discoloration of sputum to a severe blood loss. Patients are always apprehensive about loss or discharges from the body, and the nurse removes any unpleasant material from the bed-side tactfully and with all possible speed.

OBSERVATION OF VOMIT

The manner in which vomit is expelled may be significant. In projectile vomiting the stomach contents are ejected with force at intervals, for instance every one to four days. The amount is copious and there is a sour odour. The vomit may contain undigested food and bile (appears green). When it contains digested food following haemorrhage, it appears similar to coffee grounds.

Collection of Specimens

Collection of urine for ordinary examination
About 160 ml. of urine are collected in a glass specimen jar which is labelled with the patient's name. Early morning specimens are more concentrated and therefore abnormalities more easily detected.

To collect a 24-hour specimen the patient is given a bed-pan or urinal at a definite time, e.g. 10 am, and the urine is discarded. All the urine passed after that time is collected in a labelled Winchester bottle or special container. At 10 am the following day the patient uses a bed-pan or urinal and the urine is included in the specimen.

When the urine is to be examined in the laboratory for the presence of pathogenic bacteria, it is necessary for the specimen to be collected in such a way that the urine does not become contaminated during the procedure. Either the bladder is emptied by passing a urinary catheter using an aseptic technique and collecting the urine in a sterile specimen jar (catheterisation), or by collecting a *mid-stream specimen of urine*. In the latter technique, the area round the urethral orifice is washed with warm water and dried with a clean towel. The patient passes some urine into a clean bed-pan or urinal, then into a sterile container, and the stream is completed in the clean bed-pan or urinal. The sterile container is either a sterile bed-pan or urinal, the urine being transferred from this to the specimen jar using a sterile measure for pouring if necessary. The sterile specimen jar itself may be used, a wide jar being necessary for the female patient. Care is taken not to contaminate the inside of the specimen jar and lid.

Catheterisation of the urinary bladder is described later.

Collection of Faeces
A specimen of faeces is taken from a stool in the bed-pan on a spatula or scoop and deposited in the clean specimen jar.

Collection of Sputum
When the laboratory examination of sputum is necessary, the patient is given either a clean glass specimen jar or a waxed cardboard container in the late evening and asked to expectorate into it when he first coughs next morning. This cough is the most productive during the day and there is less likelihood of saliva being mixed with the sputum.

Vomit is transferred from the vomit bowl to a covered can or jar.

If faeces, vomit or sputum are to be examined on the ward, the material is retained in its original receptacle, covered and labelled, then discarded immediately after examination.

Other specimens to be examined in the laboratory include blood taken from the patient's vein by the doctor, cerebro-spinal fluid (see lumbar puncture) and swabs from tonsils, nose or wounds.

Labelling of Specimens
The following details are written or printed on an adhesive, preferably self-adhesive, label: patient's name with one forename in full, his age, and suspected disease, the nature of specimen, the name of the ward and the date.

Matthew CLARK	Ward 4
48 years	7.11.72
Dysentery	
Specimen of FAECES	

The label is fixed to the container, preferably at the bedside, immediately after obtaining the specimen. Then the labelled specimen and the laboratory form, signed by the doctor, are placed in the collection box for the laboratory. It is necessary for certain specimens of urine and cerebrospinal fluid to be delivered to the laboratory *immediately* after the specimen has been obtained. This will be indicated on the form and the nurse attends to this.

Changes in the Patient's Condition

The nurse observes the patient's condition on admission and uses this as a guide for future observations:

Skin—colour, whether warm or cold, moist sweating.

Behaviour—unconscious, irrational, apathetic, nervous, suffering from pain.

Temperature
Pulse
Respiration
Urine
Faeces
Vomit
Sputum

Observations of these have been referred to earlier in this chapter.

The day or night nurse sees her patients when she comes on duty and, as she completes her day or night shift, will have observed changes in their conditions and reported these. Further points may be noted:

whether he has slept; his appetite; degree of pain, and if this were relieved by medical or nursing treatment; his reactions to drugs; state of wounds; and his interest in his surroundings.

It is useful to be able to assess whether the patient's condition is improved or has worsened during the previous twelve hours, and if he is very ill during the previous two or three hours, or even within the last few minutes.

Reporting observations, either verbally or in writing, on a patient's condition and his treatment is an essential part of a nurse's training, for by this means she learns to be accurate, clear and concise in her reports. The doctor relies on the nursing staff who attend the patient day and night for information which together with his own findings will assist him in forming a diagnosis and ordering treatment. Training in observation also produces a rapid assessment in an emergency situation and can be a life-saving measure.

Giving, Receiving and Writing Ward Reports

Reports of the patient's condition and treatment are given and received in the ward sister's office where the matters spoken of will not be overheard (the knowledge of a patient's condition and his personal affairs is professionally confidential). It is not always convenient or tactful to discuss treatment at the patient's bed-side. The sister may use the giving and receiving of ward reports as an opportunity for teaching her nurses.

Reports on observations and treatment are written twice daily in a ward report book, or, as they occur, on individual cards in a *Kardex file*. These reports are stored on the ward for two years as a source of reference should enquiries be made regarding the patient and his nursing treatment, or they are filed with his medical notes and retained in the Registration Department of the hospital.

Matters of minor and temporary importance are discussed in a verbal report, and this is frequently combined with the reading of the written report.

Writing a Report

The nurse or pupil nurse makes her entry *in ink*. Different colours may be designated for different purposes, e.g. dangerous drugs in red ink. The date and time are entered and the report signed. The remarks are brief and to the point, but also explanatory and accurate. Comments and exaggerations, 'slang' and dialect are not permissible, and handwriting must be clear and legible. Abbreviations may be allowed but these must be agreed upon by all members of the nursing and teaching staff and they are kept to a minimum.

The nurse reports, under the guidance of the sister, new observations and changes in the patient's condition, nursing and medical treatment which has been carried out, the drugs administered and the patient's response to these and special examinations or surgical operations performed. Accidents and complications such as bed-sores are included.

The person writing the report is responsible for its accuracy, and if in doubt should check a statement before she writes it.

Minor reports are made verbally by the nurse to sister at a convenient time, e.g. on the completion of a treatment. She will pass on relevant information to the doctor during his ward round, and also to the staff nurse or the night nurse as she goes off duty. These latter reports may include information on the patient's attitude to his diagnosis, treatment, operation or the hospital routine, whether he has visitors, or requires some special service from the minister of religion or the medical social worker, the safe custody of his clothing and valuables when these have not been transferred to a relative, any idiosyncrasies to food or drugs. At the same time, minor complaints are reported such as rattling windows or dripping taps, and the minor repairs requested.

Reports on treatment and drugs are written immediately following the procedure.

If the ward routine includes major reports, these are written twice a day, e.g. 8 pm and 7.30 am and are given with a detailed verbal report from the day to the night staff and vice versa. Very brief reports (or Bulletins) are sent to the Matron's office once or twice during twenty-four hours, and these show admissions, discharges, deaths, major treatment and operative surgery. These are used by the Administrative staff and night sisters.

Methods of giving reports vary between hospitals, and may change as different ways of making communications are devised. Research is being made into various methods of communication with regard to ward reports e.g. by tape recorder and computer.

CHAPTER 18 | NURSING CARE OF
THE UNCONSCIOUS PATIENT

The patient may be deeply unconscious (in coma) or responds to some stimuli. The nurse assesses the depth of unconsciousness and reports any change.

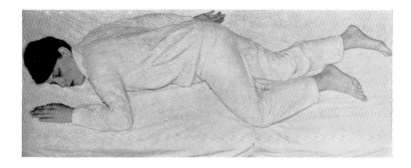

Figure 13. Position for an unconscious patient (by courtesy of the Board of Governors, Charing Cross Hospital, London).

The problems in nursing an unconscious patient are:
1. Maintenance of an adequate airway.
2. Prevention of pressure sores.
3. Prevention of broncho-pneumonia.
4. Prevention of damage to blood vessels and nerves due to pressure over the relaxed muscles and abnormal movement at the joints.
5. Nutrition—the swallowing reflex disappears in deep unconsciousness and the patient cannot be fed by mouth.
6. The bladder and the bowels do not function normally.
7. He cannot describe any symptoms to the nurse, who must therefore make frequent and accurate observations and report these.

1   Maintenance of an Adequate Air-way

The patient lies in the left or right lateral position with the face directed slightly downwards so that secretions or vomit may flow out of his mouth and the tongue remains forward in the mouth, *not* relaxing backwards into the pharynx. A pillow is placed *behind* the patient to maintain his position. A third pillow beneath his neck may prevent his face rotating too much towards the mattress. The nurse prevents bed-covers from covering the patient's face. Small vomit or anaesthetic cloths are unsuitable as they obstruct the nose and mouth. If it is necessary for the patient to lie on his back, the head is turned to one side but it is difficult to maintain this position. The head may be held by the nurse so that it is bent slightly backwards. She places her fingers along the jaw line, pressing the lower jaw forward and upward. This prevents the tongue from blocking the throat. An artificial airway in the mouth and throat (pharynx) is used after operation until the patient is conscious. An intratracheal (into the air-passage) tube may be introduced through the mouth by the doctors to maintain an open air-way, and sometimes in coma, a tracheostomy tube is inserted.

Should there be any possibility of food in the stomach, a naso-eosophageal tube is passed and the contents aspirated. This prevents vomit entering the pharynx from whence it may be inhaled into the lungs. An unconscious patient is *not* given any fluids by mouth for the same reason.

2   Prevention of Pressure Sores

Pressure sores are prevented by changing the patient's position from right lateral to left lateral and vice versa every two hours. A loose open-back gown is worn by the patient so that he does not lie on folds of material.

Bed-linen is changed whenever damp or creased, and the bed-linen pulled tight beneath him in making the bed. His skin is kept clean and dry, and his nutrition must be adequate.

3 Prevention of Broncho-pneumonia

Broncho-pneumonia is prevented by changing the patient's position every two hours. This movement aids in emptying the lungs of excess secretions and increasing lung ventilation. Inhalation of vomit is prevented by emptying the stomach, placing the mouth lower than the stomach in his bed-position or by the introduction of endo-tracheal or tracheostomy tubes. If the patient has a previous respiratory infection such as chronic bronchitis, the doctor may order a course of antibiotic therapy. Physiotherapy to empty the lungs of secretions and improve lung ventilation is of great value.

4 Prevention of Damage to Blood Vessels and Nerves Due to Pressure

Relaxed muscle offers no resistance to pressure and therefore gives little protection to underlying structures. So pressure on limbs, e.g. from bed accessories, is avoided. In addition, the muscles in this condition decrease the stability of joints, and gross normal movements can take place. These are prevented by supporting head and limbs during lifting and transport, and while treatment is being carried out. As an example, if the upper limbs were allowed to hang down while the unconscious patient was being transported on a stretcher trolley, the shoulder joint would be grossly extended and the blood vessels and nerves passing through the axilla might be stretched and consequently damaged. For this reason, the patient's hands are placed under his buttocks with fingers and thumbs outstretched, and, to make one more point, if the patient is a woman she does not wear a ring with a stone set into it because on this occasion the stone would damage the skin of the buttock and pre-dispose to a bedsore. The feet are maintained in dorsi-flexion, i.e. with the ankle flexed to prevent stretching of the muscles at the front of the leg resulting in 'drop foot'.

5 Providing Adequate Nutrition

Nutrition continues even if the patient is unconscious, but as the swallowing reflex is absent an oesophageal tube is passed to the stomach and a fluid diet is administered by a funnel at two-hourly intervals. The diet is of adequate amount, nutritious and well balanced. Between the feeds of

30 ml. each, the tube is closed with a clean spigot, and the nurse checks that the end of the tube is still in the stomach and *not* the upper part of the oesophagus where fluid may pass into the pharynx and be inhaled.

Cleaning the mouth is necessary at frequent intervals, usually every few hours. As soon as the patient becomes semi-conscious and can swallow, tube-feeding is discontinued and the patient is given small, very frequent fluid feeds. Unless the patient receives skilled nursing care, dehydration and starvation can occur.

6 Ensuring Bladder and Bowel Function

At first the patient may have retention of urine, and the abdomen is examined for distention of the bladder. If this is present the doctors may request catheterisation of the urinary bladder to be carried out, and the urine is tested for abnormalities. Later there may be incontinence of urine, and continuous drainage of the bladder may be considered with aseptic technique of catheterisation, scrupulous hygiene of drainage receptacles, adequate intake of fluid and chemotherapy to combat urinary infection. The semi-conscious patient will be very restless if the bladder is distended with urine so steps should be taken to relieve this. He can often be persuaded to use a urinal. Constipation is common though not serious as the intake of food is limited. Glycerine suppositories are useful, and two administered per rectum will often result in a bowel action.

7 Special Observations

Special observations include:
    (a) depth of unconsciousness,
    (b) fluid intake and output, sometimes electrolyte balance,
    (c) food intake,
    (d) condition of skin and mouth, pressure areas, hair and nails.
As the patient recovers consciousness, he begins to respond to being touched or called by name.

The first sense to be lost and then to return is that of hearing so the nurse is careful what she says, particularly at the bed-side of an unconscious patient or that of a patient being anaesthetised or who is recovering consciousness, and does not make any comment either on this patient's or any other patient's condition or treatment.

The unconscious patient is more helpless than at any other time and can take no responsibility for his own life or safety. The nursing staff assume this responsibility for him and learn to prevent any harm which may threaten him. On this account he is under continual observation either by one special nurse or in full view of nurses passing to and fro in a general ward. The nurse bears in mind also that this is a person whose individuality and dignity are to be preserved during a time when his powers of self preservation and self-assertion are at a minimum.

CHAPTER 19 | CARE OF THE DYING AND LAST OFFICES

Most nurses have very natural fears about seeing a dead person for the first time and need the emotional support of a senior nurse. In some cultures and religions there are superstitions and taboos associated with the dying or dead, and these must be respected as far as possible.

For many patients death comes slowly and peacefully and the physical signs are easy to recognise. The skin becomes cold, especially the extremities, and sweat appears on the face. The temperature falls below normal and the pulse feels thin and the rate gets very slow. Breathing becomes slower and the rhythm alters and there may be long pauses between each inspiration. The patient loses consciousness and this becomes deeper until the heart and lungs fail to work any longer.

Whether death comes peacefully or otherwise the patient should never be left alone for long periods and should receive all the emotional and spiritual comfort possible. This may come from his family, his priest, and medical and nursing staff.

Many dying patients appear to be in physical discomfort or pain which is not relieved by analgesics. This usually indicates that they know that they are dying and need mental and spiritual help to face this great experience. The patient should not be left alone at this time.

Sudden death can occur in hospital from such causes as haemorrhage, cerebral thrombosis or pulmonary embolus. The shock to nurses and other patients, as well as to the relatives, can be very great and it takes really good nursing to see that the unhappy and unexpected incident is dealt with in such a way that the effect on staff and patients is kept within reasonable bounds.

All dying patients should have the maximum amount of privacy and nursing care. They should be kept clean and dry, their pressure areas attended to regularly and their mouths kept moist and sweet.

Every facility should be offered to the relatives including food and rest and the opportunity to stay in the hospital until death occurs. Their wishes should then be complied with about the personal effects of the dead person. This is particularly important with regard to wedding rings. All property handed to the relatives must be signed for in spite of the unhappy circumstances. In fact, these routine matters, if done with sympathy, often help the relatives to regain their composure.

Laying Out
It is usual for two nurses to perform this last service for their patient, but they do not start until about an hour after death has been certified by a doctor. This is to make certain that life is extinct. Orthodox Jews may not be touched by Gentile hands after death. The instructions of the Rabbi should be sought and followed implicitly.

As soon as death has been certified, the body should be laid flat in bed, with arms straight and the dentures inserted if normally worn. The jaw should be supported by a flat, flock pillow—a tight jaw bandage will mark the flesh and cause distress to the relatives. The bed is stripped of all top clothing except the sheet.

A trolley should be set with all the requisites needed, and once the nurses have started, they should not leave the bedside until they have finished. The aim is to prepare a clean and peaceful-looking body for the relatives to see, as soon as possible.

The body should be washed all over, the anal orifice packed with white wool, the bladder emptied by catheter if necessary and the legs tied together at the ankles with a bandage—a wool pad protecting the skin. A clean bottom sheet should be put on the bed, wet compresses should be placed on the eyelids and only if there is discharge from the nose should it be lightly and inconspicuously packed. All tubes, stitches and appliances (excluding Ryles tubes, intravenous and bladder catheters) should be left in position unless otherwise instructed. The vagina should not be packed. Finally the shroud should be drawn up over the body and fastened lightly at the neck; it must be labelled clearly with the patient's name. Some hospitals write the patient's name on the thigh with Biro in addition to a label on the shroud. The hair should be brushed and combed into the usual style. A crucifix may be held if desired by the relatives. A clean sheet is then draped over the bed and body and folded beneath the chin. The head is left on a clean flat pillow. All apparatus and equipment is cleared away by the nurses, who have refrained from speaking, unless absolutely necessary, throughout. The relatives are then invited to visit the bed-side for the last time.

After they have gone, the body is removed on a special trolley which has a cover to the hospital mortuary. It is usual to screen all the beds of patients who might see the mortuary trolley and to remove the body as quickly as possible so that the least possible amount of distress is caused to others. In some hospitals the relatives visit the mortuary chapel to see the body.

Where there is to be a post-mortem the body is only straightened, the jaw supported and the eyes closed with wet compresses. It is labelled and removed to the mortuary.

FURTHER READING

Basic Nursing Care

Basic Principles of Nursing Care prepared by V.Henderson. International Council of Nurses.

Routine Nursing Procedures

Law Notes for Nurses by S.R.Speller. R.C.N.
General Textbook of Nursing by E.Pearce. Faber & Faber
Modern Nursing by W.Hector. Heinemann
Care of the Dying by Cicely Saunders. *Nursing Times* Reprints
Nursing Care of the Anaesthetised Patient by Frank Wilson. Blackwell Scientific Publications
Nursing Care of the Unconscious Patient. P.Mountjoy & B. Wythe. Ballière, Tindall & Cox

PART 5 | PAEDIATRICS, GERIATRICS AND YOUNG CHRONIC SICK

CHAPTER 20 | PAEDIATRIC NURSING

PAEDIATRIC NURSING

This chapter is written as an introduction to a very demanding branch of nursing. The nursing of sick children has a very special appeal to most nurses and it calls for high levels of technical skill, emotional control and personal relationships.

There are many excellent textbooks available which deal with specific illnesses. Some of these are listed at the end of this chapter, which is concerned mainly with the psychological and physical surroundings of the sick child and the development of the normal child.

In recent years a great number of studies have been made of the effect of hospitalisation on children. Their behaviour both in hospital and afterwards has been watched most carefully and there is now sufficient evidence to show that most children suffer far more from their hospital stay if the visiting of their parents is restricted. This applies to babies and children between the ages of nine months to eight or nine years and is especially important to the $2\frac{1}{2}$-3 years group.

Many hospitals now allow free visiting and the more enlightened ones encourage the mothers who wish to do so to nurse their own children, supported and guided by the medical and nursing staff.

The physical surroundings of the children's ward should be bright and cheerful and the area divided into small units so that cross infection can be controlled and children of the same age groups can be together. There should also be play rooms and single rooms for those children who need quiet surroundings, and adequate facilities for mothers to 'live-in'.

A few hospitals now employ play-therapists to help convalescent children with this important part of their development. In long-stay hospitals it is usual for the children to undertake part-time education and qualified teachers carry out this work by arrangement with the Local Education Authority.

Radio and television are very important to most children, but their use must be thoughtfully controlled as the noise of these coupled with the usual noise that children make can be most disturbing for the really sick child.

The safety of the children has to be carefully maintained. Windows and balconies are danger spots as are restrainers in cots or beds. Hot-water bottles are not usually used as they are considered too dangerous. Medicine cupboards and trolleys, sterilisers and the ward kitchen are also danger zones. The children must be suitably clothed both in bed and when they are up. Young children especially, love to sleep on top of the bed-clothes—usually face down—and they can quickly catch cold if they are not warmly clad.

Admission

Great care should be taken not to aggravate an already unhappy situation by the application of any unsympathetic routine on admission. Mother and child should not be separated, unless the child wants to wander off to see the other children, whilst his mother gives the necessary details to the nurse admitting her child. These details should include the terms which the young child uses to describe bladder and bowel functions. Mother and child should then be shown round together and the mother encouraged to stay for the first meal and the putting-to-bed stage. Unless it is obviously essential the child should not be bathed until the normal afternoon or evening toilet time and the mother can then help. Except in the case of emergency admissions, medical examinations should not take place until the child has had time to get used to his surroundings. Babies and young children should be held on either the mother or nurse's lap whilst the doctor conducts his examination. Alternatively they can all sit round the bed or cot—unfamiliar adult figures towering over a toddler can be very frightening. Unpleasant procedures such as rectal examination should be left as long as possible.

It is important where there is free visiting for the nurses not to make the mother feel guilty, if for good reasons she cannot visit as frequently as other mothers. It is wise then to ask another mother to 'adopt' the lonely child.

Another danger to watch is that the nurse does not usurp the place of the mother—this is very easy to do, but the good paediatric nurse is one who learns to find satisfaction in supporting and teaching the parents of the children in her ward, and not in being a mother-substitute.

Observations and Examinations

It is usual to record the temperature, pulse and respiration rates of sick children in the same way as adult patients, but the techniques used may be different as are the normal levels for each.

Temperature
Normally the same as adults, but it fluctuates much more readily, and can reach greater heights during infection. In babies a special anal thermometer is used. This has a thicker bulb which should be well lubricated before being gently inserted into the anus. This is done whilst the baby lies on its back either in its cot or on the mother's lap. The legs are raised together and held there until the temperature is recorded. Toddlers and unconscious children should have the thermometer placed in a dry groin or axilla and held there until the time is up. Older children who are conscious may be treated like adults.

Pulse
Pulse is taken in the same way as for adults, but needs some practice before it can be counted with accuracy. The rate is usually higher and it is very easy to press too hard on the vein and so lose the rhythm. The use of a stethoscope is advocated for babies. Another difficulty is to find the convalescent child at rest for long enough to make the observations worth while.

Respiration
Again slightly higher than in adults but easy to count.

Blood Pressure
As with all other nursing procedures the child should be told what is going to happen and the proper-sized sphygmomanometer cuff should be used. The blood pressures of children are not taken as frequently as those of adults.

Skin
The skin of children should be unblemished and have great elasticity. It soon shows signs of lack of fluids by becoming dry and stiff. The colour is normally pale pinkish-white after the first week; any undue redness or yellowness should be reported as should spots or lumps.

Stools
These are dark green at birth due to meconium in the intestines. As a milk diet is established they become the colour of mustard and very soft, and as a mixed diet is introduced, so the stools become darker and more solid, as in adults. Any deviation from the normal either in colour, amount, consistency or smell for the age and diet of the child should be reported.

Urine
Normally pale in colour and clear. About two-thirds of the fluid intake is passed per day as urine, e.g. a two-year-old should drink just 600 ml a day and pass 450 ml of urine.

Collection of specimens from boys is easy. The cleaned penis should be placed inside a sterilised test tube or bottle and strapped into position. Girls present some difficulty and they should either micturate into a sterilised kidney dish or, in infants, have a sterilised rubber glove fixed with strapping over the vulva. Occasionally a catheter specimen will have to be taken.

It is useful to know the approximate times of micturation so that suitable routines can be established.

Young babies pass urine every half hour and therefore need to have their napkins changed frequently. From six months onwards control can be established by the regular use of a chamber after feeds so that by one year urine can be retained from five to six hours during the night and about three hours during the day. It is wise therefore to protect the child and cot at night during this period. From two and a half years onward there should be complete control.

Infant Feeding
The importance of breast feeding cannot be too strongly emphasised not only because of all its physical benefits but for the psychological ones for both mother and child. Every effort should be made to make suitable accommodation available for the mother of any baby admitted who is still being breast fed. The mother needs privacy, facilities for rest and an adequate diet.

Under-feeding
This is the commonest difficulty in breast feeding and the main symptoms are:
    (a) Crying and restlessness.
    (b) Failure to gain weight and the baby appears ravenous.
    (c) Vomiting due to air being swallowed by sucking an empty breast.
    (d) Stools dark, sometimes green, infrequent and small.
    (e) Low urine output.
To find out the exact intake the baby must be weighed both before and after feeds for twenty-four hours and for more than one day. This is called test-weighing. It should not become a routine procedure as the mother gets over-anxious at each time and this affects her milk supply. Once the average intake is estimated it may be necessary to give a complementary feed of expressed breast milk from the milk bank, or

of artificial milk. If this is done the time spent in feeding by breast and bottle should not exceed twenty minutes, or both mother and baby will be too tired to enjoy the experience.

All breast-fed babies as well as those on artificial milk need vitamins C and D. Both should be given by spoon starting from four to six weeks after birth. Vitamin C is usually given as orange, rose hip or blackcurrant juice, and vitamin D as cod liver oil. Both these can be obtained by the mother through her child welfare clinic. The amounts of each will be prescribed.

Artificial Feeding
Unlike breast feeding the preparation of an artificial feed is fraught with difficulties and dangers. The weighing of the powder and the measuring of the liquid for mixing must be absolutely accurate and all the utensils used as well as the bottle and teat must be sterilised. Most children's wards have a separate room for this procedure known as the milk kitchen. Some paediatricians prefer modified cow's milk to dried milk preparations and the making-up of these feeds calls for a high degree of accuracy and aseptic technique. The need to modify cow's milk can be seen by comparing its composition with that of breast milk:

	BREAST MILK	COW'S MILK
Protein	1·5%	3·5%
Fat	3·5%	3·5%
Carbohydrate	6·5%	4·7%

The method of modifying cow's milk is worked out for each individual baby and is based on:
(a) Amount of fluid required per kilogramme body weight every twenty-four hours.
(b) The number of calories required in twenty-four hours according to age and weight.
(c) The calorific value of milk and sugar.
In some ways dried milks are easier to use but care must be taken to use the right type of dried milk as ordered by the paediatrician. They are sold in four grades:

Full cream	Humanised
Half cream	Special

Directions for use are always given on the tin, but sometimes these are disregarded and an individual recipe used.

The way in which an artificial fed is given is most important. The dangers of infection can be eliminated by meticulous preparation of the mixture and bottle. The nurse may wear a mask and special gown throughout this period. The baby should be given a clean napkin and held by the mother or nurse in as upright a position as possible whilst the feed is taken, to prevent milk getting into the eustachian tubes and causing ear trouble. The feed should not take more than twenty minutes and if this period looks like being extended the last amount can be given by spoon. A bottle should never be given by propping it in the baby's mouth whilst it lies in its cot.

Problems of artificial feeding
   (a) infection
   (b) allergy to milk
   (c) over feeding

Weaning
Weaning or the gradual introduction of a diet of mixed foods can start at 3 months after birth unless there are medical reasons for delaying the start.

Some babies find this beginning of independence a difficult time and resist food unless it can be sucked from a bottle. It can be a most trying time for the mother and at this period a stranger can sometimes handle the situation with the firmness required. If the baby has been used to taking vitamins from a cup and spoon from the beginning fewer problems seem to arise.

The main principles to observe are that new food should be introduced in small amounts and that each stage should take about a week before passing on to the next one. The aim is to have dispensed with breast or bottle by the time the baby is nine months old.

Infant Toilet

Normal healthy babies can be bathed every day as long as the procedure is carried out with the minimum of exposure to varying temperatures. All equipment and clothing should be collected together in a warm, draught-free area and the water prepared before undressing the infant. It is wise to leave on the napkin while the face and head are washed, the baby being securely wrapped in a towel and held under one arm, face up and head supported in the palm of the hand. Once this part of the toilet has been completed the baby should be held firmly in the lap, the towel unwrapped, the napkin removed and any faecal matter cleaned away before soaping the body all over. Once this is done the baby can be immersed in the bath (38°C—comfortable to elbow test). The head and shoulders should rest on the arm of the nurse, who grasps the baby by the upper arm farthest away from her. With her free hand she quickly rinses the soap off, paying particular attention to the groins, axilla and neck folds. The baby is then lifted with both hands onto the lap in a rolling movement towards the nurse's body so that he is face down for the first areas to be dried. This should be done with a firm patting movement rather than rubbing. Again, the skin folds in neck, axilla and groin should be carefully and thoroughly dried. Powder and cream are not necessary, but if used, a very light hand is needed! Dress quickly, starting with vest and then napkin followed by gown and coat and bootees. Very young babies feel secure if they are then firmly, but not tightly, wrapped in a cotton blanket or shawl. Feeding usually follows bathing and should therefore be done with quiet firmness and as quickly as possible so that the baby is not too tired to take its diet.

It is usually necessary to change the napkin following the feed before returning the baby to its cot and the older babies may begin to be 'potted' at this time.

Very ill babies should not be handled more than absolutely necessary and should not be bathed daily until well enough to stand the exertion. They come to no harm provided that their skin folds are kept clean and dry, their napkins and clothes changed every hour to prevent pressure sores. Special attention should be paid to their eyes and noses and fingernails. All procedures can be carried out without removing the baby from its cot.

Premature babies require highly skilled nursing care and all nurses who work with them receive additional and specialised training.

Toddlers' and Children's Toilet

Young children, even in hospital, seem to get very grubby, especially their hands and faces. In addition to a daily bath, either in bed or in the bathroom, if their condition permits this, they need to have their hands sponged before every meal and their hands and faces after every meal. As the use of a pot or the toilet is encouraged before meals a 'now wash your hands' routine can be established without difficulty.

Older Children

As with adults, it is important to give as much privacy as possible to children from eight years upwards when they are bathing or being bathed. For those who are able to bath themselves care must be taken to see that all sources of danger are eliminated, e.g. boiling water, slippery floor, draughts from windows or doors.

Other Important Nursing Procedures

Toilet Training
It is important to either start or maintain regular emptying of bladder and bowel, and all children from a year upwards should be included in a

regular toilet round. Only if a toddler makes a great fuss should he be excluded as the struggle does more harm than good.

Pressure Areas

Despite the fact that children in bed appear to be always on the move unless they are very ill, their pressure areas need watching very carefully, especially those in plaster or wearing splints.

Mouth Hygiene

Babies and toddlers can be easily infected by thrush which attacks the mucous membrane of the mouth, if the sterilising technique for feeding utensils is at fault or if barrier nursing is incorrectly carried out. The thrush, which produces milky-white patches inside the mouth and on the tongue, is treated by local application.

Toddlers and older children should be taught or encouraged to brush their teeth at least twice a day, and the eating of sweets and biscuits discouraged—particularly last thing at night.

Very ill children should have the same oral hygiene care as adults, wool buds being used instead of clip forceps.

Giving Medicines

This is not an easy or pleasant procedure for parent, nurse or patient, especially when the patient is a toddler. Much will depend on the imaginative dispensing of the medicines prescribed as they are much easier to administer or to swallow if they are liquid, coloured, odourless and sweet and non-oily.

Young children should wear a bib and sit on the nurse's lap so that the nurse can control the arms and legs whilst giving the liquid from a spoon—not a glass.

Injections are best given into the front of the thigh with a needle similar to that used for adults, but penetrating less deeply. Two nurses or mother and nurse should always do this together to prevent the limb jerking.

Normal Milestones

Because of the comprehensive maternity service in this country and the high standard of living, most babies are born in a very healthy condition. The following table shows how the average normal child develops:

AGE	WEIGHT	HEIGHT	TEETH	SLEEP	ACTIVITY
Birth	3·2 kg	51·3 cm	—	20–22 hr	Very little
6 mths	6·4 kg	61·5 cm	Lower and upper central incisors	14–16 hr	Grips articles, sits up alone, crawls
1 yr	9·6 kg	71·6 cm	Lateral incisors (9–10 mths)	12–14 hr	Stands up alone
2 yrs	12·8 kg	76·7 cm	Premolars and canines	12 hr at night plus 2 hr midday	Walking
3 yrs	15·0 kg	84·5 cm	Molars	12 hr at night plus 2 hr midday	
4 yrs	17·0 kg	91·8 cm		12 hr at night plus 2 hr midday	
7 yrs	22·4 kg	96·8 cm	Permanent begin to erupt	10 hr	
12 yrs	32·0 kg	157·7 cm	All except wisdom teeth	10 hr	

CHAPTER 21 | NURSING OLD PEOPLE AND THE YOUNG CHRONIC SICK

Special Needs of the Elderly

Most old people prefer to live in their own homes surrounded by their own possessions. They enjoy being grandparents, aunts or uncles, and dread the day when illness or increasing feebleness brings the end of independence; even those living alone and without relatives cling fiercely to their independence.

Until recently very little positive thinking or research had been done about the needs of the elderly; but with the increasing number of our population living to well past retiring age—due to our high standard of living and the help of readily available medical treatment—it became apparent that the old, rather negative care of the elderly would have to change.

In 1962 a report called 'An Investigation of Geriatric Nursing Problems in Hospital' was published by the National Corporation for the Care of Old People. Many important facts emerged from this report but there are three which should help nurses to understand the modern approach to the nursing of old people, they are:

1. *To rehabilitate* all those with potential

2. *To maintain* the infirm disabled patient

3. *To give tender, loving, skilful nursing* to those whose illness is terminal.

Rehabilitation

Many old people now recover fairly quickly from acute medical or surgical illnesses and require very little rehabilitation. They should be encouraged to regain their independence as quickly as possible and to return home, supported by as many of our Statutory and Voluntary Services as may be necessary. Good liaison between Hospital and Public Health Services is vital.

Some, however, will require, because of the nature of their illness, e.g. a stroke, to start on a long-term programme of rehabilitation. This is a combined operation of patient, doctor, nurse, physio and occupational therapists, and not least the relatives and friends. Setbacks and depression must be dealt with sympathetically but firmly so that the patient does not become apathetic and need long-term hospitalisation. Some hospitals now have a day centre where rehabilitation is continued on an out-patient basis until full independence is regained but this needs the support of good transport facilities.

Maintenance

Some patients will never regain the full use of their faculties, but nevertheless they should be encouraged to lead as full a life as possible. This may either be within the hospital or in a suitable home outside. Remedial exercises and occupational therapy can continue either in their own home through the Local Health Authority Services or in the out-patient department of a hospital. The aim is to keep the patient from becoming bedfast for as long as possible.

Terminal Nursing

Some of the most difficult nursing is in this group of patients. Incontinence and mental confusion are very trying conditions to deal with, but skilful nursing of these patients who are the 'elderly citizens of our community' can be most rewarding.

Psychological Needs of Old People

These are much the same as for other age groups and we must see that they receive from us the courtesy and respect that is their due. No elderly patient should be referred to as 'Mother' or 'Dad', but by their surname and proper title. Their hospital clothes should give them both dignity and pleasure as should the surroundings in which they are nursed.

If they are treated like children they will behave like children and their rehabilitation will take much longer and be much more difficult for patient and staff alike.

Special Needs of the Young Chronic Sick

In caring for the young chronic sick, the nurse is faced with many problems. First of all she has to adjust herself to a great deal of routine bedside nursing care, some of which may be extremely hard physical work. At the same time she will be trying to communicate with people who are having to adjust themselves to a permanently restricted life. Their adjustment needs to be watched most carefully so that it does not become a passive acceptance of chronic illness or a bitter resentment of circumstances.

The nurse has a very large part to play in helping these young disabled people to live as full a life as possible. She must become a real teamworker with the other professional men and women engaged in the rehabilitation or maintenance of her patients.

As with elderly patients, the aim is to return these people to their homes, able to be as physically independent as possible. At the same time, all the services which can help the young chronic sick to have a measure of financial independence should be brought into the picture so that any special skills or aptitudes the patient may have can be channelled into useful occupation.

For some the outlook is good, but for others, a bed-fast or chair-fast life seems inevitable. For these, home life is still better than permanent hospitalisation provided that the home can be adequately supported by both statutory and voluntary services. Where this is not possible the admission of the patient to a Cheshire Home or similar organisation should be considered. Regional Hospital Boards are beginning to build special units in selected hospitals.

Patience, tolerance and sympathetic discipline will be needed when caring for the young chronic sick, but most of all the ability to stimulate and guide reluctant minds and limbs into new avenues of thought and occupation.

FURTHER READING

Paediatric Nursing

Baby and Child Care by Dr B.Spock. Pocket Book Inc.

Practical Paediatric Nursing. Sheila M.Bates. Blackwell
Paediatric Nursing. M.Duncombe & B.Weller. Ballière, Tindall & Cox

Geriatric and Chronic Sick Nursing

The Nursing of the Elderly Sick by T.N.Rudd. Faber

SECTION 2 | CAUSES OF DISEASE AND TREATMENT

Causes of Disease may be listed as follows:
1 *Injury* or damage to tissue.
2 *Infection*, i.e. invasion of the body by harmful bacteria.
3 *Poisoning* (toxic effects) either from substances or bacteria introduced into the body or produced by the body itself.
4 *Tumours*, which are overgrowths of tissue.
5 *Deficiencies* either in the diet or due to failure in some part of the body's chemical activity.
6 *Allergy* or oversensitivity to a substance in contact with body tissue.
7 *Degeneration* or wearing out of tissue.

Treatment of Disease includes:
1 Rest.
2 Diet.
3 Drugs.
4 Surgery.
5 Radiotherapy.
6 Physiotherapy.
7 Occupational therapy.
Some aspects in the treatment of disease are discussed in the following chapters. Others are introduced elsewhere in the book.

CHAPTER 22 | FIRST AID: EMERGENCIES: MAJOR DISASTERS

This is the initial treatment given to anyone who sustains sudden illness or an accident whether it occurs at home, in hospital, at work or in the street. Many accidents are preventable and nurses as citizens should check their homes and their cars to minimise risks and set a good example to others. They also have a duty towards their patients if they work in hospital to see that the risk of personal injury to them through faulty equipment or poor ward management is eliminated as far as possible. Public Health nurses carry out similar preventive measures in the homes they visit and those who work in Industry not only act as health and safety supervisors but very often train teams of first-aiders as well.

The Objects of First Aid

1. To save life.
2. To prevent complications.
3. To prepare for medical aid.
4. To assist the doctor.

Qualifications of a First Aider

1. Theoretical knowledge of anatomy and physiology and first aid.
2. Efficiency in practical work.
3. Organising ability.
4. Calm manner.
5. Tact and sympathy.
6. Sound judgment.

Control of the Situation

1. Removal of cause of injury, e.g. switch off electric current or remove patient from cause, e.g. gas-filled room.
2. Patient told to lie still or put into most natural position.
3. Bystanders told to stand aside except those who can help.
4. Obtain permission if possible from patient before beginning examination or treatment.

5. Prevent shock.
6. Treat urgent conditions:
   (a) Cessation of breathing.
   (b) Haemorrhage.
   (c) Shock.
7. Send for medical aid as soon as possible and police in cases of street accident, suspected suicide, manslaughter or murder.

Inspection of Patient

1. General appearance including colour of lips and skin.
2. Expression.
3. Pulse and breathing.
4. Temperature, if possible.
5. Movement of limbs, head and back.

A. URGENT TREATMENT—EMERGENCIES

1. RESPIRATORY ARREST—cessation of breathing
   (a) Mouth-to-mouth breathing—see p. 312.
   (b) Pressure on chest wall
       (i) Holger Neilsen's method
       (ii) Shafer's method
       (iii) Eve's Rocking method
       (iv) Silvester's method.

2. CARDIAC ARREST—cessation of pulse
When a patient collapses and the nurse finds that
   (a) he has no pulse *or*
   (b) he has no pulse and is not breathing, she
       (i) summons help
       (ii) screens the bed
       (iii) places the patient on the floor and clears airway if necessary, i.e. removes dentures and deals with vomit.
       (iv) begins External Cardiac Massage.
       (v) if neither pulse nor respirations present alternate (iv) with mouth-to-mouth breathing—approx 25 × 1″ pressure on sternum to 5 or 6 lung inflations.

External Cardiac Massage
   (a) Strike the sternum sharply with the fist.
   (b) Press the lower end of the sternum 60–70 times a minute with the heel of the hand, the second hand being placed over the first.
   (c) 1″–1½″ is the depth of depression required for an adult: much

less for a child and only the pressure of one hand. Infants need only finger pressure.

Great care must be taken not to injure ribs and underlying organs.

Most hospitals now have a special telephone call signal for the emergency resuscitation team, who are on call day and night for the treatment of cardiac and/or respiratory arrest. Every nurse should know how to summon help and her part in servicing the team when it arrives.

3. HAEMORRHAGE

Severe bleeding can be very frightening for both patient and onlookers and unless it is controlled it can cause death. Haemorrhage is classified in four ways:
1. By the type of bleeding.
2. By the time of bleeding.
3. By the visibility of bleeding.
4. By the special sites of bleeding.

Types of haemorrhage
    (a) Arterial—bright red, spurts from end of wound nearest heart.
    (b) Capillary—red, flows briskly or oozes from all parts of wound.
    (c) Venous—dark red, flows steadily from end of wound farthest from heart.

Time of haemorrhage
    (a) Primary—occurs at time of injury.
    (b) Reactionary—within 24 hours of injury.
    (c) Secondary—24 hours to 14 days due to infection of blood vessel wall.

Visibility of Blood
    (a) External.
    (b) Internal.

Special Sites of Bleeding
    (a) Haemoptysis—bleeding from lungs—blood coughed up—bright red and frothy.
    (b) Haematemesis—blood is vomited—dark brown like coffee grounds.
    (c) Epistaxis—from nose.
    (d) Haematuria—blood in the urine.
    (e) Malaena—blood in the stools which are tarry in appearance.

Treatment
1. Lie patient down on blanket if possible.
2. If bleeding from limb, raise, unless fractured.
3. Expose wound. Arrest bleeding (see next paragraph).
4. Cover with clean dressing.
5. Bandage except in case of foreign body or fracture.
6. Send for medical help if necessary.
7. Keep patient moderately warm.

Methods of Arresting External Haemorrhage
1. *Nature's method* is to form a clot of blood which should never be removed by the first-aider, but covered by a clean pad and firm bandage.

2. *By digital pressure:*
   (a) Venous and capillary bleeding can usually be controlled by the application of a clean pad and firm bandage.
   (b) Arterial bleeding sometimes needs to be arrested by pressure on the artery above the point of injury. It is important therefore to know where the main arteries cross a bone, for it is here that pressure should be applied.

The eight most important pressure points are:
1. Temporal Artery—crosses the temporal bone at the zygomatic process (used to count the pulse rate).
2. Occipital Artery—Four fingers' breadth behind and a little below the external auditory meatus against which it should be pressed.
3. Facial Artery—crosses the jaw bone one inch in front of the angle of the jaw.
4. Common Carotid Artery—runs alongside the trachea—should be pressed against the cervical vertebrae at the level of the larynx.
5. Subclavian Artery—crosses the first rib. Pressure on the hollow above the clavicle with the neck flexed to the affected side.
6. Brachial—runs down the margin of the biceps muscle; compress against the humerus.
7. Radial and Ulna—these arteries should be pressed against the bones of the same name at the wrest level.
8. Femoral—this artery can be felt pulsating in the middle of the groin. Pressure by both thumbs is needed to be effective.

3. *By Tourniquet.* Very rarely used because of the damage it can cause to the limbs if not loosened every 15 to 20 minutes.

4. SHOCK

Shock is a condition in which the blood pressure falls to dangerously low levels. It is the result of either severe injury such as severe burns, crushing, multiple fractures or major surgery. It is made worse by fluid loss either through haemorrhage, vomiting, severe sweating or diarrhoea. Fear and pain can also affect the degree of shock.

Signs and Symptoms
  1. Low blood pressure.
  2. Pulse feeble, slow at first but becoming quicker and thinner.
  3. Temperature subnormal.
  4. Skin cold and clammy, pale with a tinge of blue.
  5. Vomiting.
  6. If the patient is conscious he will complain of thirst but otherwise appears listless.

Treatment
  (a) Keep crowds away and let patient get as much fresh air as possible.
  (b) Move the patient as little as possible but get head lower than rest body.
  (c) Arrest haemorrhage or put splints on fracture.
  (d) Whilst the patient should be kept moderately warm do not apply heat. Keep sheltered from draughts and cold.
  (e) Send for medical help.

B. Treatment for Other Conditions

1. Fractures

Fractures or broken bones may be caused by:
  1. *Direct violence*, e.g. kick, trip and fall, bullet.
  2. *Indirect violence*, e.g. falling from standing position—fractured skull.
  3. *Muscular action*, e.g. spasm of thigh muscle—fractured patella.
  There are several types of fractures which can be diagnosed by a doctor and confirmed by X-ray examination. The important points for a first-aider to remember are:
  1. The patient will have a good deal of pain.
  2. There will be some degree of shock.
  3. Bad management of the situation can cause additional damage to the bone or surrounding tissue.

Signs and Symptoms
   1. Deformity, swelling, unusual movement. Crepitus.
   2. Pain and loss of function. History of accident.

Treatment
GENERAL
   1. Treat for shock and send for medical aid.
   2. Collect materials for splinting and/or support.
   3. Cover any wounds before starting to splint.
   4. Move patient and limbs as little as possible, but get to hospital
      without delay.

SPECIFIC
   1. *Fractures of lower limbs*—use sound leg as splint and bind the two
      together above and below site of fracture or pack round with pads.
   2. *Fracture of upper limbs*—support with sling made from square of
      material or two straight scarves.
   3. *Fracture of collar bone*—support arm with sling.
   4. *Fracture of wrist*—splint wrist using roll of newspaper. Support
      in sling.
   5. *Fracture of the spine*—do not move the patient but maintain
      natural curves by putting rolled coat or cushions under lumbar
      region and neck.
   6. *Fracture of the skull*—keep patient still and quiet, raise head
      slightly, make notes for doctor on bleeding, if any, from nose or
      ears. Note condition of pupils of each eye.
   7. *Fracture of jaw*—apply jaw bandage.
   8. *Fracture of pelvis*—apply a binder to pelvis and tie legs together,
      watch for haematuria.
   9. *Fracture of ribs*—keep upper limbs still. Watch for haemoptysis.

2. Dislocations

These occur when bones are pulled out of their sockets. They are very
painful and there is usually swelling over the socket, loss of function in
the joint and deformity of the limb. The main complications are damage
to the nerves and blood vessels.

Treatment
   1. Splint and support in most comfortable position.
   2. Cold compresses help to relieve the pain and swelling.
   3. Send for medical aid and arrange for transport to hospital.

3. Sprains

These are conditions due to ligaments and muscles torn or wrenched, but there is no dislocation of the joint. As there is pain and swelling they are sometimes difficult to diagnose correctly and it is safest to treat as a fracture or dislocation until medical advice is given.

4. Burns and Scalds

Burns are caused by DRY heat, scalds by MOIST heat.
There are three degrees of burns and scalds:
1. Scorching or reddening.
2. Blistering (nerve endings exposed, resulting in pain).
3. Damage to deeper tissues (no pain if nerve endings destroyed).

Danger of Burns
1. SHOCK—this is the 'killing' element in severe burning where large areas of skin are involved.
2. SEPSIS—infection due to air-borne organisms.
3. Contractions of skin during healing. Plastic surgery very often required later.

Treatment
1. Get medical aid or ambulance as quickly as possible.
2. Cover burnt area with clean dressing and bandage lightly or wrap whole body in clean sheets.
3. Treat shock.
4. If medical help is not available quickly soak sheet in solution of soda bicarbonate (1 dessertspoonful in 1 pint warm water).
5. If face involved, make mask of linen and soak in solution; keep moist.
6. Burns due to *corrosive acid*, flood thoroughly and quickly with warm water.
7. Burns due to *corrosive alkali*, treat as for acid but add vinegar to water if available.
8. In case of *clothing on fire*, approach victim from behind and cover with rug or blanket and smother flames.

5. Poisoning

A poison is any substance which, when taken into the body in sufficient

quantities, will produce death. It may be taken accidentally or intentionally by:
  (a) swallowing,
  (b) inhalation,
  (c) injection.

Types of Poison
  1. Corrosives—burn the mouth and lips—strong acids and alkalies.
  2. Irritants—do not burn—metallic poisons, poisonous fungi, berries, decomposing food.
  3. Hypnotics—do not burn—opium, barbiturates.
  4. Deliriants—do not burn—belladonna, chloroform, alcohol.
  5. Convulsants—do not burn—strychnine, prussic acid, potassium cyanide.
  6. Analgesics—do not burn—Aspirin.

Treatment
  1. Send for medical aid or arrange to get patient to hospital.
  2. Get as much information as possible about the patient and the poison.
  3. *If lips and mouth not burned*—make the patient vomit by:
     (a) Giving an emetic—2 tablespoonsful of salt in tumbler of water.
     (b) Inserting fingers into throat of patient—protect hand whilst doing this.
  4. *If lips and mouth are burned*—do not make the patient vomit, but give antidote if available.
  5. In all cases keep the patient warm and quiet; be prepared to give artificial respiration. Save all vomit, urine and receptacles which may have contained the poison.
  6. If the circumstances are suspicious—inform the police.

6. Unconsciousness

There are two degrees of unconsciousness:
  1. *Stupor*—the patient can be roused, but with difficulty.
  2. *Coma*—the patient cannot be roused.

Observation of Patient
To assist the doctor it is helpful to make a note of the following:
  1. The time the patient has been unconscious.
  2. What caused the unconsciousness.
  3. Pulse and respiration rates.
  4. Condition of the pupils—contracted or dilated.

5. Any odour of the breath.
6. Type and number of convulsions.
7. Any paralysis.
8. Degree of incontinence.

Treatment
1. Send for medical aid.
2. Treat haemorrhage or asphyxia if present.
3. Put patient in best position flat, head to one side, jaw supported. If face pale, lower head; if flushed, raise it.
4. Loosen all tight clothing.
5. Keep patient warm, but give plenty of air.
6. Give nothing by mouth until fully conscious.
7. Do not leave patient alone.

7. Fits

The commonest cause of a fit in an adult is epilepsy, so it is important to recognise the three stages of an epileptic fit.
1. *Aura*—the warning period which is very short, patient usually has time only to cry out before.
2. *The Tonic Phase*—when the muscles contract and respiration may be suspended—the patient usually falls to the ground.
3. *The Clonic Phase*—when the muscles relax and contract producing violent movements of trunk, limbs and jaw. Incontinence may occur and sometimes the tongue gets bitten at this stage.

Treatment
1. Remove all obstacles from the area where the patient has fallen to prevent him injuring himself further.
2. Keep bystanders back so that there is plenty of room and air.
3. If possible get a pad of material between his teeth during a period of relaxation but do not force the jaws apart.
4. Cover patient after fit and support head on pillow. Mop face and hands and clean mouth.
5. Get to hospital if the fit happens in a public place, or advise him to see his doctor if it occurs at work or at home.

8. Foreign Bodies

The removal of most foreign bodies requires medical skill, therefore the first duty of the nurse is to arrange for medical help as soon as possible.

All the natural orifices are excellent receptacles for foreign bodies, i.e. beads in the nose or ears: hairpins and dentures in the throat: wire in the urethra.

If the foreign body has entered through the skin the wound should be thoroughly cleansed, the foreign body, if visible, strapped to prevent it disappearing altogether and a sterile dressing applied.

It cannot be too strongly emphasised that the removal of foreign bodies from any part of the body is a highly skilled surgical procedure in most cases.

C. MAJOR DISASTERS

A major disaster may be said to be an accident involving a large number of seriously injured casualties, e.g. 30 or more. Arrangements for dealing with the situation are agreed between Regional Hospital Boards and City or Town Authorities. Instructions regarding the procedures to be adopted are issued to all members of the services likely to be called in to help, e.g. Police Force, Ambulance Service, Fire Service, Hospitals, and voluntary organisations such as St. John Ambulance Service, British Red Cross Society and the Women's Royal Voluntary Service.

It is the duty of nurses to be sure that they are familiar with the procedure covering arrangements current in their own hospitals.

Nurses off duty are expected to return at once if they hear of a major disaster occurring in an area covered by their own hospital. They will be allocated duties by the senior nursing officer on duty.

Some hospitals are designated to receive casualties and others to send out emergency teams to the area of the accident. Nurses in Wards and Departments will know what they are expected to prepare for and will make the necessary arrangements as quickly, quietly, efficiently as possible making a minimum amount of fuss.

CHAPTER 23 | MEDICINES AND POISONS

MEDICINES are substances other than diet given to the patient in the treatment of disease or to relieve its symptoms.

DRUGS are medicines but the term 'medicines' usually refers to simple remedies taken by mouth.

POISONS are those substances which if taken in sufficient quantities are dangerous to health or life. A label on the bottle states 'POISON'. They are stored in a locked cupboard.

A number of poisons which are harmful if taken in excess of the prescribed doses are included in the lists of SCHEDULE POISONS. There are regulations concerning the use of these in the Poisons Act, which is an Act of Parliament. The names of Schedule drugs used in medical treatments are contained in Schedules 1 and 4. Amongst these are the barbiturates, sulphonamides and digitalis. These drugs are given to a patient only on the prescription of a qualified medical practitioner. The prescription states the date, the patient's name, the drug, the dose to be given, and in some cases when the drug is to be repeated. The signature of the qualified medical practitioner is necessary. A label on the bottle or box states SCHEDULE POISON. Usually records are kept of these drugs when they are administered, either on the patient's report card, in a report book or in a Poisons Record Book.

Certain Schedule poisons are habit-forming drugs (drugs of addiction). This means that some people may become accustomed to the drug and feel they cannot manage without it even though the reason for having the drug has since disappeared. A craving for the drug leads to many complications for the individual and his family. Supervision of the custody of some of these drugs is controlled by the *Dangerous Drugs Act*, which is an Act of Parliament; for example:

Opium and substances prepared from it—morphia, papaveretum (omnopon), diamorphine (heroin).

Cocaine.

Indian hemp

Pethidine hydrochloride.

A label on the bottle or box states POISON. D.D.A. These drugs are stored in a locked cupboard labelled D.D.A., the key of which is kept on the person of the ward sister or a member of staff appointed by her. (This latter person is *not* authorised to pass the key on to any other person without the ward sister's instruction.) A drug which is controlled by the *Dangerous Drugs Act* is administered to a patient only on the prescription of a qualified medical practitioner which has been signed by him.

Records are made of the drugs received on the ward and of the drugs administered to patients. These may be inspected at any time by the pharmacist, who may also check with the ward sister the supplies in the Dangerous Drug Cupboard.

There are other habit-forming drugs (drugs of addiction) such as barbiturates, which are sedatives, some tranquillisers and some stimulants.

These are *not* controlled by the *Dangerous Drugs Act* but in many hospitals records of supplies to the wards and administration of the drugs are kept in the same way.

Checking of Dangerous Drugs

It is customary in hospital, though not by law, for the measuring and administration of dangerous drugs to be witnessed by a responsible person, either the giver or the witness being a State Registered Nurse. This is referred to as the 'checking' of drugs. Required for this procedure are:

Prescription sheet with date, patient's name, drug and its dose, and signed by a qualified medical practitioner.

Dangerous Drug Record Book.

Drug as written on prescription sheet.

A syringe for measuring the dose.

Adequate lighting is necessary.

The person who holds the D.D.A. cupboard key unlocks the cupboard, takes out the box of ampoules containing the prescribed drug and locks the cupboard. The witness checks the name of the patient, the date, and prescription on the prescription sheet and makes sure the prescription has been signed. She then checks the name of the drug with the name on the box of ampoules *and* on the ampoule to be used. It is usual to count the number of ampoules in the box before and after the drug is given; the numbers are recorded in the Dangerous Drug Book.

The giver draws up the drug into the syringe and the witness checks that the prescribed amount is prepared for injection, by referring to the prescription sheet. Details of the drug may be entered in the Dangerous Drug Book at this point, and the box of remaining ampoules is returned to the D.D.A. cupboard which is again locked.

Both giver and witness go to the bedside of the patient, the giver carrying the injection tray and the witness the prescription sheet. The patient is addressed by name as a precaution in ensuring this is the patient for whom the drug has been prescribed. It is helpful if the giver or both she and the witness know the patient already. Her name may be on the bed and on the charts attached to the bed or locker. If she is unconscious there is a special responsibility; the charts and case notes are checked for her full name. She has on her wrist an identification band to which the witness can refer.

When the drug has been administered, the record in the Dangerous Drug Book is completed and signed by the giver and the witness. The patient is observed and the effect of the drug noted.

Storage of Medicines and Poisons

MEDICINES are stored in a cupboard which is not easily accessible to patients, and is preferably locked. The cupboard should not be in direct sunlight as this may cause some drugs to deteriorate. These drugs are stored in dark-coloured bottles. Adequate lighting is necessary either from an electric bulb inside the cupboard or in front of it, otherwise a pocket torch is required. No medicine is poured from one bottle to another, and only the dispensers fix labels to the bottles. The pharmacist may indicate an expiry date on the label and after this date the drugs should not be used, but be returned to the Dispensary. Similarly tablets which have changed colour or crumbled, and liquids in which sediments have formed, are inspected by the Dispensary staff as they may now be ineffective. Strict order and tidiness in a medicine room or cupboard are part of accident prevention procedure. Both assist in speedy administration of drugs during emergencies, and are an indication of a high standard of efficiency in the ward.

POISONS, including Schedule poisons, are stored in a locked cupboard, which in some hospitals is fixed inside the medicine cupboard.

DANGEROUS DRUGS are stored in a locked cupboard marked D.D.A. either fixed inside the medicine cupboard, or in Sister's office. The contents of this cupboard may be checked twice a day, usually at the change of duties in the morning and in the evening by the ward sister or staff nurse with a ward nurse.

Administration of Drugs

1. By mouth. These drugs are given in the form of mixtures, emulsions, oils, powders, tablets, pills, capsules and cachets.
2. Under the tongue.
3. By rectum.
4. By inhalation.
5. By hypodermic or subcutaneous injection.
6. By intramuscular injection.
7. By intravenous injection.
8. By intravenous infusion.

Administration of drugs by mouth

The medicine and its label are examined carefully and compared with the prescription sheet. The bottle containing a liquid medicine with a sediment is shaken thoroughly holding the cork firmly in with the index finger. In pouring out the medicine the label is protected from stains by holding the bottle with the label next to the palm. The cork is removed and held in the little finger so that it will not become soiled or confused with corks from other bottles. The medicine glass into which the medicine is poured is held at eye level for greater accuracy in measurement. The medicine is poured out to the exact amount.

The medicine and dose are again compared with prescription sheet. If necessary the neck of the bottle is washed as the cork is replaced. The medicine is taken to the patient on a small tray. If there is a sediment in the mixture it should be stirred with a spoon before the patient takes it. The nurse stays with the patient while he takes the medicine. He may wish to drink water or fruit juice to remove the taste.

Small amounts of drugs are measured in a minim measure.

A *powder* may be poured on the tongue from the paper in which it is contained or placed on a teaspoon or mixed with a little jam if the patient is allowed to have this.

Pills, tablets, capsules and cachets are taken from their containers with a teaspoon and not touched by hand. The patient takes them from the teaspoon.

Tablets can sometimes be crushed between the bowls of two spoons. When the patient cannot swallow pills easily he can be given a piece of bread to chew. The pill is swallowed with this.

Oils are not always pleasant to take, and the texture and flavour may be disguised by adding fruit juice or soda water.

A linctus is a sweet, thick liquid which is given in a teaspoon, *not* diluted with water. A Ministry of Health teaspoon for measuring medicines holds 5 millilitres.

Administration of Drugs under the Tongue
There are a few drugs given in this way; glyceryl trinitrate is an example. A tablet is placed beneath the tongue and is absorbed through the mucous membrane.

Administration of Drugs by Hypodermic or Subcutaneous Injection
(Both these terms mean 'beneath the skin').
This is an aseptic procedure, and the nurse's hands should be clean. The *drug* is sterile and contained in an *ampoule* or *bottle*. Its name is compared with that on the *prescription sheet* and the dose is noted. The appropriate *record book* is available when the drug is a Dangerous Drug, or a Poison to be checked and recorded.

A sterile 2-millilitre syringe and hypodermic needle are required. Disposable types are preferable. The cap is removed from the needle container and the syringe attached. The hands must not touch the nozzle of the syringe or the needle. The needle container is replaced over the needle point to protect it. If an ampoule is used it is broken by drawing a *file* round the neck, and separating the top part of the ampoule from the base with a sharp, clean snap. Most ampoules can be broken without using a file. The needle is inserted into the fluid and the plunger of the syringe withdrawn so that the drug is drawn into the syringe. The ampoule is held upside down to empty it. If the bottle is used, the top is first cleaned with a *swab and antiseptic lotion* and allowed to dry before inserting the needle. To allow an easy withdrawal of the drug, some air is injected from the syringe into the bottle (the same amount of air as drug to be withdrawn). The exact amount of drug is drawn into the syringe. The drug and the dose are again checked with the prescription sheet. Any excess would be pushed out of the syringe into the empty ampoule.

The procedure is explained to *the patient* and the nurse makes sure that his name is that on the prescription. Either she knows him as her patient and addresses him by name or she checks with his identity wrist-band. The *place for injection* is the arm on the outer aspect midway between shoulder and elbow or nearer to the elbow. Injections may also be made into the thigh between hip and knee on the outer aspect in which case screens or curtains are drawn round the bed. The skin is cleaned with a *swab and antiseptic lotion*, and then held taut with the thumb and finger of one hand while the needle is introduced fairly steeply into the flesh. Do not insert the total length of the needle as this puts some strain on the joint between the head and shaft of the needle, but withdraw it about $\frac{1}{8}$ inch. Hold the head of the needle firmly with the index finger. The piston is withdrawn a little to ensure the needle has not entered a blood vessel. Then the injection is given steadily and without haste. The needle is withdrawn quickly and the skin swabbed again.

The patient is made comfortable. The drug is recorded.

Disposable needles and syringes are discarded into a disposal bag. To avoid accidents from sharp needle points some defined procedure is necessary. The method to be used will be determined by the Nursing Procedure Committee in consultation with other staffs concerned with collection, transport and diposal of waste materials.

Examples:

Method 1. The needle point is pushed into the syringe through the rubber diaphragm.

Method 2. The syringe is discarded into the disposal bag. The needle is discarded into a container which is easily recognisable and is labelled 'used needles, blades and broken glass for special disposal'.

Glass syringes are dissembled, washed, dried and sterilised by the ward or C.S.S.D. staff.

Administration of a Drug by Intramuscular Injection

The procedure is similar to that in giving a hypodermic injection. The syringe may be 2, 5 or 10 millilitres depending on the amount of drug to be administered, and the needle is larger, e.g. No. 1.

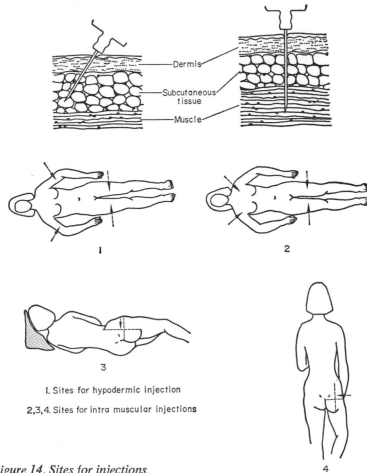

1. Sites for hypodermic injection

2,3,4. Sites for intra muscular injections

Figure 14. Sites for injections.

Places for Injection (Fig. 14)

    (a) Deltoid muscle in the shoulder.

    (b) Quadriceps extensor muscle, a little to the outer side at the front of the thigh, midway between hip and knee.

(c) Gluteal muscle in the buttock. The injection is given in the upper outer quarter to avoid the sciatic nerve.

Drugs which are thick liquids are warmed by holding the ampoule in the hand and a needle with a wider bore is used.

The patient's confidence and co-operation are needed as he should be relaxed during procedure, otherwise the muscles are contracted and become hard, so that giving the injection is more difficult.

A sharp needle is essential. It is inserted at right angles to the skin. The injection is given fairly slowly. Sometimes the area is massaged gently to assist absorption of the drug.

Intra-muscular injections can be painful and when they are to be repeated at frequent intervals the nurse varies the place for injection.

Preparation for Intravenous Injections

Drugs given by this method are absorbed immediately. They are administered only by medical practitioners.

The equipment is sterile as this is an aseptic technique and includes a *5- or 10-millilitre syringe* and an *intravenous needle* which is short and has a wide bore. *Swabs and antiseptic lotion* are necessary for cleaning the skin. The *drug* is contained in an *ampoule* and a *file* may be necessary to open it. It is checked with the *prescription sheet*. An appropriate *record book* may be needed.

The procedure is explained to the patient so that his confidence and co-operation are obtained. He is comfortable and relaxed. The injection is usually made into a vein at the elbow. If the patient is right-handed, the left arm is prepared by resting it on a pillow. If he is left-handed, the right arm is prepared. In a clinic, the patient sits with his arm resting on a table. To make the vein larger and more easily entered, pressure is applied to the arm above the elbow. This is done by tying a piece of rubber tubing round the arm with a slip knot, or by applying the cuff of a blood pressure machine or a pocket tourniquet. The rubber tubing or tourniquet are applied over a towel or the patient's sleeve, *not* next to the the skin (Fig. 15).

The doctor has drawn up the drug into the syringe and cleaned the skin. He introduces the needle into the vein. The rubber tubing or tourniquet is released gently or the cuff of the blood pressure machine deflated. He injects the drug. The needle is withdrawn and the skin swabbed. A sterile swab is pressed over the puncture, the patient's arm is raised above his head keeping the elbow extended for a moment or two to allow the drug flow into the circulation. A swab may be secured over the puncture with adhesive tape.

The patient is made comfortable. The equipment is cleaned, syringe and needle either sterilised or discarded. Any special effect of the drug is observed in the patient and reported.

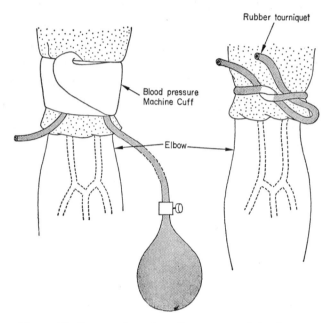

Figure 15. Preparation of an Intravenous Injection

Lotions, Powders, Liquids, Ointments
When intended for external use these are stored in a cupboard separated from the medicine cupboard. They are labelled 'For External Use Only' or 'Not To Be Taken'. Those which are poisons are labelled 'POISON'. Bottles containing poisons such as antiseptics, disinfectants and liniments, are ridged. Lotions and liquids which lose their strength in strong light are stored in dark blue or green glass containers.

Bottles should be wiped carefully after use so that the fluids do not come into contact with the hands to cause skin irritation and burns. Liquids are not poured from one bottle into another, stoppers and caps are replaced immediately and the labels are kept clean and intact.

A nurse should learn the habit of checking all the substances she uses. This method is an example:

Read the label (in a good light).
Measure the liquid, or lotion . . . etc.
Read the label again.

Some concentration is always necessary and when a nurse is measuring lotions (or checking drugs) she should not be disturbed. If this cannot be avoided, it is wise for her to repeat the procedure from the beginning.

Abbreviations in prescription are best avoided but examples of some abbreviations are:

t.d.s.·	means	three times daily.
b.d.	means	twice daily.
o.m.	means	every morning.
o.n.	means	every night.
p.r.n.	means	whenever necessary.
s.o.s.	means	once when necessary.
stat.	means	at once.

Measurement of Liquid Medicines in the Home
Patients are given a plastic measure or teaspoon as required with the medicine. In this way the amounts are standardised. The teaspoon holds 5 millilitres.

Metric System

Length	1000 millimetres	=	1 metre.
	100 millimetres	=	1 centimetre.
	100 centimetres	=	1 metre.
Fluids	1000 millilitres	=	1 litre.
Weight	1000 grammes	=	1 kilogramme.

English and Metric Equivalents

1000 millilitres	=	1 litre	=	$1\frac{3}{4}$ pints.	
600 millilitres	=	1 pint.			
30 millilitres	=	1 fluid ounce.			
4 millilitres	=	1 fluid drachm.			
1 millilitre	=	15 minims.			
30 grammes	=	1 ounce.			
1 kilogramme	=	$2\frac{1}{4}$ pounds.			

Nurses are advised always to use ARABIC NUMERALS when writing reports or completing records. Abbreviations also are of no use unless everyone who reads the report or record understands the meaning of the abbreviation.

Lotions and their Measurement

Lotion 1 in 20 means 1 part of the pure substance made up to 20 parts with water.

Example: 10 millilitres of Izal made up to 200 millilitres with water makes Izal lotion 1 in 20.

Lotion 1 in 300 means 1 part of the pure substance made up to 300 parts with water.

Example: 10 millilitres of pure Izal made up to 3 litres with water makes Izal 1 in 300.

To measure a lotion which is a different strength from the lotion in stock, the calculation can be stated thus:

Take the strength in stock, multiply by the amount required, divide it by the strength required.

Example: in stock—Glycothymoline mouthwash 1 in 2.

Required—120 ml of Glycothymoline 1 in 8.

Calculation—2 multiplied by 120 is 240. 240 divided by 8 is 30.

Take 30 ml of stock solution and make it up to 120 ml with water.

In most hospitals, the Pharmacy issues lotions to the wards in the strengths required for use. Should any dilution be necessary, instructions may be found on the label. Otherwise the details are stated by the Ward Sister or are in the Ward Procedure Manual.

Pure Izal is issued in a labelled can. One squirt of Izal from the can is 10 millilitres. One squirt of Izal made up to 3 litres with water makes Izal lotion 1 in 300.

CHAPTER 24 | INFLAMMATION AND INFECTION

INFLAMMATION is the normal reaction of body tissues to injury. *The sources of injury* are: heat, wounds, friction, acids and alkalies, irradiation (e.g. X-rays) and disease-producing micro-organisms.

Immediately following the injury the tissue, e.g. the skin, becomes white due to the release in the damaged cells of a substance which constricts the blood vessels in the area and localises the effect temporarily. After this action the INFLAMED AREA becomes *reddened* as the arterioles and capillaries dilate, so that more blood is available supplying the tissues with additional oxygen, foodstuffs and white blood cells, thus providing for recovery and healing. The increased blood supply leads to excess of fluid in the tissue spaces, and causes *swelling*. Blood distributes heat round the body, and more blood brings more heat to the area. There is also increased local cell activity, and *heat* is a symptom of inflammation. Swelling means pressure on nerve endings and the patient complains of *pain*, and there is *loss of function* in the organ affected.

Treatment. The cause, the injurious or irritating factor, is removed. The increase of blood is encouraged by *local application of heat* which dilates the blood vessels. Local applications of cold are sometimes applied to prevent swelling and relieve pain.

To localise the damage to the affected area, provision is made for the inflamed part to have *rest*. Limbs may be kept still by bandages or slings or splints. The same principle applies in inflammation of organs other than skin, bones and joints. In acute appendicitis (inflammation of the appendix), the intestines are rested. Diet is suspended, the intake confined to small amounts of fluids and no aperients or enemas are administered. When the kidney is grossly inflamed (acute nephritis) and no urine is passed, the patient's fluid intake is limited to 500 millilitres of water a day and protein is omitted from the diet. *As the tissue recovers* from infection new cells replace those which have been destroyed. The remains of the latter are removed through the lymph vessels and are disposed of in the lymph nodes before the lymph enters the bloodstream. When healing is rapid the new cells are the same as the original tissue and scarring is minimal. Where there is gross damage, dead tissue, foreign objects or persistent infection, the inflammatory reaction is prolonged and replacement is by inelastic fibrous tissue producing a well-marked scar.

When tissue dies the condition is known as *gangrene*. The area becomes greenish black, and finally separates from the healthy tissue. It is kept quite dry and clean. If it becomes infected then the surgeon considers its removal to prevent generalised infection in the body.

INFECTION is the entry of disease-producing micro-organisms into the body and the body's reaction to this.

Disease-producing micro-organisms are called pathogenic bacteria. They enter the body through a break in the skin, i.e. a wound, or through an opening (orifice) into the body, i.e. mouth, nose, urethra, vagina.

The local effects of infections are those of inflammation—redness, swelling, heat, pain and loss of function.

The general effects include a rise in body temperature (pyrexia). This may take place very rapidly to discourage the bacterial activity and is achieved by involuntary contraction of voluntary muscles. The patient feels cold and may shiver uncontrollably, his temperature rising in a few minutes to between 38°C to 40°C and then returning to normal by sweating. This is a *rigor*.

Taking the temperature every four hours in infection reveals irregular rises in temperature during the day. The pulse and respiration increase in rate. The skin is hot and dry and later becomes hot and moist. The patient complains of headache, thirst, loss of appetite, a dry mouth and he feels ill. He is constipated and passes less urine as sweating increases. At night he may become restless and confused or delirious.

On investigation the blood count will show an increase in white blood cells.

Classification of Bacteria

Bacteria can be identified by their appearance unders the microscope (Fig. 16). STAPHYLOCOCCI are spherical-shaped organisms in clusters. One type is found normally on the skin and is harmless but *staphylococcus aureus* causes infection of the hair follicles (boils), tissues (abscesses), bones (osteomyelitis) and wounds. Strict cleanliness and an aseptic technique are necessary to prevent the infection of wounds by these organisms. Several strains of staphylococci are now resistant to penicillin, which makes treatment of this infection difficult and is the reason why precautions to prevent infection are essential.

STREPTOCOCCI are spherical-shaped micro-organisms in chains. These do not produce such serious effects since the use of sulphonamides and penicillin, but cause tonsillitis and nephritis. Some children become hypersensitive to this organism and react by showing symptoms and signs of rheumatic fever. They are treated by continued administration of penicillin to prevent a further streptococcal infection. Heart valves damaged by rheumatic fever can become infected by streptococci and bacterial endocarditis then develops. *Pneumococci* can cause pneumonia, *meningococci* cause meningitis, and *gonococci* cause gonorrhoea.

BACILLI are rod-shaped micro-organisms. *Bacillus coli* is a micro-organism found in the bowel normally but it can cause disease when introduced into another part of the body, e.g. through the urethra into the bladder and kidneys. This is one reason for aseptic technique in urinary catheterisation. *Salmonellae bacilli* cause typhoid fever, and sometimes food poisoning. *Tubercle bacilli* cause tuberculosis and were difficult to destroy in the body before the discovery of drugs such as streptomycin.

CLOSTRIDIA are pathogenic bacteria which survive without air (oxygen) and are therefore found in soil and in the intestines of animals who eat soil with their food. In surroundings unsuitable for their growth and reproduction they change, forming spores which are resistant to ordinary methods of destroying bacteria.

One type of these organisms can cause gas gangrene, a serious infection of wounds.

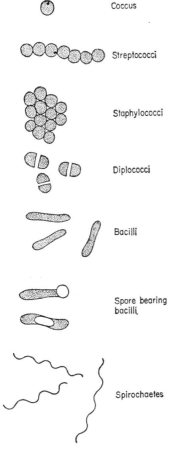

Coccus

Streptococci

Staphylococci

Diplococci

Bacilli

Spore bearing bacilli

Spirochaetes

Figure 16. Bacteria.

Another type causes tetanus (lockjaw). These infections may occur after the contamination of wounds by soil and are more commonly seen in country districts or after injuries which have taken place on playing fields.

Protection against tetanus is provided in Accident-Emergency Departments of hospitals immediately after the injury. Injections of tetanus toxoid and penicillin are prescribed and administered. The penicillin destroys any tetanus bacilli which may have entered the wound. The toxoid stimulates the body to produce anti-toxins against possible tetanus toxins. People whose occupation exposes them to injuries and in whom the resulting wounds are likely to become infected by soil, should be immunised against tetanus.

VIRUSES are extremely small and cannot be seen through an ordinary microscope but are visible through an electron microscope. They do not thrive until they enter young living cells for they require special substances (enzymes) within the cells for their existence. They cause a variety of diseases including several of the infectious fevers, e.g. chicken-pox, small-pox, measles, influenza, the common cold.

The Main Sources of Infection

Human beings are sources of infection when they are:

    (a) suffering from an acute attack of a particular infection with well-marked symptoms and signs (infections include food poisoning and septic wounds as well as the 'infectious fevers');

    (b) exposed to a mild attack with no obvious symptoms and signs, but bacteria are present in the body tissues, e.g. polio-myelitis, tuberculosis;

    (c) recovered from an acute attack but have retained the causative organism within the body, e.g. typhoid bacilli.

Both (b) and (c) would be 'carriers' and as such are dangerous to susceptible members of the community.

ANIMALS can be a source of infection unless strict regulations are enforced. The milk from a cow with tuberculosis can cause tuberculosis in human beings. Hides can transmit anthrax, an infectious disease, to man.

SOIL is the natural home of bacteria causing tetanus and gas gangrene and if soil is in contact with even minor wounds it may act as a source of infection.

The methods by which infection may be spread are by:

    1. direct contact with the infected person;

    2. contact with his secretions when speaking, coughing or sneezing (droplet infection);

3. excreta as in typhoid and dysentery.
4. discharges of mucus or pus.
The hands of those in contact with or attending to the patient can spread infection unless the appropriate routine and strict personal cleanliness are observed.

The Body's Defences Against Infection

Healthy Tissues and a Normal Body
Tissue damaged in injury or disease is likely to become infected. Malnutrition or starvation may predispose a person to infection. An inactive organ becomes infected more easily than a normal one, for example when the bladder cannot contract and urine remains in it for a period of time, infection of the bladder is a possibility.

White Cells in the Blood
The special white cells produced in the bone marrow but circulating in the blood are able to move out from the capillaries into the tissue spaces. There they surround and ingest the pathogenic bacteria which have invaded the tissue. Remains of tissue cells, white cells and bacteria are removed by absorption into the lymph vessels (Fig. 17). If the collection is too large for this method of removal, it becomes liquefied into a thick yellow fluid known as *pus*, which eventually escapes from the skin surface. If it is well below the skin surface, it may be removed by surgical incision and drainage. The discharge probably contains pathogenic bacteria and is therefore a potential danger where there are other wounds, so it is immediately burned.

A lack of white cells in the blood lowers the patient's resistance to infection. ANTIBODIES are protein substances in the blood plasma which act against pathogenic organisms and anti-toxins act against their toxins. There are different antibodies to deal with different organisms.

Immunity

Immunity is the resistance of the body to infection and depends largely on antibodies in the blood.

NATURAL IMMUNITY to some diseases is present at birth. This is inherited and because of it man is immune from many diseases of animals and birds.

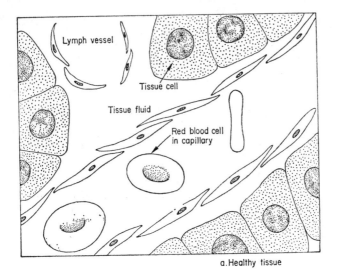

a. Healthy tissue

b. Infected tissue

Figure 17. Tissue in infection: diagram shows damaged cells and white cells ingesting bacteria and dead cells in the tissue spaces.

During life natural immunity is acquired as the result of:
(a) an acute attack of the disease, *or*
(b) minor attacks of the disease even though symptoms and signs are not evident, *or*
(c) being in contact with the disease.
The person produces his own antibodies against the disease and is able to resist infection which may occur later.
Examples: diphtheria, small-pox, measles.
This active immunity in which the person makes his own antibodies may also be acquired by artificial means. Bacilli can be treated chemically so that they are effective but safe and a solution of these injected. Toxoids can be prepared from the toxins of bacteria and used in the same way. This form of artificial immunity is difficult to procure in the virus infections, and in small-pox the fluid from a cow-pox lesion is applied to a minute wound in the skin to stimulate the body to produce antibodies against small-pox (cow-pox and small-pox are similar).
Examples of artificial immunisation: Diphtheria toxoid, small-pox vaccination, B.C.G. immunisation against tuberculosis.

PASSIVE IMMUNITY
The serum used to produce passive immunity is obtained from the blood of a horse which has previously been inoculated and developed an immunity. It is given to patients suspected of having an infectious disease which may have serious complications, e.g. tetanus. This immunity is of short duration but helps the patient until he can make his own antibodies in sufficient amounts to overcome the infection.

Prevention of Infection

Public Health Regulations
Port medical authorities in this country can prevent any person suspected of having a serious infection such as small-pox from entering the country until he and any contacts are clear of infection. Animals infected by serious disease or carrying fleas or lice are not allowed to leave the ship. Hides and furs are inspected and guarantees required regarding their source.

Local Authority Regulations
Medical practitioners who diagnose an infectious disease notify the Medical Officer of Health for the area. Isolation of the patient may be arranged either at home or at an infectious disease unit in a special or general hospital. Susceptible contacts are protected by immunisation.

Speedy diagnosis is important in prevention of spread. Pyrexia, skin rash and an abnormal discharge are suggestive of infection and if there is a history of contact with infection a provisional diagnosis may be made to enable the necessary measures to be undertaken without delay. Bacteriological examination of swabs of nose and throat, secretions or wounds may be necessary to confirm a diagnosis.

Prevention of spread of infection at home and in hospital is by these methods.

1. The maintenance of a high standard in:
   (a) personal cleanliness, including the avoidance of droplet infection;
   (b) domestic cleanliness using modern equipment and methods.
2. Prompt diagnosis of infectious conditions. The observation of correct techniques in the nursing of any patient thought to be infectious (isolation nursing).
3. The practice of aseptic technique in dressing wounds and in other surgical procedures.
4. The nursing of babies in cubicles while they are being treated in hospital so that infection from other patients is avoided.
5. The use of clothing and bed-linen which withstand frequent laundering and can be boiled, such as cotton cellular blankets.
6. Hygienic methods of storage, preparation, cooking and serving of food, and in dealing with crockery and utensils after meals.
7. Medical treatment of 'carriers'. If this treatment is not entirely effective the person may be barred from certain occupations. For instance, a carrier of organisms causing dysentery does not handle food.
8. The use of appropriate drugs such as antibiotics.
9. Immunisation when this is possible.

Infection can be avoided by preventing the methods by which transmission takes place.

DROPLET INFECTION. The micro-organisms in the nose and throat are coughed, sneezed or breathed into the air. Correct behaviour is an asset; a handkerchief is used during coughing or sneezing, and the head is turned away from any other person in the vicinity. The nurse does not talk while dressing an open wound, and a mask over the nose and mouth is an added precaution to prevent droplet infection of wounds or sterile equipment.

DUST is removed from all surfaces of furniture and equipment by damp-dusting, a method of cleaning in which the cloth is wrung out in water or an antiseptic in an oil base, so that the dust sticks to it easily. A disposable cloth with a small amount of liquid polish may be used, but it is preferable for this to be destroyed after cleaning. Damp dusters are washed and boiled daily otherwise these articles become vehicles for the spread of infection.

Dust is removed from floors by vacuum cleaners to prevent it being circulated through the air of the ward. In a hospital general cleaning is carried out each day with more extensive cleaning like thorough cleaning of ward floors, lights and wall ledges each week. The ward and its equipment has an intensive cleaning programme once a year. A high standard of domestic cleanliness is an important aid to prevention of infection in any situation, but becomes of great value in a hospital when patients may be possible sources of infection. In departments where infection is a real danger (such as a Burns Unit or operating theatre), ventilation may be by artificial means, and the air is filtered to remove dust as it is drawn into the room or department.

To reduce the amount of dust in hospital wards, wool blankets have been exchanged for the cotton cellular type which produce no fluff in bed-making and which can be boiled frequently.

FOOD is prepared and served by personnel who are healthy and have no infections such as sore throats and boils. Utensils for cooking, transport and service are cleaned after each time of use. The foodstuffs are fresh and wholesome, waste food is not used for human consumption and infected food is burned. Ward refrigerators keep milk and perishable foods cool and fresh. Food should be covered to prevent dust, droplet infection and insects from contaminating it.

Cleanliness of crockery and cutlery is essential, and is ensured by careful washing in a detergent and hot water, then rinsing in hot water, followed by drying in a rack round which air circulates. When dry, they are stored in a clean, dry cupboard. Dish-cloths and mops need to be boiled or disinfected after every usage, and tea-towels also if these are used. Washing-up machines are an advantage providing no food has been allowed to congeal on the dishes and utensils. Infectious patients use disposable dishes and cutlery.

PERSONAL CLOTHING is washed, sometimes boiled, then ironed. All these procedures destroy most pathogenic organisms.

BED-LINEN, including cotton cellular blankets, is washed and boiled, then ironed or dried by heat.

Infected personal and bed-linen is dealt with in a special way, e.g.:
1. Collected directly into a polythene bag which is sealed and placed in a coloured, e.g. red nylon, bag for transport to the laundry.
2. Disinfected in the ward before being transported to the laundry, e.g. in a galvanised-iron bin containing Izal 1 in 300 for 12 hours.

Care is taken *not* to contaminate the outside of bins or bags and these are clearly labelled INFECTIOUS to avoid any risk to transporting personnel.

MATTRESSES AND PILLOWS are protected from contamination by plastic covers which can be washed with disinfectant or are disposable. Otherwise the mattresses and pillows are autoclaved.

TOILET ARTICLES are carefully cleaned, then either boiled, autoclaved, disinfected in chemical solutions or destroyed. In the interests of personal hygiene, toilet articles are best reserved for each individual and these include flannels, towels, soap, combs and linen. In hospital this is most important and the nurse avoids any possibility of soap, hair-brushes, towels and bath-mat being used by more than one patient.

Special measures are taken with the patient's *personal property* when he is infectious or has died. Then any disposable article is placed in a strong paper bag at the bed-side and burned in the incinerator or furnace. Articles of value are autoclaved or disinfected. When advice is needed regarding a suitable method this is sought from the ward sister or a member of the staff responsible for the autoclaves or other methods of disinfection. Materials like leather and rubber cannot be autoclaved at maximum heat.

When a single ward or room in a private house has been used in the treatment of an infectious patient, the whole of the contents together with walls and floors can be disinfected by fumigation with formaldehyde gas. The windows are sealed with adhesive paper tape and the equipment spread out round the room for easy circulation of the gas.

The vapour is produced by heated tablets in the room, and when the apparatus is prepared the door is closed and sealed. After twenty-four hours, the paper seals are removed, and the room well ventilated as the vapour is unpleasant. Then the walls, floor and equipment are washed and the linen sent to the laundry.

EXCRETA is ordinarily disposed of by emptying into the bed-pan washer or toilet, and from there it is flushed by the water carriage system into the sewerage system which is an efficient method of disposal on a large scale. It may be considered necessary as in cases of enteric (typhoid and paratyphoid) fever to treat faeces and urine with a strong disinfectant like white fluid 1 in 10 for twelve hours, after which the contents are discharged into a bed-pan washer or toilet.

Bed-pans and urinals after ordinary use are washed thoroughly by a hot-water spray in the bed-pan washer (cold water for glass urinals), or with a mop and disinfectant (white fluid 1 in 10), and rinsed. Sterilisation is by means of boiling for five minutes, or subjecting them to super-heated steam in a bed-pan steriliser. In some hospitals disposable bed-pans and urinals are used. Covers for these sanitary utensils are quickly infected and can prove a method of spread of infection; it is therefore an advantage to use disposable paper covers for bed-pans and these are discarded into the bed-pan washer. Commodes and toilets are more widely used as patients are ambulant as soon as possible during treatment, and the cleanliness of these is as important as that of the receptacle used by the patient when he is confined to bed.

DISCHARGES. Those from the nose and mouth are collected on medical wipes or paper handkerchiefs and placed at once into a covered container or strong paper bag which will be burned during the day. Sputum is expectorated into waxed cardboard containers with screw lids and these are collected once or twice a day and burned.

Vomit is disposed of in the same way as urine and faeces.

Discharges from wounds and orifices are collected on gauze or wool dressings. On removal from the discharging area these are placed in a strong paper bag which is closed and then burned.

Equipment contaminated by discharges is disinfected or destroyed, the latter being considered preferable.

DRESSINGS which have been applied to the skin are destroyed by incineration. Where possible, bandages are also destroyed by incineration. Crepe pressure bandages are expensive and it may be considered necessary to wash and boil these; the elasticity is decreased but sometimes remains sufficient for a firm bandage. Domette many-tailed bandages, calico and cotton roller bandages are washed and boiled in the laundry. These bandages, when contaminated with pus, blood or serum, are burned. Adequate wool dressings frequently replaced will avoid staining of the bandage.

DRESSING TOWELS are dealt with as infectious linen. The disposable type are burned after use with the soiled dressings.

INSTRUMENTS are disinfected after every use as these are most likely to become infected during the dressing of wounds and in other procedures. They are dropped immediately after use into a receptacle containing water or an antiseptic. At the end of the ward dressings session, the pail is removed to the instrument cleaning sink where the instruments are washed in detergent, and the hinges, crevices and serrated edges are cleaned with a brush. The person cleaning the instruments wears gloves. The instruments are rinsed, dried, packed and autoclaved. If an autoclave is not available they are boiled for 5 minutes but this method is not entirely satisfactory. Some instruments are disposable Intricate equipment needs special care in cleaning and sterilisation.

Each part of a SYRINGE is washed and cleaned with an appropriate brush, then sterilised in a water steriliser. Alternatively the parts are reassembled and the syringe sterilised in an autoclave, infra-red cabinet or hot-air oven. Most syringes and needles now are disposable.

G

For method of disposal see page 165.

Special needles are syringed through to clean them, washed in detergent, rinsed well, dried, points sharpened if necessary. The stilettes are cleaned and replaced. The complete needles are then packed and sterilised.

HANDS. The patient washes his hands at least twice a day, also after going to the toilet or using a bed-pan. He avoids contact with any wound discharges or dressings on his wounds.

In addition to ordinary personal cleanliness of the hands and keeping the skin healthy and free from cracks, abrasions, pricks and minor infections, a nurse washes her hands after any procedure in which the hands may become contaminated, such as emptying bed-pans or giving an enema. She washes her hands before a clean procedure like preparing food and feeding the patient, and before performing aseptic procedures such as giving an injection or changing the dressing over a wound. When complete asepsis of the hands is required as in assisting at an operation, sterile gloves are worn. If the hands might come into contact with highly infectious material, then rubber gloves are worn to prevent heavy contamination of the hands, the skin of which cannot be cleaned and disinfected in the same way as equipment.

It is because of the impossibility of ensuring that the skin is free from pathogenic bacteria that the nurse is expected *not* to allow the hands to become contaminated by infectious material but to use forceps in handling it, and if these are unpractical, disposable plastic gloves.

During isolation of an infectious patient, the nurse prevents her uniform from becoming infected by wearing a cotton gown which covers it completely.

Aseptic Technique

Aseptic technique is a method of procedure by which sepsis is avoided. The purpose of aseptic technique is the prevention of infection during:
  (a) surgical operation;
  (b) dressing wounds;
  (c) techniques involving a puncture in the skin, e.g. injections;
  (d) introduction of equipment into parts of the body which are easily infected, e.g. catheterisation of the urinary bladder and suction to clear a tracheostomy tube.
In preparation for aseptic technique, bacteria present on instruments are destroyed by the application of heat or chemical agents. The articles are then said to be sterile.

Methods of Sterilisation

BOILING WATER, which is moist heat, can be used. Clean instruments, bowls, receivers, syringes and needles, are boiled in a water steriliser, the temperature of the water being 100°C. This will destroy many bacteria in a few seconds, and all of them in five minutes except spore-bearing bacilli (the anaerobic bacilli which cause tetanus and gas-gangrene). These organisms are unlikely in a hospital ward where equipment is clean and free from dirt and soil. The articles should be separated from each other and sharp blades or points protected by sponge rubber. These are immersed in the water in the steriliser and boiled for five minutes. Timing is by a 'pinger' as used in a kitchen for cooking, or a five-minute sand-timer. A card which states 'Sterilisation in progress' may be useful to ensure no further articles are placed in the steriliser before the present session is complete. The nurse, wearing a mask, removes the equipment from the steriliser with large forceps. The instruments and syringes are placed in sterile dishes covered by sterile lids to prevent contamination between the steriliser and the bed-side where the aseptic technique is to be performed.

STEAM UNDER PRESSURE. The temperature of *steam* can be raised above boiling point by confining it within a space under pressure. The sterilising machine in which this is done is an *autoclave* and consists of an inner chamber with an outer chamber or jacket. The articles are packed loosely into unsealed drums, or special bags which allow steam to flow in and out of them but through which bacteria cannot pass from outside. The drums and packages are placed in the inner chamber and the steam-tight doors are closed. The air is withdrawn from the chambers and then steam passes through the outer jacket into the inner chamber. This takes about fifteen minutes. As the autoclave doors are tightly closed and steam continues to enter, the pressure of steam rises and at the same time its temperature rises. At the required pressure, e.g. 15 lb per square inch, and temperature, 120°C, the steam is turned off and the pressure and temperature are continued for thirty minutes. Then the steam is driven off to be replaced by dry filtered air which dries the articles in about twenty minutes. By that time the drums are still hot but can be taken out. They are sealed and dated as they are removed. The tight packing of drums prevents adequate circulation of heated steam through them, and damp articles after autoclaving soon become unsterile. A test is made by the bacteriological laboratory staff from one drum or package in every sterilising session, and temperature and pressure charts on the auto-clave indicate the degree of heat to which the articles have been subjected.

High-pressure autoclaves are used in large sterilising units for linen, instruments and dressing packs, the pressure being 32 lb per square inch, temperature 135°C, for 4½ minutes. The advantage of these is that several sterilising sessions can take place on one day.

Packets sterilised in a Central Sterile Supply Department are sealed with a tape which changes colour during an efficient sterilising process, e.g. pink to brown. Should a nurse find a packet sealed with a tape which has not changed colour she should not use the packet but return it to the department or the C.S.S.D. staff visiting the ward.

Low-pressure autoclaves are useful for delicate rubber goods and some glassware (17 lb per square inch at 120°C, for 14 minutes).

DRY HEAT is not as efficient as moist heat for sterilising articles, but glass and metal instruments like syringes are placed in a *dry oven* heated by electricity to 160°C for one hour. Rubber and plastics are unsuitable for exposure to such a high temperature. It is a lengthy procedure but useful where syringes and needles are in frequent use and an autoclave is not available.

INFRA-RED CABINETS are used for sterilisation of syringes. A cabinet is built like a small tunnel with batteries of heaters in the roof, the syringes passing through the tunnel on a steel mesh conveyor belt at 200°C for 18 minutes. As this heat is 'penetrating' it is possible to seal syringes in their container *before* sterilisation. This equipment is large and expensive but it is very suitable in a Central Sterile Supply Department.

ANTISEPTICS are not satisfactory as a general method of sterilisation, for individual solutions have varying effects on different bacteria. Strong antiseptics are harmful to the skin and if used to sterilise an article, this should be well rinsed with boiling water before being used. A considerable length of time is required for exposure of an article to the *weak* solution of an antiseptic.

Instructions regarding the sterilisation and disinfection of articles in a hospital are usually issued from the Nursing Procedure Committee after consultation with the Prevention of Infection Committee, which includes a bacteriologist. Each nurse carries out the instructions carefully, and the measurement of lotions must be accurate.

Examples of Methods used in the Sterilisation of:

Syringes and needles. Infra-red cabinet, hot-air oven, autoclave, or boiling in a receiver for five minutes after dismantling the syringe. Needle points are protected by their stilettes or small squares of lint or sponge rubber.

Instruments and surgical equipment. Autoclave or boiling for five minutes. Cheatle's forceps for handling sterile equipment are stored in white disinfectant, e.g. Izal 1 in 320.

Plastic equipment varies. Polyvinyl can be boiled and autoclaved. If in doubt when sterilising unfamiliar equipment the Instrument Curator or Supplies Officer is consulted unless directions have been included with the equipment.

Rubber equipment. Tubing is cleaned immediately after use by syringing through with cold water, hydrogen peroxide 5 volume or cetrimide solution 1%. Autoclaving or boiling.

Clinical or lotion thermometers. Chlorhexidine solution 0·5% in water.

Infant feeding bottles and teats. Bottles can be autoclaved. Both are suitable for boiling for five minutes or immersion in sodium hypochlorite solution 1% (Milton) 1 in 80 dilution for two hours.

Skin Antiseptics

Cleaning the skin:
    Savlon 1%.
    Cetrimide 0·5%.

Before operation or injection:
    Tincture of Iodine 2·5%.
    70% industrial methylated spirit.
    Tincture of chlorhexidine (hibitaine) 0·5% in 70% industrial methylated spirit.

The Main Points in an Aseptic Technique for Dressing Wounds

A. Ventilation in the ward is reduced to a minimum and no ward cleaning is in progress. By these means dust is prevented from circulating in the air.

B. Nurses wear clean aprons or overalls and caps which preferably cover the hair. To prevent droplet infection of the wound or equipment or dressings the nurses either do not speak during the dressing or they wear masks.

C. The dressing trolley is thoroughly clean and no soiled article is allowed to contaminate it or the equipment it carries. The nurse does not handle any article, such as lotion bottles, on this trolley unless her hands are clean.

D. The dresser washes and dries her hands before she uses sterile instruments. She picks up these by the handles so that the blades remain sterile. Her hands do not touch the wound. If this cannot be avoided she wears sterile gloves.

E. Dressings and equipment which come in contact with the wound are sterile when they touch the wound. Dressings are handled by sterile forceps.

F. Used instruments and equipment are placed at once in a bin containing water or an antiseptic or in a paper bag. Soiled dressings are discarded into a thick paper bag which can be sealed. Later the instruments and equipment are washed in detergent, scrubbed if necessary, then sterilised and dried before being stored or repacked. Bags of soiled dressings will be burned. Unused dressings are collected in a clean bag as salvage.

G. The nurse washes her hands after making the patient comfortable, and her assistant washes her hands after cleaning the dressing trolley.

The technique is repeated for each individual wound, even though more wounds than one are being treated in the same patient.

Disposable Equipment

Use of this type of article in hospital reduces laundry costs and saves time which would otherwise be spent in cleaning and sterilising. These goods are not inexpensive, and the nurse needs to exercise care in ordering only the amount required and to avoid the unnecessary opening of packages and exposure of their contents. In homes where facilities for preparing equipment are inadequate or unsuitable, general practitioners and domiciliary nurses and midwives find disposable and pre-sterilised equipment an asset.

There has been an increase in penicillin-resistant staphylococcal infection in hospital wards and the disposal of articles immediately after use assists in preventing infection. Dressings and inexpensive cotton bandages have always been destroyed after contamination by discharge from a wound, but industrial firms have now developed and enlarged the range of goods which can be disposed of after use.

EXAMPLES

Paper hand towels lessen spread of infection and cost is offset by reduction in laundry expenses.

Paper masks are efficient for one and a half hours. When damp they are no longer of any value.

Disposable *theatre caps* are thin paper gathered on to an elastic band and *uniform caps* are made in a traditional pattern.

Rubber gloves are now obtainable in sterile packs for use in special aseptic ward techniques and the operating theatre.

Thin loose *rubber gloves* are used for the examination of patients, and also when attending to an incontinent patient.

Bed-pans and urinals of a compressed paper material can be disposed of after use in a special destructor cabinet.

Some *disposable instruments* have been devised, e.g. suture removers, instrument forceps, also razors.

Paper dressing towels. These can be water-repellent for use in protecting bed linen in major dressings and irrigations, and to cover a dressing trolley prepared for a ward dressing. Others are absorbent.

Gauze and wool swabs. Cotton wool rolls and absorbent paper pads are purchased ready cut and folded.

Paper handkerchiefs or medical wipes remove secretion and discharges and have replaced cotton handkerchiefs and swabs of gauze wool or lint.

Tube gauze bandages and Netalast bandages are easily and quickly applied and efficient. They are discarded after use.

Wooden applicators and tongue depressors are alternatives to the metal varieties and forceps.

Plastic oxygen masks and *nasal catheters* are light in weight and easy to wear and use, efficient and reasonably inexpensive.

Plastic drainage bags which hang at the side of the bed assist in preventing infection in bladder drainage.

Pre-sterilised disposable equipment is purchased from industrial firms and received in sealed paper or paper bags which are barriers against bacterial infection.

Gauze *dressings*, wool or paper absorbent pads, paper dressing towels, metal foil gallipots and compressed paper trays are packed singly or in combination, e.g. dressing pack.

Syringes made from polystyrene in various grades, propane or polypropane are sterilised in transparent bacteria-barrier packets.

Injection needles are packed separately in transparent containers. The patient is assured of a *sharp* needle by this method.

Plastic catheters and tubes such as intra-gastric feeding tubes are pre-sterilised, and after use are discarded.

Blood transfusion and intravenous therapy equipment is pre-sterilised and disposable.

Major equipment such as the cannulae in cardio-pulmonary by-pass for open-heart operations and dialysis coils in artificial kidney treatment are prepared and sterilised by the industrial firm which produces them.

Pre-sterilised mucus extractors consisting of a plastic tube which can be inserted into the pharynx of a newly born infant and a transparent plastic vessel into which the mucus can be collected together with another plastic tube placed in the midwife's or nurse's own mouth for gentle suction to be applied.

STORAGE OF EQUIPMENT STERILISED BEFORE ITS ARRIVAL IN THE WARD
Packages are transported in strong boxes on a trolley reserved for this purpose. In the ward they are stored in cabinets, preferably in a small room reserved for these. The room may also contain the dressing and

injections trolleys, bottles of lotions, etc. The equipment is used in rotation and most packets and tubes are stamped with the date, or a coloured disc shows the time after which the article should not be used. Orders are made each day or there is a regular basic issue, and no permanent stocks are retained in the ward.

Damage to plastic or paper cases is prevented by orderly arrangement in compartments and they are inspected for flaws immediately prior to use. Any article out of date or package thought to be unsatisfactory is returned to the Superintendent of the c.s.s.d., or the Instrument Curator or Supplies Officer.

The nurses's hands are clean when she handles the packages and these are not opened except at the bed-side.

COLLECTION OF DISPOSABLE EQUIPMENT is into covered bins or thin plastic bags supported in a carrier or in strong paper bags. Metal staples, elastic bands or adhesive paper strips are used to seal the bags immediately after they are three-quarters filled. Needles, suture removers, scalpel blades can penetrate a thin material and cause injury, therefore it may be wise to collect these separately in a thick paper bag or box or carton. As the bags are destroyed without inspection it is important that the nurse should not include any *non-disposable* equipment in these bags, boxes or cartons.

DISPOSAL OF DISPOSABLE EQUIPMENT is by the ward incinerator, the hospital incinerator or the town or city refuse department. Dressings and paper burn easily, but metal foil melts and either this or a mass of injection needles can block a small ward incinerator. Plastic materials also melt and are unsuitable for ordinary incineration.

There should be no possibility of disposable equipment being removed from the collection bag between its use in procedure and its disposal; this could be dangerous when the articles are infected by antibiotic-resistant organisms.

Isolation Nursing

When the patient has an infectious condition which may be transmitted to other people he is isolated until risk of infection has disappeared. Depending on the type of infection and the number of people affected, isolation is arranged in:

    (i) Infectious Diseases hospital.
    (ii) One ward of a general hospital into which a number of patients with the same disease are admitted.
    (iii) Side ward with one bed.
    (iv) Cubicle as in children's admission unit.

(v) Bed in a general ward.

As infectious fevers like diphtheria, whooping cough and scarlet fever are less common, most infectious fever hospitals are now General Hospitals with some wards reserved for patients in the town or city who develop complications of an infectious disease like measles, or conditions such as severe gastroenteritis, enteric fever, poliomyelitis, or influenzal pneumonia. Some wards are reserved for patients with pulmonary tuberculosis, though the need for beds is less than ten years ago.

Principles of isolation nursing are similar in different situations, but some details follow concerning the nursing of an infectious patient in a side ward or in the general main ward.

ISOLATION NURSING IN A SIDE WARD (Fig. 18)
The room is ventilated by opening the windows, but the door is kept closed and on it is a notice to say that visitors are not allowed to enter without permission from sister or the charge nurse.

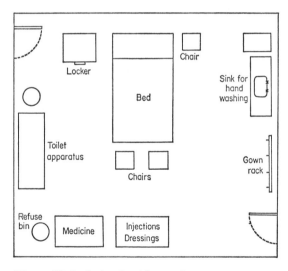

Figure 18. Isolation in side ward

All equipment for nursing the patient is kept within the room, and any article leaving the area is disinfected.

Nurses entering the room cover their uniform with a cotton gown which fastens at the back. If this becomes soiled by discharges it is changed immediately. A red band or other mark identifies the outside of the gown, which is the contaminated surface. Gowns are reserved for one patient only. After attending to the patient the nurse washes and dries her

G*

hands and unties the gown tapes. Then she slides a coat hanger into the gown and hangs it on a hook with the outside (red band) outside. She now washes and dries her hands and is able to attend to another patient. If the patient has droplet infection (pneumonia, tuberculosis, meningitis), the nurse wears a mask. Disposable towels and masks are convenient. Contamination of door handles is prevented by washing the hands before opening the doors. Wash basins are equipped with elbow taps, otherwise they are turned on by covering them with a piece of dry paper over which the hand is placed. Permanent charts and papers are kept outside the room, and at the bedside are temporary charts, etc., completed in pencil so that the patient's records and nurses' pens are not contaminated. The room is cleaned by the nurses and the necessary equipment is reserved within the room. For damp-dusting, disposable cloths are used and the floor is mopped with white fluid 1 in 600 morning and evening. Twice a day clean linen and stock are taken into the room. Disposable articles are useful.

Food is served on disposable paper or plastic plates and transferred at the door to the patient's own tray. The plates with any waste food are placed in a strong paper bag which will be burnt. Disposable plastic cutlery of an inexpensive type is also available.

Used linen is sealed in a bag to be transported to the laundry. Medical and surgical equipment is disinfected before being used elsewhere in the ward.

At the end of the period of isolation it may be considered advisable to destroy a number of personal articles when these are difficult to sterilise. For this reason unnecessary and valuable property is not usually brought into the ward. Visitors may be unfamiliar with the routine of wearing gowns and perhaps masks, and when they spend some time with the patient the procedure and the reasons for it are explained to them before they are assisted with the protective clothing. They are warned not to sit too close to the bed and the patient, and the visit is limited to about ten minutes. Only a few close relatives or friends are permitted to visit.

The isolated patient is at first likely to be very ill and he appreciates the quiet and privacy of a side ward but there should be means by which he can contact the nurse if she does not remain in the room. As he begins to recover, he may find the seclusion very lonely when there are no other patients and few visitors. Treatment and nursing care can be spread over the day so that he receives some attention at frequent intervals, such as each hour or half hour. Inexpensive books and newspapers can be provided, and later these can be burned. When he writes letters it may be possible for these to be disinfected before being posted, e.g. by an infra-red cabinet.

When the patient is pronounced free of infection by the doctor, he is bathed and his hair washed. Clean clothing is provided, and when dressed he lies on a clean sheet, and is lifted onto a clean bed, by which he returns to the general ward. The side ward with its furniture and general equipment is sealed by adhesive paper tape and formaldehyde vapour released within it. After twenty-four hours the tape is removed, and the room and its contents are cleaned.

BED ISOLATION IN A GENERAL MAIN WARD
This was known as 'barrier nursing' when a chalk mark on the floor indicated the extent of the isolated area (Fig. 19).

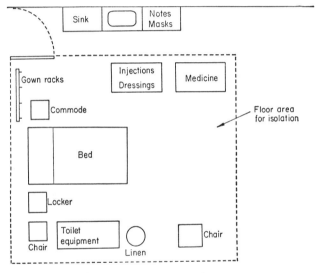

Figure 19. Isolation in general ward

The disease for which this patient is being treated is *not* spread by droplet infection, otherwise he would be isolated in a side ward or infectious diseases unit.

The principles are the same as those employed in side-ward isolation. Nurses attend to other patients in the ward, but put on gowns when they attend to this patient, remove them as they leave the bed-side, and wash their hands before attending to other duties in the general ward. No article used elsewhere in the ward is allowed inside the isolation area, and as far as possible the patient's equipment is retained inside the area.

A nurse serves him with his meals, receiving them from a tray outside the area. Soiled linen is received at the bedside into a polythene bag.

This is sealed with a rubber band and placed in a strong nylon bag (un-contaminated on the outside) for transport to the laundry. It is important to gather up the used linen carefully so that it does not touch the floor, the nurse's gown or the outside of the bag. If the bag is filled too full it will burst open and cause an infection hazard.

Faeces and urine are disinfected as previously described in prevention of infection, and the sanitary equipment is disinfected. Other patients are re-quested not to visit the isolated patient but there is no reason why they should not converse from an adjacent bed. There is no need to place screens permanently round the bed unless it is necessary to remind people visiting the ward as well as those working in it that the patient is isolated. Screens or curtains become contaminated and are drawn round so that one surface is always on the inside. They are washed daily or sprayed with an antiseptic like chlorhexidine. The floor in the area is mopped twice daily with disinfectant and care is taken not to place furniture etc. against the wall.

During isolation the patient's treatment and nursing care continue as at any other time. Should recovery not take place, thorough disinfection procedure is undertaken and articles which cannot be disinfected ade-quately are destroyed.

Similar methods are used in an ambulance, casualty station or operating theatre where an infectious patient has been treated.

Public Health Department Officials supervise fumigation in the patient's home when this is necessary, and Health Visitors advise rela-tives of people with chronic infections on methods of prevention in spread of disease.

Communicable Diseases

MEASLES is caused by a virus and is spread by droplet infection. It is common among children and begins, following an incubation period of ten to eighteen days, with a respiratory catarrh like a common cold and then white spots appear inside the mouth and a brownish rash on face and trunk. The illness itself is not severe but complications such as broncho-pneumonia, and otitis media, can be serious. A second attack is uncommon, as immunity is long lasting.

GERMAN MEASLES or RUBELLA is also caused by a virus and is *not* a serious disease but during early pregnancy the virus can damage the foetus and be the cause of congenital defects, such as deafness, cataract and congenital heart conditions. Serum from a convalescent patient can be given to a pregnant woman exposed to infection. Immunisation is be-ing offered to girls of 13 years of age through the School Medical Service.

WHOOPING COUGH or PERTUSSIS occurs usually in the first three years of life and is serious in infants and small children who have not been immunised. The causative organism behaves like a virus and is spread by droplet infection. After an incubation period of about seven to fourteen days, a respiratory catarrh develops followed by paroxysms of coughing. Several short coughs terminate in a 'whoop' as the throat contracts. The patient usually vomits and easily becomes exhausted, though recovery from the attack is rapid. Nutrition suffers as a result of the vomiting. The complication of broncho-pneumonia is serious. The disease is prevented by the immunisation of infants.

DIPHTHERIA is a disease which can occur at any age, but due to immunisation the disease should not be common today. It is caused by the diphtheria bacillus, an organism which attacks mucous membrane in the throat, forming a thick, white 'false membrane' which can obstruct the air passage in an infant. The poisons from the organism may affect nervous tissue, causing paralysis of soft palate, throat or eye-muscles and the heart muscle may be affected, causing cardiac failure. The incubation period is short and the disease is spread by droplet infection.

MUMPS is caused by a virus which produces a general acute infection and the salivary glands enlarge, so that the patient has difficulty in opening the mouth. In a few male patients the testes are affected by the virus and this complication is treated. The incubation period is three weeks. There are no carriers.

CHICKEN-POX occurs at any age but usually under ten years. The cause is a virus and the incubation period is ten days. The rash is mainly on the trunk and is seen in all its stages at the same time, i.e. red spots, blisters and scabs. Complications are rare. Adults in contact with chickenpox occasionally develop Shingles (Herpes Zoster) in which a painful rash appears on the body or face. The skin is painful and tender for some time after the rash disappears.

SMALL-POX affects cattle and human beings. The cause is a virus and it is the most serious of all infectious diseases. It is spread by contact with the patient or any article which has been in contact with him. The incubation period is ten to fourteen days and the patient is extremely ill with a rash mainly on the face and limbs. Small red spots appear on the fourth day of illness; these become blisters on the seventh day, pustules on the eleventh day and are scabs by the fifteenth day firmly adherent to the skin. Serious complications include broncho-pneumonia and cardiac failure. When the scabs separate from the skin, scars may remain. There are regulations in this country which prevent a person suspected of having the disease from landing after arrival by ship or plane until he has been examined by a medical practitioner. Vaccination by cow-pox serum is available for every citizen, beginning at six months of age, through the general practitioner service or child welfare clinics. The immunity becomes less effective after a few years and revaccination, particularly for those who may be exposed to infection, including hospital staffs and people travelling abroad, should be considered every three years. All people who have been in contact with a suspected case of small-pox are vaccinated at once. The patient is nursed in strict isolation and the nurses caring for him volunteer to remain in isolation until he has recovered.

SCARLET FEVER is caused by the haemolytic streptococcus, and the incubation period is short—two days. Infection by this organism is less serious now. Sulphonamides and penicillin are effective in the treatment. Carriers can be a problem and the organism causes a number of diseases amongst which are otitis media, acute tonsilitis, puerperal fever, and erysipelas, which is an infection of the skin. Signs of scarlet fever are an acute sore throat with a bright flushed skin with myriads of tiny points of deeper red. The illness is short but complications may occur and these include nephritis, endocarditis and rheumatic fever.

The ENTERIC GROUP of fevers are caused by typhoid and paratyphoid bacilli. The organisms are excreted by the patient in the stools and can survive in sewage and contaminated water. These diseases may be spread by carriers who contaminate food and water. In untreated cases fever may be pronounced and the patient can be very ill with delirium and sometimes lapses into coma. The small intestine is inflamed and ulcers may form. Pneumonia, haemorrhage from or perforation of the bowel are possible complications. The diet is important in preventing the latter conditions and consists of food containing no roughage and of high nutritional value, with a concentrated food such as Complan in order not to irritate the inflamed intestine. Convalescence is necessary as the patient is very weak. These diseases are prevented by a high level of personal hygiene, efficient methods of sanitation and treatment of known carriers. In areas where contaminated water is a possibility, the water is boiled or treated with chlorine on a large scale. Potassium permanganate is added when amounts of water are small. Bottled water from elsewhere may be procured for drinking. Fruit and salad vegetables are washed before eating raw.

Immunisation is available for people who intend to travel in countries where satisfactory methods of sanitation are not available. Dysentery and salmonellae food poisoning are other infectious diseases of the gastro-intestinal tract causing acute attacks of vomiting and diarrhoea.

POLIOMYELITIS affects any age and is caused by a virus spread by droplet infection. The disease varies in form from a short acute feverish illness to one in which groups of voluntary muscles are paralysed, causing permanent disability. When the diaphragm is affected, the patient's respiratory function is continued by an artificial respiration machine. The disease is prevented by immunisation.

EPIDEMIC INFLUENZA is caused by a virus and the disease varies in symptoms from time to time. The respiratory form is serious, leading to pneumonia within a very short time. A vaccine is available.

TUBERCULOSIS is caused by the tubercle bacilli and can affect most body tissues. The bacteria are breathed in or taken in through the mouth. There is a bovine type of tuberculosis, and drinking milk from an infected cow can cause disease in humans, resulting in bone and joint disease or peritonitis. For this reason tubercular cows are removed from herds and milk is heat-treated (pasteurisation).

Inhalation of tubercle bacilli causes pulmonary (lung) tuberculosis. Many people have a very slight attack when they are young with no symptoms and they form antibodies against the bacteria.

Complications for which the patient may seek medical advice before the disease is recognised are pleurisy (pain in the chest on breathing), pleural effusion (collection of fluid in the pleural cavity) or haemoptysis (coughing up of blood).

In more severe infections lung tissue is destroyed leaving a cavity in which pus collects. This contains tubercle bacilli and is discharged from the lung during coughing and expectoration. The sputum is infectious and disposal is preferably by collection in a waxed container with a screw lid which is then burned.

Unfortunately the disease becomes chronic and when not sufficiently severe to demand medical treatment causes continuous ill-health in the patient and spread of infection to others. This latter may occur particularly when coughing and expectoration in older patients are already present due to chronic bronchitis or broncho-pneumonia.

Treatment is mainly by drugs—streptomycin, sodium aminosalicylate (P.A.S.) and isoniazid. These are the 'first-line' drugs. 'Second-line' drugs are available. A vaccine affords protection against tuberculosis in the susceptible individual.

SYPHILIS is a communicable disease caused by a spiral-shaped organism which is transmitted during sexual intercourse, and because of this the infection is referred to as a *venereal disease*. Following an incubation period of 3 to 4 weeks, a small ulcer forms at the site of infection, the penis in the male and the vulva in the female, which eventually heals. The ulcer is infectious. A few months later there is a rash and fever. Infection of another person can occur in this stage. The symptoms eventually disappear and the patient may think he has recovered. The organisms remain inactive in the body tissues until some years later when they cause a disease which is localised as chronic inflammation in the skin or the central nervous system and the cranial nerves. At this time the patient is not infectious.

The syphilitic organism can also be transmitted from an infected mother to the foetus and the child will be born with *congenital syphilis*.

Treatment is by penicillin, which is effective. It is possible for a patient, however, to become reinfected and treatment may be prolonged because of this. Hospital treatment is rarely necessary and most of this work is accomplished in clinics.

Prevention of syphilis is attempted by a social medicine programme which includes:

1. Convenient and confidential facilities for speedy investigation and treatment which are offered to any person who suspects he or she has been infected.

2. Tracing of contacts and encouraging them to attend for treatment.

3. Health education emphasising that to prevent infection it is necessary to avoid sexual intercourse with any person known to be or likely to be infected.

GONORRHOEA is caused by gonococci. It is usually transmitted during sexual intercourse and is therefore classed as a venereal disease. The infection produces inflammatory reactions throughout the reproductive tract in either sex and a purulent discharge is produced which is highly infectious.

Treatment by penicillin is effective in most cases but the organism appears to be showing signs of becoming penicillin resistant. The number of young people with this communicable disease has risen during the last few years. The programme for prevention is similar to that which combats syphilis.

TRICHOMONAS is caused by a microscopic parasite which can invade the reproductive tract in both sexes. It is transmitted during sexual intercourse and also by infected towels etc. Although the disease itself does not have widespread effects in the body, it causes an irritating discharge and, consequently, a degree of discomfort. Treatment is by Flagyl, an oral drug.

Nursing Care of the Feverish Patient

Fever is the term given to the general reaction of the patient to infection. Fever causes the patient to feel ill, but in spite of its discomfort it is a normal defence process in the body and indicates that the patient is resisting the disease to the best of his ability. Bacteria pathogenic to man prefer, for complete activity and reproduction, an environment of 37°C (98·4°F). It may be to discourage their habitation that the body raises its own temperature to between 38°C to 40°C (101°F to 105°F) in an acute infection by involuntary contraction of voluntary muscle, which can be sufficiently severe to cause the teeth to chatter and the bed to shake. This is a *rigor* and the temperature rises quickly.

As the patient improves the fever lessens. When the temperature is normal convalescence begins, providing other signs also indicate recovery. At the present time infection is much less common than it was before improved standards of hygiene and education, discovery of the drugs sulphonamides and antibiotics, and the practice of immunisation. The care of the feverish patient which was so much a routine and familiar procedure is necessary now for only a few patients but in basic principles it has changed very little.

Symptoms of fever include headache, thirst, nausea, loss of appetite, constipation, and a general feeling of not being well. The patient may complain of general pains and disturbed sleep.

Signs of fever are hot dry skin which is flushed and later becomes damp, visible sweating, unnaturally bright eyes, restlessness and delirium, particularly in children. If sweating continues, signs of dehydration appear in the patient. His eyes sink back into his head, and the skin is loose. His temperature is raised, usually the highest recording being in the evening. The pulse rate increases, e.g. from 70 to 90 or even more. The respiration rate is also increased, e.g. from 18 to 24, depending on the type of infection. For example, the rate rises considerably in chest infections.

In severe infections such as septicaemia the patient looks grey and is unaware of his surroundings. He may collapse due to heart failure when this organ is exposed to an infection in the blood. A continued fast pulse rate can cause fatigue in the heart muscle, particularly when this already is not very efficient. If the brain is affected by the infection of toxins, the patient may show signs of meningeal irritation with severe headache, delirium, stiff neck and back, or he lapses into coma.

When fever is prolonged the patient begins to lose weight even though dehydration is prevented. This is because his appetite is much less than normal, his digestion is temporarily weakened and he uses up his stores in fat and muscle in increased metabolic activity.

NURSING CARE OF THE PATIENT

This is the basic bed-side care needed by every ill patient, but the nurse ensures that the feverish patient makes no unnecessary physical effort. She and a colleague lift him gently on and off a bed-pan and during bed-making. His head and back are well supported by pillows in the position in which he is likely to be most comfortable. Any article he may require is placed by his hand on the locker or bed-table. The nurse is available especially during the night, and if he is nursed in a side ward he is provided with a bell. A feverish child is often afraid in the night and someone should be with him.

To maintain nutrition as far as possible he is given glucose and sugar in fruit drinks and small, easily digested meals, including for example, soft-boiled or coddled eggs, thin bread and butter, a little milk or sponge pudding, small amounts of steamed fish or casserole chicken. He usually dislikes milk drinks but prefers tea, orange and lemon drinks, meat extracts in hot water, or clear soups. Vitamin C is necessary, and can be given in orange or lemon juice or blackcurrant syrup. Drinking clear fluids and chewing a little fruit frequently prevent his mouth from becoming dry and uncomfortable. Fresh or tinned pineapple and savoury aspic jellies may encourage an interest in food as he begins to recover.

The mouth needs careful attention to prevent dryness, loss of the sense of taste, and later infection of the mouth, salivary glands and stomach. Adequate fluid intake is the most important preventive. Pressure areas are exposed to damp from sweating and friction in restlessness, and need special care. If he is allowed to lie in one position pressure sores, bronchopneumonia or venous thrombosis may occur. Therefore his position is changed every two hours.

The effect of the raised temperature may distress the patient or cause loss of sleep and rest. This can be relieved by clothing him in cool, loose garments with adequate ventilation in the room and the temperature not more than 18°C. The application of a cold compress to the head, iced drinks and simple sponging of the skin with warm water are comforting. Tepid sponging is beneficial to the patient during the evening, when his temperature is highest and he is most restless. The patient must not be exposed to strong, cool draughts or the skin uncovered for more than a few moments, otherwise his temperature will fall too rapidly and he will collapse.

The physician may prescribe drugs such as salicylates which promote sweating and in so doing lower the temperature. It is unwise to give alcohol to a patient who is restless and mentally confused while feverish; he will most likely become excitable and irrational. This patient may be restless because he wants to pass urine, and if the nurse can persuade him to do this he will usually become quiet and co-operative. When mental confusion is severe and the patient may be harmed, the doctor may prescribe a barbiturate or paraldehyde as sedation.

Dehydration is prevented or treated by the administration of water either by mouth, naso-oesophageal feeding or intra-venous infusion.

Fluid by mouth in very frequent small amounts is preferred as use of equipment may predispose further infection, and drinking maintains a healthy mouth. Fluid replacement is assessed from the fluid balance chart and the extent of the patient's sweating. He may require three litres a day. He loses salt in sweating and this can be replaced by introducing one teaspoonful of salt to one litre of drinking fluid. The taste will not be obvious when sugar and fruit juice have been added. In intra-venous therapy salt is included as 0·9% or 0·18% sodium chloride.

Fever leaves the patient feeling very weak, and a period of convalescence is necessary with nutritious diet, moderate then increasing exercise in the fresh air when possible, adequate sleep and rest, and a change of surroundings.

CHAPTER 25 | SURGERY: BANDAGING

In surgical treatment of disease a wound is made. This procedure can be complicated by *pain and haemorrhage*. As the skin, which is the body's first defence against *infection*, has been cut, sepsis may follow.

These have been three great problems in surgical procedure, and in the past the prospect of such treatment caused the patient apprehension and fear. Advances in knowledge and skill have resulted in *anaesthesia and analgesics* to abolish the pain associated with surgical operation. Instruments to clamp and seal bleeding points and catgut to ligature blood vessels with replacement of lost blood by *blood transfusion* have removed much of the fear of haemorrhage. Infection is prevented by a strict *aseptic technique* and a high standard of *cleanliness* in the operating theatre and its equipment.

Although hospitals and operations are now discussed more freely and details of treatment are not so unfamiliar, it is natural that every patient admitted to hospital for surgical treatment should feel some measure of *fear*. Many do not show what they feel and the nurse should be as considerate to these people as she is to one who can talk about it. The *surgeon will explain the operation* to the patient and the nursing staff may be able to answer simple questions about the preparation for operation, the visit to the operating theatre, who will be with him, in which ward he will be nursed afterwards and so on. Admission a few days before the operation gives the sister or charge nurse an opportunity to talk with the relatives, gain their confidence and co-operation, and arrange for telephone inquiries and visits after the operation. The patient is helped to understand what the operation involves when he can meet another patient who has recently recovered. His morale is kept high by the cheerful optimistic atmosphere of the ward, the loyalty and confidence between the members of medical and nursing staffs and the unshakeable sense of team-work throughout the ward and operating theatre.

When the operation has been explained to the patient, he gives his *consent* by signing appropriate forms: for the surgeon to carry out the operation required as treatment, for any procedure necessary afterwards and for the administration of an anaesthetic. This is a legal formality. The consent of a parent or guardian is required before an operation on a person under sixteen years of age. When the consent to operate has not been obtained the surgeon is informed. On any occasion when surgical operation is suggested or intended the patient's next-of-kin is informed by the hospital. The police give valuable assistance in tracing relatives when illness or accidents occur unexpectedly.

EXAMINATION AND INVESTIGATIONS

A *history* of the patient's illness is obtained. During a *general examination* of the patient the surgeon notes the nutrition of the patient. If there is malnutrition for any reason this is put right before operation, and additional feeds of Complan and vitamin medicines may be ordered. The patient's blood pressure is measured and the heart and lungs are examined by the doctor. A cough is reported, also whether or not the patient is a smoker and if he has a cold.

Investigations depend on the patient's illness and the type of operation to be performed. The more common procedures include *X-ray of the chest* and *blood tests*, e.g. haemoglobin, blood count, blood groups. *The urine is tested* for the presence of sugar, albumin and ketones. A fluid balance chart is recorded so that dehydration may be avoided.

Preparation of the Patient for Operation

The Skin

The patient goes to the bath or is bed-bathed after admission with special attention to the area of skin likely to be involved in the operation. Septic spots or abrasions are reported. The site of operation is indicated by the surgeon. Hair on or near to the area is removed by shaving and this may be more convenient if completed before the patient's bath. Permission from the patient is sought before the head is shaved.

Further preparation of the skin is now rarely carried out in the ward.

Lotions are applied to the skin immediately prior to the operation by aseptic technique:

    (a) to remove natural oils from the skin, e.g. methylated ether. Cetrimide is a detergent which prevents the growth of bacteria;

    (b) to act as skin antiseptics, e.g. methylated spirits, iodine.

Sterile towels are placed round the area and the lotions are applied on swabs held in forceps. The area is swabbed methodically in strokes across the skin and then allowed to dry.

The Alimentary Tract

Pre-operative diet is easily digested food with very little fat and residue. The last meal is 4 to 6 hours before operation, but small amounts of water can be given to within 4 hours of surgery. The anaesthetist may give instructions.

If a naso-oesophageal tube has been passed at the instructions of the surgeon, the aspirated fluid is recorded on the fluid balance chart. An aperient such as Senokot or Dulcolax may be necessary to ensure a satisfactory bowel action the day before operation. Before surgery of the bowel more extensive preparation is necessary, including rectal or colon washouts.

The Bladder

The patient passes urine just before he leaves the ward. If this has not been possible the surgeon is informed. Catheterisation of the bladder is usual before pelvic operations and sometimes the catheter remains in position until after the operation.

Clothing

The patient wears a white cotton gown which ties at the back with tapes. In operations which do not involve the trunk and lower limbs, pyjama trousers can be worn beneath the gown. A disposable theatre cap is worn over the hair. Watches and rings (except wedding rings) and ear-rings are removed and Sister places these in a special cupboard or drawer which can be locked for safety. Loose wedding rings can be secured to the finger by adhesive tape. Chains round the neck are discouraged. If a patient is anxious to wear a religious medallion, the anaesthetist is in-informed so that he knows it is there and can deal with it should it cause pressure if the patient's position be changed. Hair grips are removed and lastly the dentures are taken out and placed in a denture carton to be kept in the patient's locker. It may be routine for a band with the patient's name to be placed round his right wrist (if intravenous therapy will be introduced in the left upper limb) or some other suitable place.

Sedation and Pre-operative Drugs
The evening before operation the patient may be prescribed a sedative such as a barbiturate to ensure a satisfactory night's sleep.

Pre-operative drugs are given half an hour before the administration of the anaesthetic. These normally include a *sedative* which causes the patient to relax and eases his fears, e.g. papaveretum or pethidine (both are Dangerous Drugs), and a drug to reduce secretions in the upper respiratory tract, e.g. atropine or hyoscine depending on the type of anaesthetic used. If for any reason the administration of these drugs is likely to be delayed the anaesthetist is informed of this, as he may wish to give further instructions. Valium, a tranquilliser, is sometimes used as a preoperative drug.

The patient is lifted carefully on to the operating theatre trolley, covered by a clean cotton blanket and given one or two pillows, or he is transported to the theatre entrance room on his own bed. All notes and X-rays will be required. He is accompanied by a nurse from his ward who can reassure him by remaining by his side until he is anaesthetised.

IN AN EMERGENCY, many details of this preparation may of necessity be omitted. When the surgeon has stated that he will operate immediately:

1. The operation is explained to the patient if he is conscious and his consent obtained.

2. The near relatives are informed. It is useful to know his religion.

3. His urine is tested.

4. A quick examination of the skin (and hair) show standard of cleanliness and the theatre staff are told of any problems. The skin will be prepared in the theatre.

5. He is asked when he last had a meal. The surgeon may request the passing of a naso-oesophageal tube and aspiration of stomach contents.

6. He is dressed for operating theatre, passes urine, dentures are removed, etc.

7. The pre-operative drug which has been prescribed is given.

A sample of blood may be obtained for cross-matching with blood in the Blood Bank in case transfusion be required.

Post-Operative Treatment and Care

Preparation for the Patient's Return from the Operating Theatre
The *operation bed* is prepared with clean sheets, and extra waterproof protection is provided when necessary. One pillow with waterproof under-cover is placed on the bed, the remaining pillows are on a chair at the bed-side. The top bed-clothes are folded back so that they can be removed easily. Bed-blocks or an elevator are available when none is

incorporated in the patient's bed. Should there be some degree of shock raising the foot of the bed may be part of the treatment.

If the patient is likely to be unconscious *mouth gag, tongue forceps, damped dental squares, swab-holding forceps* and *anaesthetic cloth* are on a tray at the bed-side. Special post-operative equipment may be needed such as *oxygen apparatus,* and a *stand or holder for blood or intravenous fluid bottles. Drainage bottles* or bags and tubing are other possible requirements. *Charts* for recording pulse, blood pressure, or fluid balance are prepared.

The patient's RECOVERY FROM THE ANAESTHETIC and immediate effects of operation may take place in a room joined to the operating theatre or attached to his ward (recovery room). On many occasions he is conscious or almost conscious as he leaves the operating theatre. He is taken on the theatre trolley or in his bed to the general ward. DURING TRANSFER FROM THE THEATRE TO THE WARD, the theatre orderly manages the trolley or bed. Having received, in the theatre, information regarding the operation performed, and instructions for any immediate treatment to be carried out in the ward, and, observing the patient's condition before he leaves the theatre, the ward nurse accompanies him to the ward, walking by his head to observe any changes. She carries a mouth gag, tongue forceps, vomit bowl and towel.

A mechanical air-way may have been placed in the patient's mouth and throat, and this will remain until he coughs it out. If there is no mechanical air-way and he suddenly becomes blue, the nurse supports his jaw by pressing it forward, with the head turned to one side. If this does not relieve the condition she uses the tongue forceps while the trolley attendant obtains medical assistance. The mouth is opened, using the mouth gag, and the points of the tongue forceps are passed through the under part of the tongue at the centre near the tip. The forceps are closed and the handles outside the mouth are held firmly so that the tongue is well forward and flattened. The handles may be secured to the patient's clothing or by a tape if some other emergency procedure is required of the nurse. When breathing is established, the forceps are removed.

Post-operative Nursing in the Ward

As the patient arrives in the ward the top bed-clothes are removed from the operation bed. He is lifted slowly and carefully to prevent a sudden fall in blood pressure which would pre-dispose a state of shock. If the *lateral position in bed* is used a pillow is placed behind him so that he does not roll onto his back. A pillow is placed under his head and the bed-clothes are returned to the bed. The nurse notes his appearance, general condition and pulse rate. A patient who is unconscious on his return to the ward is observed continuously for cessation of breathing or cyanosis. For this reason adequate lighting is necessary at all times when watching such a patient.

DIET after operation depends on the type of operation which has been performed. When the patient is fully conscious he is given fluids for the first 12 to 24 hours. To prevent dehydration 100 millilitres each hour should be sufficient. Large amounts of fluid, especially milk, can produce a feeling of nausea. The fluid diet is followed by small, easily digested meals, and dry foods such as biscuits and bread and butter can relieve a tendency to vomit. Within 3 or 4 days the diet is increased to ordinary meals. Vitamin C given as fresh fruit or fruit juices assists in the healing process and these drinks are refreshing when the mouth is dry. Following operation on the oesophagus, stomach or duodenum, diet may be delayed for a few days. Water, and later milk and water are given in small amounts frequently and the diet increased as the patient's condition improves.

Intravenous therapy may be in progress for one of the following reasons:

to replace fluid or blood loss during or after operation.

to adjust electrolytes to correct level;

when the patient cannot have fluid by mouth following an operation on the alimentary tract;

because the patient is unconscious.

The rate of flow is indicated by the surgeon, e.g. 20 drops per minute or 70 millilitres per hour.

This treatment prevents *dehydration*. This condition would be indicated by the urine being dark and small in amount and the mouth dry.

Electrolytes in the blood may also have been assessed. The doctor prescribes the particular fluid to be given intravenously such as sodium chloride 0·9% solution or 0·18% solution. There are also special solutions containing electrolytes in various amounts; one of these is Butler's solution.

Blood transfusion may be in progress replacing blood loss during operation.

When the patient is ill following operation, the amount of urine passed is recorded on a *fluid balance chart* together with the intake of fluid. This ensures that *dehydration* does not occur and is a guide to kidney and bladder functions.

ASPIRATION OF THE STOMACH CONTENTS may be a procedure performed at intervals following a gastric operation or to prevent vomiting. A naso-oesophageal tube has been passed and remains in position with the lower end in the stomach. The upper few inches of the tube are secured to the patient's cheek in front of his ear by a piece of adhesive tape. A spigot is unnecessary and indeed unsuitable as it prevents gastric contents and gas escaping from the stomach and this can cause some discomfort.

The stomach contents are withdrawn, using a millilitre syringe. Any abnormalities of fluid such as blood are reported. The amount is entered on the Fluid Balance Chart.

Continual suction is sometimes necessary using a low-pressure suction machine attached to a drainage bottle which in turn is connected to the naso-oesophageal tube.

ORAL TOILET. The patient is receiving no food and probably no fluid by mouth and oral toilet is essential at least every two hours.

BLADDER AND KIDNEY FUNCTION. The nurse observes when the patient passes urine after operation, and reports when there is any delay after about eight hours. If the bladder is distended, the patient is encouraged to empty the bladder by such measures as turning on a water tap, or changing his position in bed so that he sits more upright. It may be possible for him to stand by the bed supported by the nurse or be taken in a chair to the toilet, but this depends on the operation, and the ward sister will give instructions. If these attempts prove unsuccessful the surgeon may prescribe a drug which causes the bladder to contract. When the operation involves the pelvic organs, catheterisation may be necessary. Should the patient *not* have passed urine and the bladder is *not* distended, the surgeon may wish to investigate the kidney function by blood tests including electrolytes and blood urea estimations.

BOWEL ACTION. It is expected that the patient will be constipated following an operation as he has had little to eat and is inactive. As soon as he begins to take ordinary food, defaecation is likely to take place at the usual times.

Being able to sit out of bed on a commode or visit the toilet assists in producing a normal bowel action. An aperient may be required the day following operation and occasionally two glycerine suppositories or a simple enema are ordered.

THE WOUND. The cut edges of the skin are drawn together by *stitches* (sutures) of nylon or strengthened silk. Some skin wounds are closed by small clips, e.g. Michel clips.

When a wound involves deeper layers of tissue as in the abdomen, deeper sutures of nylon are used. These are called *tension sutures* and they are tied over the skin sutures.

Tissues beneath the skin are sutured with catgut produced from sheep's intestine. The advantage of this suture is that it is *absorbed in the body.*

A wound which is completely closed by sutures or clips rarely requires a large dressing as there is no discharge. It may be sprayed with an antiseptic liquid which solidifies over the wound and prevents entry of infection. One such liquid is Nobecutaine. Otherwise a small dressing is placed over the wound secured by adhesive tape. Skin sutures are removed in 5 to 7 days on the surgeon's instructions.

REMOVAL OF SUTURES. The equipment required is a *basic dressing trolley* with the addition of *sterile suture scissors* or *suture removers* and a gallipot in which to place the sutures. An aseptic technique is employed. The dresser grasps a free end of the suture with plain dissecting forceps and with the other hand cuts the suture where it leaves the skin beneath the knot. She then draws the part of suture in the skin through until the suture is free. It is placed in the gallipot. This method ensures that no unsterile part of the suture passes through the skin. The sutures are removed in turn and the wound inspected carefully if the sutures are very fine to make sure that all have been removed. The skin is swabbed with an antiseptic. A patient can sometimes be very apprehensive about having sutures removed. The procedure rarely causes pain but it is helpful for the patient to be reassured that it is likely to be painless so that he relaxes. He is told when the removal of sutures is completed.

Sterile clip removers are required to remove clips. The lower part of the blade fits beneath the clip. As the forceps are closed the clip flattens and releases its hold on the skin edges. Tension sutures are removed usually on the 10th day.

Discharges from Wounds and their Drainage

(*a*) *Blood.* The surgeon may leave a rubber tube drain in the wound, and through this blood will appear should reactionary haemorrhage complicate the operation within 24 hours. The nurse from time to time observes the dressing into which the tube drains. If bleeding occurs beneath a closed wound, there is swelling and the patient complains of discomfort. The surgeon removes a suture to release the blood or clot.

(*b*) *Tissue fluid.* This discharge is from beneath the skin or a cavity which remains after removal of an organ or part of an organ.

(*c*) *Pus* is a thick yellow discharge from infected tissue. It may be produced in a septic wound or is the discharge from an abscess which has burst or been incised by the surgeon.

(*d*) *Other fluids* such as stomach contents, bile, and cerebro-spinal fluid may also be discharged.

Drainage from the skin is absorbed by sterile dressings secured by clean bandages. If the bandage becomes damp from the discharge infection will enter the wound through the moist patch. For this reason it is important to redress such wounds or bandage more sterile wool over the dressing whenever necessary.

Drainage from below the skin is mantained by the insertion of a piece of ribbon gauze, a rubber tube or corrugated rubber drain into the wound. The discharge is collected into sterile dressings or a bottle. A drainage tube is usually held in position by a skin suture. To prevent the tube slipping into the wound cavity, a large safety pin is passed through the tube, then closed. The tube is removed when the surgeon instructs. Those draining blood and tissue fluid are usually removed on the second day. Tubes draining fluids from a cavity, e.g. pus and bile, are removed when the drainage is reduced to a very small amount.

When healing of tissue is taking place slowly beneath the wound, the surgeon may request that the tube should be shortened at intervals. The tube may be rotated slightly each day to prevent the skin growing close to the tube. (Tubes are shortened or removed by the ward sister or her deputy on the instructions of the surgeon.)

Drainage from a cavity through a tube into a bottle is the method sometimes used in removing the bile following cholecystectomy (removal of the gall-bladder), and in draining tissue fluid from beneath a mastectomy wound (removal of the breast). A small amount of suction from a machine may be used to assist the flow. The suction machine is attached by pressure tubing to the bottle, and the bottle is connected to the rubber tube in the wound by pressure tubing.

Drainage from the chest takes place into water in a large bottle. This is called underwater seal drainage, and the bottle must not be lifted from the ground unless the tubing has been clamped off, otherwise some of the water may flow back into the chest.

It is customary to measure drainage and observe any discharge in amount, appearance, etc.

In shallow wounds where there is likely to be some discharge and it is necessary to keep the wound open for this to escape, a *corrugated rubber drain* is inserted. It is removed in 24 to 48 hours.

EXERCISE. The patient is encouraged to move in bed, particularly when his bed is made. He sits out of bed and walks about in the ward as soon as possible after operation, in many cases the following day.

In some wards the *physiotherapist* arranges class exercises at the surgeon's request. This is in addition to an exercise programme for individual patients after certain operations, for example in orthopaedic surgery.

An *occupational therapist* teaches and supervises the making of articles, painting, etc. During these activities the patient uses muscles and joints in his hands and arms besides releasing creative energy and preventing boredom.

Breathing exercises improve the lung ventilation and assist in preventing post-operative pneumonia. They are particularly useful after chest surgery and abdominal operations near the diaphragm. The nurse can encourage the patient in these when she makes his bed or attends to him. He should be able to push against the nurse's hand placed over his lower ribs when he breathes in.

COUGHING is necessary to remove mucus from the air passages, but is painful for the patient who has had a chest or abdominal operation. The nurse shows him how to support his wound by slight pressure from his hands, or she places her own hand over the dressing. He coughs while she supports him in a sitting position with the head slightly forward. A sputum carton is held for him while he expectorates. Then the nurse makes him comfortable supported by pillows.

Some Possible Complications of Operations

ASPHYXIA (choking). This is prevented by the maintenance of an efficient air-way.

To summarise the points already made:
1. A lateral position is most suitable but not always possible.
2. Mucus is removed from the mouth and throat using damp dental squares held firmly in sponge-holding forceps.
3. A mechanical air-way assists breathing and will be coughed out when no longer required.
4. The nurse can support the jaw, pressing behind the angles of the jaw to bring it forward, so that the tongue does not block the pharynx.
5. When this is not effective and the air-way is obstructed by the tongue, the tongue forceps are used, though this is rarely necessary.

HAEMORRHAGE. Bleeding occurring within 24 hours of operation is referred to as *reactionary haemorrhage*. This is a possible complication as the blood pressure rises to normal.

Pallor, perhaps some restlessness and a rising pulse rate are signs of bleeding. There would be a fall in blood pressure also. Blood may appear through the wound drain should one of these have been inserted.

Treatment is to stop the bleeding and this may necessitate a further operative procedure. Blood by transfusion replaces blood loss.

SHOCK is a serious complication of surgery. Should it occur, the patient becomes pale, almost grey in colour. His extremities are cold, his skin may be clammy. The pulse is quick and weak. The patient collapses and his temperature and blood pressure are low.

When shock is present, treatment begins at once. Slowly and with care the patient is placed flat in bed. The doctor may request bed-blocks or elevator to *raise the foot of the bed* immediately.

Moderate *warmth* is applied using extra blankets, and perhaps a flannelette sheet next to the patient, but *no* hot-water bottles (these would cause a burn on the patient). Windows and doors are closed to prevent a cooling draught.

Oxygen is administered using nasal catheters, with flow rate of 4 to 6 litres per minute. Frequently no drugs are ordered, and morphia is avoided as it depresses the nervous system.

Fluids used in *intravenous therapy* depend on the situation. If haemorrhage has occurred, blood will be given. Otherwise plasma or a prepared solution which restores blood volume is used.

Further surgery may be required but this is usually delayed until the patient's condition has improved.

While the treatment is in progress the nurse disturbs the patient as little as possible. She is quiet and does not fuss. If the patient's mouth is dry it is wiped with damp swabs or tissues, and sweat can be mopped from his face with a towel.

PAIN during 12 to 24 hours following operation is relieved by analgesic drugs prescribed by the surgeon. Examples of these are papaveretum and pethidine (Dangerous Drugs). The drug is more effective when given as soon as the patient shows signs of some restlessness. The nurse reports to sister when the patient she is observing becomes more aware of pain and discomfort immediately following operation and anaesthetic.

After 12 to 24 hours the post-operative pain is usually much less and these drugs are not required. The nurse can relieve many types of *discomfort* such as that resulting from creased night-clothes, pressure of a pillow against a drainage tube, an unsuitable position in bed, or thirst.

When the patient cannot *sleep* for a few nights after operation the surgeon may prescribe a sedative but this usually becomes unnecessary in a short time.

Retention of urine sometimes occurs after any abdominal or pelvic operation. The doctor orders a drug which causes the bladder to contract, or may pass a catheter in a male patient or requests a nurse to catheterise the female patient. If there is no urine in the bladder the surgeon investigates kidney function by blood tests.

Distension of the abdomen following an abdominal operation is usually due to retention of flatus in the alimentary canal. The patient is extremely uncomfortable. It is more likely to occur if the patient is unable to move about in bed or he becomes constipated. Passing a flatus tube (a long tube with a slightly narrowed opening at one end) may relieve this condition. For this proceaure the following *equipment* is required:

a flatus tube or long rectal tube;

swab with lubrication for the tube;

towel to protect the bed;

paper towel to clean the anus after the procedure;

a bowl of water.

Screens or curtains are used round the bed.

Method. The patient having been told of the procedure lies on his left side if possible. The bed is protected, the patient is covered except for the anal area.

Having lubricated the narrowed end of the tube, it is passed through the anal canal into the rectum to about four inches. The other end of the tube is held beneath the water in the bowl. Flatus will escape as bubbles through the water.

Following the procedure the patient should feel more comfortable, and his abdomen is softer.

Depending on the operation area, the patient may be moved in bed and this may assist him in passing flatus, for example, lying face downwards for a few minutes.

Problems arise in elderly patients who are very ill. Constipation can be severe, necessitating an olive-oil enema followed by a soap and water, or salt and water (2 teaspoonfuls to 1 litre), enema.

In cases of faecal impaction manual removal of faeces is carried out by a skilled person. This is followed, when the patient's condition allows, by aperients and enemas to establish a normal daily bowel action.

VENOUS THROMBOSIS is a clot in a vein and can be caused by pressure on the vein behind the knees as the patient lies in bed. For this reason knee pillows are avoided after operations. This condition may be the cause of pyrexia. The calf of the affected leg is tender and there may be slight swelling. Treatment includes rest with no movement in the limb, which is protected by a bed-cradle.

Should part of a clot separate it may move in the circulation to a major blood vessel in the lung (pulmonary embolism). The patient becomes suddenly very ill with pain in the chest. He coughs blood-stained sputum. The doctor is informed immediately.

COMPLICATIONS OF WOUNDS

1. *Wound infection.* This would be indicated by a rise in the patient's temperature with other signs of fever. The wound would be examined by the surgeon or ward sister. It may be necessary to remove one or more sutures and the surgeon would usually prescribe appropriate antibiotic

treatment. A musty smell or a greenish colour observed in pus is reported at once as these are signs of further infection.

2. In abdominal surgery, the skin of a debilitated or very ill patient may not heal easily. Occasionally *the wound gives way* and part of the small intestine appears through the opening. This complication may cause the nurse a great deal of anxiety when it occurs but treatment is quite straightforward. She covers the protruding intestine with small towels or muslin mops wrung out in hot water and obtains medical aid. The surgeon will re-suture the wound in the operating theatre.

When this complication is suspected, the wound is strapped firmly and an abdominal binder is frequently applied. The patient remains in bed until the wound is satisfactory.

Routine Nursing Attention

ATTENTION TO THE ILL PATIENT after operation may be arranged at intervals, e.g. two-hourly, and would include:

1. *Relief from pressure on the skin*, by raising him while the draw sheet is pulled through or by changing his position in bed. The sacral area and heels may need massage.

2. *Movement.* Flexion and extension at the wrists and ankles by the nurse prevents stiffness at those joints. Bending the lower limbs slightly at hip, knee and ankle as the patient is moved helps in the same way.

3. *Deep breathing* is encouraged when the patient is able to make the effort.

4. Being given a drink or feed.

5. Attention to his mouth.

6. Observing his general condition, also his wound, his skin over pressure areas, and listening to any comments he wishes to make.

7. This last procedure provides an opportunity for the nurse to be with the patient for a few minutes to give him confidence and encouragement, and prevent the sense of loneliness which can occur in every serious illness.

This periodic routine of attention should not be prolonged as the patient becomes very quickly exhausted. He rests after being made comfortable and will probably sleep for a time.

General Basic Nursing Care for the Patient after Operation
In the first few hours after anaesthetic and operation, the patient appreciates the nurse being close at hand but prefers not to be disturbed. This is partly due to his drowsiness following the administration of an analgesic which relieves pain or a sedative which soothes him.

Depending on the type of operation and the condition of the patient, he may be supported in a *sitting position* a few hours after operation.

When he becomes completely conscious, his face and hands are washed, his clothing changed and he is made comfortable. Next day *bed-baths* begin as normal routine. *Pressure area*s are relieved from pressure by changing the patient's position at intervals and are treated by massaging, using skin talc or cream on the skin. He is taking little food or fluid on the first day, and his *mouth* needs attention by frequent mouthwashes or by cleaning with swabs until he is able to eat a small, easily digested diet. A clean and moist mouth assists in preventing infection of the mouth and possible inflammation of a parotid salivary gland (parotitis). Dentures are replaced as soon as recovery from the anaesthetic is complete.

The *hair* is arranged in a comfortable manner and male patients are shaved by the barber.

The patient is allowed to *sleep and rest* as much as he cares to during the first day or two, but then sits out of bed and walks in the ward.

Visitors

The patient quickly becomes exhausted, and only a very near relative is allowed to visit him on the first day after operation. The visitor remains only a short time and arrangements are made for enquiries by telephone.

When the condition of the patient or some special situation concerning near relatives (such as travelling long distances) necessitates the visitors staying in the hospital during the recovery of the patient from anaesthetic, they are usually accommodated in a room reserved for visitors and made as comfortable as possible. They are given frequent bulletins about the patient's condition and the ward sister arranges the times when they may see the patient.

Sympathetic friends and relatives often bring flowers for the patient after his operation, and he appreciates being able to see some of these as he lies in bed either in a small posy bowl on his locker or on the table in the main ward.

Day by day the patient's activity increases, and with this his independence. He washes and baths, eats his diet, has no difficulty with bowel or bladder function, can perform his exercises and he can enjoy occupational therapy, television or chatting with his colleagues. He sleeps well at night. His interest begins to be centred on other people in the ward rather than on himself, and many patients at this stage offer to do little services for those who are more ill and sometimes for the nurses. Occasionally some tact is needed here, for the patient may be a little too optimistic about his physical progress and over-activity can lead to fatigue and sleeplessness at the end of the day.

This is the time of *convalescence* when he needs no medical and nursing supervision throughout the day, but enjoys nutritious meals, plenty of sleep at night, increasing exercise during the day, mental stimulation in a change of environment, with sunshine and fresh air if possible.

REHABILITATION means preparing for the routine (or habit) activities of day-to-day living and of work, and includes dressing oneself, cooking meals, shopping in a busy town, using public transport, gardening, manipulating machinery, playing games and so on. Often there is no problem but in some cases the patient needs help from his family and friends, physiotherapists, occupational therapists, medical social workers and employers.

After certain operations, he attends his medical practitioner or the consultant in the hospital out-patients' department who will check his progress.

BANDAGING

Bandaging used to be a most necessary skill for all nurses, but with the introduction of tubular gauze and Netelast which is quickly applied and stands up to the early ambulations of patients, the old methods of bandaging are rapidly being replaced by new techniques. It is necessary, however, to have a knowledge of the basic facts about bandages and bandaging and to acquire skill by practice in applying the ones in common use.

Bandages

These are applied to any part of the body for one or more of the following reasons:
1. To keep a dressing on a wound in place.
2. To give support to a limb.
3. To prevent swelling.
4. To keep splints in position.
5. To control circulation in a limb.

The main types of bandages are:
1. Roller—made of cotton, calico, stretch or crêpe, plaster.
2. Manytail—made of calico or domette.
3. T-bandage—made of cotton or calico.
4. Triangular—made of calico.
5. Tubular—tube gauze and Netelast.

ROLLER BANDAGES can be bought in various widths and the nurse chooses the one to suit the size of the area to be covered. They can be applied to any part of the body.

H

MANYTAIL BANDAGES are usually made of five lengths of 5-inch wide and 56-inch long calico or domette. They are sewn centrally on to an 8-inch square of the same material with each length overlapping its predecessor by one-third. They are used to keep abdominal or chest dressings in place and are easy to apply and comfortable to wear.

T-BANDAGES are made in the shape of the letter from which they take their name and are used to keep perineal dressings in place.

TRIANGULAR BANDAGES are used open as a sling, folded as an improvised supporting bandage, or to bind a splint in position.

TUBULAR BANDAGES

      (i) Tube gauze—made by special firms who supply detailed instructions and applicators. Careful practice is needed as there is some danger of pressure sores if the bandage is incorrectly applied. It is not easily usable on the trunk.

     (ii) Netelast—this is rapidly replacing the old-type bandage. It is made of cotton and elastic made into a wide-mesh tubular net. It can be easily and safely applied to all parts of the body without applicators. It is light, comfortable and hygienic to wear.

RULES FOR BANDAGING

A. Roller Bandaging

1. Select the right width and appropriate number required.

2. Make the patient comfortable, explain what is to be done. Support the affected part if necessary.

3. Always have a dressing or layer of wool between skin and bandage.

4. Hold the head of the bandage uppermost.

5. Unroll short lengths at a time so that the procedure can be controlled.

6. Begin to bandage from within—outward and from below—upwards.

7. Keep an even pressure but avoid looseness as this will neither hold a dressing in place or give support, and beware of tightness as this will interfere with the circulation.

8. Cover two-thirds of the preceding bandage.

9. Keep joints *flexed* when bandaging them to allow some movement and free circulation of blood. N.B. The foot should be at right angles to the leg when being bandaged.

10. Fasten end securely with a safety pin, taking care not to prick the patient or to leave it in a position where it will cause pressure.

B. *Manytail Bandaging*
1. Roll all the tails from each side into the centre and pass this behind the patient's back. The first tails to be used should be the lowest.
2. Two nurses are better (but not essential) than one in order to bandage the patient firmly and securely.
3. The last tail is placed diagonally across the others and pinned.
4. If the bandage rides up it can be kept in place with groin straps made of cotton bandage.

C. *T-bandages*
1. Tie waist ends first.
2. Bring other two ends between legs and pin to waist band.
3. Make sure the bandage is not cutting into the groin.

D. *Triangular Bandages (used as a Sling)*
1. Stand in front of the patient.
2. Position arm with hand higher than elbow.
3. Place one corner of bandage over *sound* shoulder and apex of it just above the elbow on the injured side and under the arm.
4. Bring over corners of bandage across forearm and fasten with a *reef* knot in the hollow above the clavicle. Put a small pad beneath it to prevent pressure.
5. Pin the apex at the elbow so that the joint is enclosed.
6. Inspect to see that the whole arm including the wrist is supported and that the shoulder is in a natural position.

E. *Tubular Bandages*
Special instructions are supplied by the makers for the use of these together with the necessary applicators.

PATTERNS IN BANDAGING
There are four main patterns used to help the bandages to be applied neatly and securely to the varying widths and angles of the body. They are:

1. *Simple Spiral*—for uniform widths, e.g. finger.
2. *Reverse Spiral*—for shaped limbs, e.g. leg.
3. *Figure of Eight*—for applying pressure or where movement is allowed, e.g. knee or elbow joints.
4. *Divergent Spica*—for joints, but does not exert pressure.

THE MAIN SPECIAL BANDAGES

1. Eye Bandage

Although some surgeons prefer knitted eye shades the eye bandage is an important roller bandage to have skill in applying. The rules are:

(a) Face the patient, who should be sitting comfortably and ask him to hold the pad.

(b) Start from affected side to good side across the forehead, making one complete round to fix the bandage.

(c) Continue round but this time bring the bandage up *under* the ear and across the eye-pad on the nasal side.

(d) Each succeeding turn overlaps the bandage on the pad but crosses the fixing turn and passes under the ear at the same point.

(e) The final turn should be round the head and the bandage secured in the front with a safety pin.

2. Ear Bandage

The pattern here is the same as for the eye, and the rules for application exactly the same. A crêpe bandage is more suitable than a gauze one, but care must be taken to keep the eyes clear.

3. Breast Bandage

When pressure is required use a 3-inch to 4-inch cotton or crêpe bandage. Stand in front of the patient and starting on the affected side alternately encircle the waist with the bandage and carry it across the dressing on the breast to the opposite shoulder. By covering one-third of the preceding row of bandage each time a firm and comfortable support can be given with about four turns in both directions.

4. Varicose Veins

Bleeding from these can be sudden and severe. Swift, efficient first aid is essential.

(i) Lay the patient down.

(ii) Raise the affected leg.

(iii) Cover bleeding area with firm hand pressure. As soon as bleeding is controlled, apply a clean dressing to the area and a firm bandage from below upwards.

(iv) Send the patient to hospital for urgent treatment.

CHAPTER 26 | TUMOURS

A tumour is a mass of tissue of any kind and the term is used to mean a collection of cells.

BENIGN OR SIMPLE TUMOURS are localised to the tissue in which they form, the mass of tissue being enclosed in a capsule. They grow slowly and the cells function in the same way as the original tissue cells. As they enlarge they may cause pressure on other organs, for example, a tumour of the thyroid gland presses on the trachea. For this reason they are removed. When removed they do not grow again.

MALIGNANT TUMOURS are *not* enclosed in a capsule but infiltrate into tissue. The cells spread in the body by means of the lymphatic system and occasionally by the blood. They grow rapidly and do not have the function of the parent tissue. The secondary growths from a malignant growth are called *metastases*. Diagnosis of a tumour is by examination of a small section of the tissue under a high-powered microscope. The section of tissue is a biopsy and is obtained during examination, for example, during bronchoscopy in suspected malignant tumour (i.e. carcinoma) of the bronchus, or during surgical operation. The tissue is placed in a small jar, labelled immediately in the operating theatre, then despatched with the request form to the histology laboratory.

The cause of tumours is not yet understood but the change of tissue is produced by a number of factors including lengthy exposure of the skin to certain compounds of tar and oil, irritation of the lung by cigarette smoking, imbalance of hormones affecting the breast, uterus and prostate gland.

Types of Tumours

A benign tumour of epithelial tissue is named an *adenoma* and the malignant tumour of the tissue or glandular tissue is called *carcinoma* (cancer). Benign tumours of connective tissue are given names according to the tissue in which they form, such as *fibroma* (in fibrous tissue), *lipoma* (in fatty tissue) and *osteoma* (in bone). A malignant tumour occurring in connective tissue, for example, in bone is a *sarcoma*.

An early diagnosis of carcinoma means that treatment can begin immediately, and be more effective. For this reason a woman with a lump in the breast or irregular bleeding about the time of the menopause, and any patient who has some bleeding from the lungs, bladder or rectum, and loss of weight is advised to consult his or her general practitioner. When there is any possibility of malignant tumour, the patient is admitted to hospital at once for investigation and treatment.

Treatment is by various methods:
1. Surgery in which the tumour is removed.
2. Radiotherapy.
3. Hormones. Carcinoma of the breast and prostate gland are sometimes treated in this way.

Certain drugs are being developed which will destroy malignant cells, e.g. nitrogen mustard. These are called cytotoxic drugs.

CHAPTER 27 | RADIOTHERAPY

The rays in this form of treatment are from substances which occur in nature, such as radium, or are from substances made radio-active artificially, such as cobalt or iodine. Similar rays are also produced electrically in an X-ray tube (deep X-rays). People come in contact with a small amount of this radiation in their daily lives. In treatment large doses are used which injure unwanted and harmful cells permanently or prevent their reproduction.

Radiotherapy is used in some cases of carcinoma to destroy the malignant tumour or cells of tissues to which it has spread. This treatment will also reduce the size of simple tumours which cause symptoms by pressure on vital organs.

Methods used in Radiotherapy

1. X-ray treatment by means of machines which give out rays from:
    (a) radio-active sources, e.g. cobalt as in the Orbitron;
    (b) electrically generated sources as in the Linear Accelerator and Marconi Deep X-ray.
2. Radio-active Isotopes in solution, e.g. gold used by injection, iodine given by mouth.
3. Radio-active substances inserted into tissues, e.g. gold grains. (These remain in position permanently.)
4. Radio-active substances inserted into cavities, e.g. radium in the vagina. (This remains in position only a limited time.)

Side-effects of Radiation

(i) RADIATION SICKNESS may be due to the toxic effect of the breakdown of tissue. Diarrhoea is more usual when the trunk is treated. The patient is given plenty of fluids and rests in bed. Treatment is slowed down. Sometimes the patient responds to encouragement and help combined with general nursing care. Prochlorperazine (Stemetil) may be prescribed to counteract nausea and vomiting, and codeine phosphate for pain and diarrhoea.

(ii) White cells may be reduced in number, lowering the patient's resistance to infection; for this reason care is taken to avoid infection.

(iii) Reproductive organs, the testis or the ovary, may be affected by exposure to radiation, resulting in sterility. Menstruation ceases.

(iv) Skin effects take some time to appear and the patient is warned of this before he goes home if any changes are likely to occur. They include redness and itching of the skin, which may also be shed, and the falling out of hair.

In the nursing care of a patient being treated by radiotherapy it is necessary to prevent a moist and unhealthy skin. The skin is not washed while it is red following treatment and starch powder is applied. Zinc and castor oil ointment is used if the skin blisters or breaks. No heat (hot-water bottles or fomentations) should be applied to the skin. Adhesive strapping is also harmful. Friction on the area by tight clothing should be avoided. An unhealthy mouth is also avoided. Regular mouth washes and brushing the teeth and gums with a soft brush, are part of the nursing treatment. Members of staff who work in radiotherapy wards and departments use long-handled forceps when assembling the radium and the substances are transported in lead-lined carriers with a long strap supported by the shoulder. Doctors and nurses are quick and neat in their movements and the time spent near the radio-active substances is kept to a minimum. On the beds of patients who have radium inserted is a

sign The bedside care is shared between members of the

staff, and the nurse does not remain with the patient more than is necessary while radium is in position for the prescribed time.

Ward and department personnel wear an exposure plate or disc which is checked every two weeks and shows the amount of exposure to radiation.

FURTHER READING

First Aid

First Aid Manual. British Red Cross Society & St John Ambulance
  Brigade
Principles of First Aid for the Injured. Proctor & London. Butterworth
Nursing Emergencies. P.London. Blackwell

Medicines and Poisons

Modern Medicine for Nurses. J.Gibson. Blackwell
Medicine for Nurses. M.Toohey. Livingstone
A Guide to Drugs in Common Use. Trounce. M.T.P.

Surgery

Guide to Medical and Surgical Nursing. Bendall & Raybould. Lewis
Nurses Guide to Common Surgery. Cooke

Tumours and Radiotherapy

Handbook on Cancer for Nurses. R.Raven. Butterworth
Care of Patient in Diagnostic Radiography. D.N. & P.O.Chesney.
  Blackwell

SECTION 3 | STRUCTURE AND FUNCTIONS OF ORGANS: COMMON SIGNS AND SYMPTOMS: CLINICAL INVESTIGATIONS: SOME MEDICAL AND SURGICAL CONDITIONS WITH RELEVANT NURSING TECHNIQUES

CHAPTER 28 | STRUCTURE OF THE HUMAN BODY

CELLS

The body is made up of millions of tiny units of living substance called CELLS, which can be seen only with the aid of a microscope. All cells are surrounded by fluid (two-thirds of the body weight is water). From this fluid the cells obtain food and oxygen and their waste products are discharged into it. Within each cell is a *nucleus* which is responsible for the cell's life, growth and reproduction. The cell reproduces by dividing into two cells and these divide into four cells and so on.

In the human body some cells are quite simple but others are highly specialised.

A *tissue* is a collection of cells with the same shape and which behave in the same way. The fluid surrounding the cells is called *tissue fluid*.

An *organ* is a structure composed of various tissues which serve some special purpose, e.g. brain, liver, lung.

Types of Tissue in the Human Body

Epithelium is a covering or lining tissue and there are variations depending on the function of the issue. It forms the skin and lines the heart and blood vessels, the air passages, the food canal, the bladder, and the uterus in the female.

Connective tissues include the supporting adipose (fatty) tissue beneath the skin, fibrous and elastic tissue, and also cartilage (gristle) and bone.

Muscle tissue is of three types.

(a) *Striped* muscle which is red in colour, attached to the skeleton and is under the control of the will, i.e. it is voluntary muscle. An example is the biceps, a muscle of the arm.

(b) *Unstriped or plain muscle* which is involuntary. It is slower in action than striped muscle. An example is the muscle wall of the bladder.

(c) *Cardiac (heart) muscle* which is striped, red in colour and involuntary.

Nerve tissue is made up of cells which are called neurones.

Blood is a fluid tissue, the fluid part being plasma, the solid part being composed of red and white blood cells.

Germinal tissue produces mature germ cells during the reproductive phase in life. In the male, the testis produces the male germ cells (spermatozoa) and in the female, the ovary produces the egg cells (ova).

The Framework and Contents in the Human Body (Fig. 20)

The skeleton and muscles form the framework of the body with the skin as a covering. The bony structure of the head is the SKULL or CRANIUM which contains the brain. The spinal column contains the spinal cord.

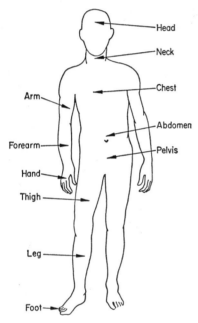

Figure 20. Main structure of the body.

In the trunk are three cavities:

The CHEST or THORAX containing two lungs, the heart, large blood vessels entering and leaving it, and the oesophagus.

The ABDOMEN containing the stomach, small and large intestines, the liver, gall-bladder, pancreas, spleen and two kidneys.

The PELVIS in which are situated the bladder and urethra, the rectum and anal canal, and in the female the uterus and vagina.

The upper and lower limbs project from the trunk and enable the individual to move and be in contact with his surroundings.

Membranes

Cavities and hollow organs are lined by membranes formed from epithelium. They secrete lubricating fluids which prevent friction between organs in which some movement takes places.

1. *Serous membranes* secrete serum, a slightly sticky fluid. These are found in the thorax as the *pleura* covering the lungs and heart, and in the abdomen as the *peritoneum* surrounding the organs in this cavity.

2. *Mucous membrane* secretes mucus and lines the food canal and air-passages.

3. *Synovial membrane* secretes synovial fluid in freely movable joints, e.g. knee, elbow.

The Systems of the Body

The cells of the body require food and oxygen in order to live and carry out their work. These substances are used in the cell, producing energy for work (function) and heat. Left behind after this activity are waste products: carbon dioxide, water and urea. From this point of view the body is like a motor engine. It needs petrol (like food) and air (oxygen) to work, producing power (energy) and heat. The waste products of the motor engine are a mixture of gases in the exhaust fumes. Like the motor engine the body can become very hot when it is active and needs to be cooled down. The motor engine is cooled by a draught of cool air or cool water (this latter is in the radiator). The body is cooled by its own production of water on the skin (sweat) and moving air round the body drying this.

The human body, however, encompasses a soul and mind; it can feel and think. When a person suffers injury, disease, ill-health, or disability, his reactions are not only those of the body tissues but also of feeling and thinking.

Some people suffer illness or disability of the mind (these are psychiatric conditions) and there are others who suffer crises of feeling (emotions) like fear, grief and guilt. These people may react by becoming ill in their bodies. It is this combination of reactions in a person who is very ill which makes nursing the sick a privileged and responsible type of work.

The work in the different systems of the body is divided as follows:

The *skeleton and muscles* enable the body to move about whilst finding food, providing shelter, protecting the weak and working for society, etc.

The *respiratory system* takes in the air and passes oxygen into the blood. It also rids the body of carbon dioxide and water.

The *digestive system* takes in food, breaks it down into tiny particles which dissolve in water and can be absorbed into the blood.

The *urinary system* rids the body of some waste products.

The *blood* carries food and oxygen to the tissues and waste products away from them. It also transports heat round the body. This fluid tissue reaches the cells through tubes called blood vessels and is pumped through these by the heart.

The *nervous system* organises and controls the body's activities by messages which pass from its cells along nerves to the different organs.

Control is also affected by means of chemical substances called hormones which are formed in special glands (endocrine glands) and circulate in the blood.

The body is aware of its surroundings through its sense organs, the *eyes, ears, nose* (smell), *skin* (touch) and *tongue* (taste).

The *skin* with its hair and nails covers the body and protects it.

Reproduction in the human takes place by the union of two different cells. The male reproductive organs produce one type of cell and the female the other type. In the two sexes the reproductive organs are different. The female reproductive system is also equipped for protecting the very young offspring until he is able to survive as a separate human being.

Function in these systems is disturbed in disease. Medicine is the study of disease and the practice of its prevention and treatment.

CHAPTER 29 | THE SKIN

This tissue covers and protects the body, and is continuous with the tissues lining the body cavities, e.g. the mouth. It is important as a characteristic of the individual's appearance; people of different races have skins which differ in colour, whilst some have scars resulting from wounds which may cause them some distress. A clear and healthy complexion is a physical and mental asset.

In health the skin is warm and soft to touch, and neither very moist nor very dry in average air temperature.

Frequently the skin is one of the first parts of the body to be observed and examined by the doctor and nurse when the person becomes ill. The signs then noted may assist in the forming of a diagnosis and in determining the patient's progress.

The Structure of the Skin

The part of the skin we see is the EPIDERMIS (epi=outer, dermis=skin) and this is made up of layers of cells. The deepest layer is the germinal or basal layer and it is from this layer that the cells above grow. The cells in the upper layers have no nuclei (the nucleus is the essential living part of a cell), and have changed into a horny substance which is waterproof. The epidermal cells on the surface are being continually rubbed off, and are replaced by more cells which grow from the basal layer. This layer also contains the pigment which gives colour to the skin. In fair-skinned people there is little colour in the basal layer of epidermal cells but in those with a dark skin or who have become tanned in the sun the cells contain various amounts of the pigment or colouring matter. The colour in dark-skinned races is permanent, being due to a characteristic inherited from the parents, but the tan from the sun's rays disappears when the exposure to the sun ceases.

The epidermis varies in thickness and is thickest on the soles of the feet and palms of the hands where friction is greatest. There is a network of ridges below the epidermis forming a pattern and this may be seen as a fingerprint.

The DERMIS or true skin lies below the epidermis and contains many small blood and lymphatic vessels. These blood vessels can dilate and then contain a large amount of blood (the skin appears flushed), or constrict, causing the circulation to the surface of the body to be lessened (the skin appears pale). Tiny blood vessels (capillaries) surround the sweat glands and hair roots (Fig. 21).

Apart from the cells forming the dermis there are also fat cells (adipose tissue). Usually there is more adipose tissue under the skin in women than in men and for that reason women are more resistant to cold. Excess fat in the body is stored here, and this helps to protect the structures below the skin.

Within the skin structures are hairs, special oils glands (sebaceous glands which secrete an oily substance called sebum), sweat glands and the nails.

The NAILS are formed from epidermal cells which have no nuclei and are horny in texture. They grow from the nail root, but the dermis forms the bed of the nail and this has many nerve endings of pain so that, although there is no pain or discomfort when the nails are cut, damage or infection of the nail-bed is extremely painful.

HAIRS grow from the epidermal cells. The hair root is nourished by the blood in the capillaries surrounding it, but the hair itself is kept healthy by the oily substance from small glands lying close to the hair (Fig. 22).

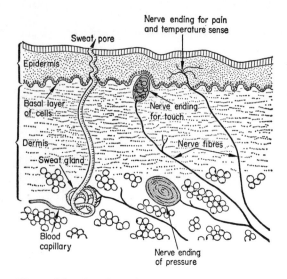

Figure 21. The skin, showing a sweat gland and nerve endings.

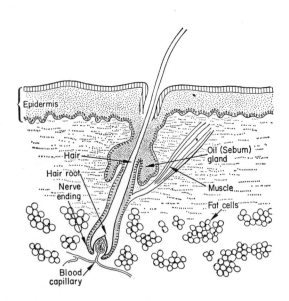

Figure 22. The skin, showing a hair and its oil glands.

Nerves enter and leave at the hair roots and most people have a sensation of pain when the hair is pulled. The hair itself has no blood vessels or nerves, so does not bleed or cause pain when cut.

The colour of the hair, as in the skin, depends on inheritance of the characteristic from the parents (but there are artificial means of colouring or bleaching hair).

Hair covers the whole of the body but is of two types, that which grows long and is replaced infrequently, and that which is short and replaced by new hair frequently. Hair on the scalp grows long except in some men in whom it is replaced by very short hair (baldness). After puberty hair growth develops in the axillae and pubic area in both sexes. In men it grows thick and long on the face as a beard.

In animals the hair (or fur or wool) is important in protecting the animal's body, but in man this is not so, and he wears clothes to keep warm.

Hair can be very beautiful and then adds to an individual's appearance.

SEBACEOUS GLANDS produce sebum, an oily substance, and are found close to the hair tube. The sebum protects and nourishes the hair and also prevents water from entering the body through the skin.

SWEAT GLANDS. These are coiled tubes and special cells in the tiny organs make sweat from the blood in the capillaries surrounding them. They are large and most numerous in the arm-pits, on the palms of the hands, soles of the feet, forehead and upper lip.

SWEAT is mostly water with some salt (sodium chloride) and a few waste products from the blood. The average amount produced in twenty-four hours is about one pint (540 millilitres).

When sweat flows on to the skin through the pores, it evaporates in the air, and does this very quickly when there is a draught of air. This evaporation cools the body. As the sweat dries the salt and small amount of waste products are left on the skin. If sweating is excessive or the body is not washed often enough, there is a characteristic odour.

Functions of the Skin
1. The skin protects the body
    (a) against friction and some injury, e.g. slight burns;
    (b) from water surrounding it;
    (c) from disease-producing bacteria (i.e. germs);
    (d) from harmful rays of the sun.
2. It is a sense organ connected by nerves to the brain, and through the skin we can touch, feel pain, and know whether articles or the air or water in contact with the skin are hot or cold.
3. The body loses heat by the drying of sweat on the surface of the skin,

and by heat passing out from it into the clothing which then becomes warm.

4. Fat, water and salt (sodium chloride) are stored in the skin.

5. Vitamin D produced by action of sun's rays on skin.

General Care of the Skin in Health

NUTRITION (i.e. enough of the right kind of food) is very important to the skin as the cells need to be replaced continually as they wear out. In the diet it is necessary to have protein, i.e. meat, fish, cheese or eggs—two portions a day, and then as much variety as possible but especially some fresh fruits and vegetables.

For foodstuffs digested in the body to reach the skin there needs to be a satisfactory blood CIRCULATION and this in the healthy person is maintained by *exercise*. The circulation of blood to the scalp is improved by hair-brushing, combing and massaging with the finger-tips.

PROTECTION against injury, friction, chemicals, burns and pressure is necessary, otherwise a wound may occur and through this, other structures are damaged, or disease-producing bacteria may pass through and cause infection. The body is protected against harm in these ways:

(a) by preventing the danger situation from occurring;

(b) by using special clothing or equipment as protection;

(c) by using first-aid treatment quickly and efficiently after an accident.

CLEANLINESS of the skin greatly reduces the number of disease-producing bacteria on the skin and so aids protection. However, at the same time, it is necessary *not* to harm the skin by using strong alkali soaps, or remove all the natural oils from the skin, or leave the skin damp, especially where two skin surfaces touch, e.g. between the toes.

The skin is kept clean by washing all the skin surfaces every day with soap and warm water in a bath, or large bowl or under a shower, and rinsing and drying thoroughly with a dry towel. Parts of the body exposed to dust and dirt (hands and face) and the parts near excretory orifices, e.g. anus, are cleansed more frequently as necessary.

When the skin is dry, i.e. lacks the natural oils, then these are replaced by application of a grease (e.g. lanolin) or a skin cream. The hands, especially in the winter, need special attention such as frequent use of hand cream. Barrier creams are helpful when the hands are exposed to water.

It is sensible to ensure that the clothes, especially those next to the skin, should also be clean.

Young children, especially boys, do not always appreciate being washed with soap and water, but most people of all ages find the contact of water on the skin pleasant and enjoy baths, showers and bathing in the sea, rivers or the local swimming baths. Fear, however, can remove this pleasure, so it is wise to avoid a situation in which a child learns to become afraid of water. This may happen when he is exposed to too much, too hot or too cold water, or he is splashed with water.

General Care of the Skin During Illness

The same principles in caring for the skin apply in illness as in health, but modifications are made as special problems arise and the nurse expects to give the patient's skin more attention at this time. In health, the person thinks little of the care for his skin and most of it is carried out in his daily habits, but these are interrupted when he is ill.

NUTRITION. The diet is frequently smaller in quantity than usual, because the patient's appetite may be less, he may be unable to eat or digest the food, or his treatment may not allow it. Even though the patient eats less, he needs protein in the diet except in special cases. If he can take only a fluid diet there are proprietary foods which can be added to milk, such as Casilan (protein). Complan is a preparation which contains all the nutrients in suitable proportions. It is made up with water. Vitamins A and C are important in healthy skin; vitamin A is in fatty foods and vitamin C in fresh fruit, orange juice or blackcurrant syrup, and fresh vegetables.

CIRCULATION OF THE BLOOD through the vessels in the skin is different when the patient cannot move. Then the nurses change his position at least every two hours, day and night, and it is beneficial to massage the skin at the same time with a dry, powdered hand or with a little moisturising cream.

Often the doctor requests the physiotherapist to exercise the patient's joints to prevent them from becoming stiff and the skin over them from becoming sore. She encourages and assists the patient in performing movements himself.

PROTECTION (a) *Against dampness.* If the patient is sweating or incontinent of urine or faeces or both, then as soon as the skin becomes wet it is washed clean and dried thoroughly and gently with a dry towel. Skin surfaces which touch each other are likely to become sore unless the skin is kept quite dry. A barrier cream (e.g. anhydrous lanoline, zinc cream and castor oil, silicone cream or spray) is useful as it forms a waterproof covering over the skin. The clothing and bed-linen are also changed.

(b) *Against friction.* If the knees or toes are rubbed by the bed-clothes, a cradle in the bed will raise these from the legs. Ankles may need to be wrapped in soft wool and lightly bandaged. Socks, comfortable but not tight, are useful for elderly patients, but must be removed at least twice a day and the feet, especially the heels, inspected for redness and then massaged well. A special type of sock has a foam rubber lining. A small piece of sheepskin bandaged over the heel can be helpful.

(c) *Against pressure.* This may be due to the pressure of the patient's body on the bed, especially if he be very heavy, or unable to move or be moved. Then special mattresses are considered, e.g. Dunlopillo or a water bed, or an additional appliance such as a ripple bed. This latter is in sections and, by means of a machine, contains varying pressures of air which are continually changing. This means there is no long-continued pressure against one particular part of the skin. Another type has sections the length of the bed which inflate and deflate alternately by means of a machine every 15 minutes. Beds which can be modified to fit the patient's contours, such as plaster of paris and block-pillow beds, also assist in the problem. Air-rings, water pillows, or foam rubber cushions are useful for various patients.

Pressure may be due to equipment in the bed. The bar of a cradle may be placed so that it presses against the leg, or there are wrinkles in the draw sheet or the patient's night clothes. Appliances in treatment also can cause pressure, including bandages applied in folds or twists over pressure areas, or an inadequately padded splint. Even crumbs left in a bed can cause a small area of pressure, and a bed-sore can easily form in skin which is already not in good health and subjected to pressure from the weight of the body on the bed.

CLEANLINESS. This is so much more important during illness when the individual has less resistance to infection. In fever or in pain he needs the comfort of a clean and comfortable skin.

If it is possible, the patient is bathed in bed once a day. The time varies according to the ward timetable but it is usually during the morning or early afternoon. He is washed or washes himself in the early morning or evening, and the hands are washed before meals if possible, and always after using a bed-pan.

If the patient is allowed out of bed, he may be taken to the bath by the male nurse or may be well enough to bath himself with some supervision. Besides washing and drying the skin, the hair is brushed and combed, the nails are trimmed as necessary and the teeth cleaned.

Female patients appreciate an attractive hair arrangement, and those in hospital for a long period of time need a hair shampoo every week even if they are helpless in bed. A visiting hairdresser may be able to give her a 'home-perm', and trim or re-style her hair. Long hair is best arranged in two plaits so that the patient does not lie on the bulky hair. Gentle brushing of the hair can be very soothing to a patient who does not rest easily. Most women, unless they are very ill, also appreciate being able to use some cosmetics and in most cases this is permissible, though it can be misleading when applied creams and powders, etc. disguise a very pale skin.

Male patients shave or are shaved every day, and a visiting barber will also trim their hair and beard, should the patient have grown one.

A patient who, for some reason, may have lost his or her hair, wears a wig or toupée. These are expensive and need special handling. The nurse remembers that the patient may be sensitive about this and she respects his confidence by her discretion.

The state of the skin and hair has a great effect on the patient's morale and is especially important for this reason in convalescence and in long-term illness.

Observations on the Skin

On Admission to Hospital
Colour: the patient's skin may be pale, or flushed, or yellow (jaundiced) or blue (cyanosed).

Moist or dry: sweating occurs readily on the forehead and palms, so the nurse can place the back of her hand (which is dry) against either of these areas.

Warm or cold: the skin can be hot and dry or warm and moist, or dry and cold, or cold and moist (clammy).

After an accident, the nurse inspects the patient's skin for *wounds*, however small and insignificant, and any bleeding is noted and reported at once.

When a patient has been ill for some time it is useful to know on admission whether his pressure areas are in a satisfactory condition.

Rashes, also scars from previous injuries or operations are noted; the former are especially important in infants and children for there is the possibility of an infectious fever causing the illness.

The nurse observes also the general cleanliness of the skin. A rapid examination of the hair, either by looking at it carefully or if in doubt fine tooth-combing, will show any head-lice if the hair be infested. Occasionally a patient may have body lice but these are found in the seams of clothing. Pubic lice are found in the hair of the body.

Observations of the Skin while the patient is in hospital are usually made while the patient is being bathed in bed or in the bathroom or during bed-making. He may complain of discomfort, itching, etc. and the nurse will then examine the skin. The skin is also examined if she wishes to note the progress of treatment, e.g. for a rash, or for the prevention of bed-sores.

Problems can arise for the patient who sits in a chair during the day. This patient is likely to suffer from pressure and the lack of blood circulation in the skin as much as the patient in bed, so his position is changed at intervals. This may be done by moving his weight from one hip to the other and altering the position of his arms and legs. The chair should be a suitable size and height with a high back and arm rests. Pillows, cushions and foot-rests are available aids.

Conditions Affecting the Skin

WOUNDS. A wound is a break in the skin. It may be extensive, e.g. in burns. It is painful because nerve endings of pain in the skin are stimulated during injury. Structures below the skin may be damaged at the same time, e.g. muscle, bone, internal organs. Part of these may appear through the skin (as bone in a compound fracture), or an object may have entered through the wound from outside, e.g. clothing, knife-blade, or pellets from an airgun.

Dangers and Problems of Wounds
A blood vessel may have been ruptured causing *haemorrhage*, and bleeding from an artery is very serious. Where much skin surface is involved or the skin is well supplied with nerve endings of pain (see Anatomy of Skin) there will be severe *pain* and this is a factor in producing the state of *shock*. Loss of fluid from the wounds, e.g. as tissue fluid in burns, can also bring about the condition of *shock*. Disease-producing bacteria can enter the body through a wound and give rise to *infection*. If the wound affects the epidermis only, healing will take place, the destroyed cells being replaced from the basal layer; but if the wound affects the dermis and basal layer cells are destroyed, then the epidermal cells are not replaced by their own kind of cells, but by fibrous tissue. This is a *scar* and it may extend the full depth of the wound into dermis and the tissue below it. The scar, unlike normal skin, is inelastic and contractures may form, often causing disability or alterations in the person's appearance.

Delay in healing is another problem which may be encountered. Normal healing of the skin takes place in five to ten days, depending on the site of wound and favourable conditions. If a wound does not heal normally then the cause may be due to poor nutrition of the patient, a foreign body retained in the wound, friction over the wound or too much muscle activity below it, or infection introduced through the wound or from below the surface of the skin (e.g. an abscess or blood-borne infection).

Wounds do not heal quickly when the person is or has been exposed to *irradiation*.

Prevention of the Dangers and Problems of Wounds

Haemorrhage. A wound and the dressing over it is observed frequently if necessary for bleeding. If severe haemorrhage begins, methods of arresting haemorrhage (*see* First Aid) are applied quickly, efficiently and without fuss. The patient is laid flat, disturbed as little as possible physically and mentally, and medical aid is summoned at once. If the amount of bleeding is small but tends to continue over a period of time it may become as serious as a severe haemorrhage. Pressure over the wound by thick dressings and a firm bandage is a method of preventing further bleeding of this type.

Pain. A nurse learns to recognise the signs of suffering in a patient and this is important when a patient is too ill or distressed to explain, when the patient is very young, very old, delirious or does not know the language in use. She reports the incidence of pain to the ward sister, who informs the medical officer. The nurse can relieve some pain by the application of gentle warmth and by making the patient comfortable until the medical officer orders treatment. To prevent shock from becoming severe, pain is relieved, the patient is disturbed as little as possible, and he is exposed to a temperature which is neither too high nor too low (hot-water bottles and exposure are both unsuitable procedures). Loss of fluid is assessed if possible and replacement is by intra-venous infusion.

Infection is prevented by providing a clean environment: sterile dressings applied securely over the wound and a non-touch technique of dressing the wound, whilst drugs such as antibiotics may be ordered by the doctor.

Scars are prevented by removing all the factors which delay healing, and sometimes by replacement of the skin loss by skin-grafting.

BED-SORES are wounds resulting from a period of time spent in bed during illness. Redness of the skin indicates the possibility of a bed-sore, and the main causes of the wound are poor nutrition, pressure of the body on the bed, friction and moisture (*see* p. 231), General Care of the Skin during Illness). There are various degrees of bed-sores, from an abrasion in which the epidermal layer only is affected, to the destruction of the basal layer, the dermis and the subcutaneous tissue below the dermis. Frequently the wound becomes infected and then a *slough* appears. This is a mass including dead tissue cells which prevents healing and needs to be removed either by lotions or surgically. As with all infected wounds there is an absorption into the body circulation of toxins (poisonous substances), and this means that bed-sores can cause a patient's condition to deteriorate or prevent his normal progress in addition to causing him pain and discomfort. Every method available is used to prevent them from occurring. Sometimes it is a very difficult task, particularly in some diseases which involve the blood circulation or nervous system, and when patients are very thin or obese, or are incontinent of urine or faeces or both.

Infections of the Skin

A BOIL is an infection of a hair follicle and the organism most frequently causing it is the staphylococcus. There may previously have been friction over the area, producing first a small abrasion. Dampness can aggravate the condition. Commonly affected areas are the face and arm-pit, but tiny boils (furuncles) occur in the nose and ear and are extremely painful. Pain is due to swelling, and this decreases when the pus formed breaks out through the skin as a purulent discharge.

Treatment is as for a wound. In addition heat may be prescribed as short-wave diathermy (a treatment carried out by a physiotherapist). Antibiotics may be ordered by the doctor if the condition is severe, and when pus is formed this may be released by incising with a scalpel under aseptic conditions. A general anaesthetic may be necessary.

Any underlying cause is investigated and treated—this calls for general observation and includes testing the urine for glucose.

A number of boils close together is called a carbuncle and this can occur in the nape of the neck or on the upper lip. The latter may lead to complications and the patient requires expert attention. On no account must septic spots or boils be squeezed, especially those between nose, cheek and lip, as the pus may be pressed inward into a vein and enter the blood stream.

ABSCESSES can form in any loose tissue including subcutaneous tissue, i.e. tissue under the skin. Staphylococci, streptococci or bacilli coli can be the causative organisms and these can come either from outside the body, e.g. by using a contaminated syringe needle, or from within the patient's own body through the blood stream. They are incised so that the pus can drain away and a rubber tube will assist in this, and then healing takes place. The patient feels generally rather ill, and, as in all infections, some rest, attention to diet and care with cleanliness are necessary.

Infection at the side of the nail is called a WHITLOW and is very painful. During recovery the patient may lose his finger-nail and this will be replaced by new cells growing up from the nail root.

Infection of an eye-lash tube is a STYE.

IMPETIGO is a skin condition caused by streptococci or staphylococci. A rash appears as blisters which burst and a watery fluid flows from the affected part. This is very irritating and the patient, who is usually a child, scratches the area, which then becomes more heavily infected. The discharge dries up and becomes a scab and before the condition can be treated efficiently, e.g. by penicillin application or an antiseptic lotion, the scabs should be removed by using prescribed lotions.

FOREIGN OBJECTS, e.g. sewing needles, fish-hooks, gun-shot, gravel (after road accidents). These require surgical removal in some cases, e.g. fish-hooks. Special techniques are required so that further damage is avoided. To prevent penetration of the object into deeper tissue the limb is not moved; for instance if a sewing needle has entered the foot the patient must not walk on that foot. X-ray examination is required.

Gravel in the skin may be removed by brushing the area with a soft nail-brush and a detergent antiseptic such as cetrimide.

BURNS are caused by dry heat, e.g. strong sunlight, fire, electric current, and SCALDS by moist heat, e.g. boiling water and steam. They may affect the epidermis only, causing redness, or include part of the dermis, when blisters develop (tissue fluid collecting between the epidermis and dermis) and these burst later leaving a raw area from which tissue fluid escapes, or the subcutaneous and deeper tissues are exposed. The larger the area the more serious the burn and hospital treatment either as an in-patient or an out-patient is advisable (*see* p. 157, First Aid).

SCARS have already been mentioned (*see* p. 234).

COSMETIC DEFORMITIES OF THE SKIN include birth-marks and hare-lip. The skin specialist and plastic surgeon treat these conditions while the child is young, e.g. six to twelve months old. Skin deformities in the adult are usually due to injury, or scars following injury.

PLASTIC SURGERY. This branch of surgery has developed considerably in the last thirty years. Not only are scars and skin deformities dealt with but also other tissue loss. For instance, following severe injuries bone and cartilage and fat can be grafted on to the body in addition to the skin graft.

Skin for grafting is taken from another area of the patient's body, e.g. the thigh, but sometimes the plastic surgeon applies skin from a relative when the damaged area is large. The skin does not grow on to the patient, but beneath it the patient's own skin begins to develop over the wound, and the graft from the relative finally falls away leaving a healing area behind.

RASHES IN COMMUNICABLE DISEASES. These diseases can be passed from one person to another. Some of them are characterised by a rash and these include the infectious fevers. Observations of the skin during childhood fever can assist in making a diagnosis. For example:

In *measles* the brownish red rash first appears behind the ears and along the hair-line, and then in blotchy irregular patches over the face and trunk.

In *chicken-pox* small red spots quickly develop into blisters which become pustules and later dry up forming brownish crusts. They are seen mainly on the trunk.

Small-pox is a severe illness and extremely infectious. It is uncommon in this country since methods of hygiene improved and vaccination was introduced. The rash is severe and appears as small spots mainly on the limbs and face. Within a week the blisters and pustules following these have formed crusts which are closely fixed to the skin. The patient is very ill and requires skilled nursing while in complete isolation.

An ULCER is a small area of loss of epithelial tissue, e.g. skin, mouth. There are several causes. Most ulcers heal quickly with appropriate treatment and general hygiene. However, if a person has an ulcer which does not heal in a few weeks, he should be advised to consult his doctor as special treatment may be required and early diagnosis aids in speedy recovery.

A MOLE is an overgrowth of a small area of skin. It is present from birth, is often dark in colour and may have a few hairs. It is often merely a personal characteristic but if a mole changes in appearance the person should be advised to see his doctor.

DERMATITIS is inflammation of the skin. This condition usually results from a substance coming in contact with the skin when the individual has acquired a sensitivity to this particular substance. The skin is red, may be 'puffy' and there is itching. The doctor treats the cause when this is found and the patient is advised to avoid contact with the substance.

Nursing Procedures

HEAT APPLIED TO THE SKIN
1. To relieve pain.
2. To treat local inflammation.
The cause of the pain is treated and the application of heat may be continued until this is effective. Analgesics may be prescribed for pain but these are sometimes inadvisable or make the patient feel ill.

Infection is less common now and when it does occur is quickly treated by appropriate antibiotics.

There are various methods of applying heat:

Dry Heat
(a) By 60-watt bulb in a lamp six inches from the skin to relieve pain in earache. There should be no possibility of movement of the lamp or the patient, and the skin is observed to avoid so much exposure as to cause reddening.

(b) *Electric pads* can be thermostatically controlled at the prescribed heat. Cotton covers are disinfected after use by a patient. The pads are applied direct to the area but are not allowed to be in contact with moisture, which can conduct electricity. These are useful in relieving pain and inflammation in some eye conditions and those affecting muscles or joints.

(c) Hot-water bottles, half filled with hot water. The air is pressed out from the bottle which is then covered with *two* flannel bags so that the skin does not become reddened. In pain the patient's skin can become insensitive to heat, and his observations are of little value. The nurse tests the hot-water bottle herself and the patient is not permitted to remove the covers.

Moist Heat
Most poultices have been replaced by methods using dry heat as described or as practised by the physiotherapist in radiant heat or infra-red treatments, which are prescribed by the doctor. Short-wave diathermy is treatment by which heat penetrates the skin to the site of pain or inflammation beneath, and is most effective. Special equipment is required and a trained physiotherapist carries out the treatment.

Kaolin Poultices
Kaolin is a special clay reduced to a powder and mixed with glycerine and certain oils including peppermint. The required amount in a container is heated in a saucepan, then spread to $\frac{1}{4}$- to $\frac{1}{2}$-inch thickness on

a piece of old linen or lint cut to the required size. It is tested to make sure it is not too hot, applied to the skin, covered with wool and remains for four hours. After it is removed the skin is washed with soap and water. The poultice can be renewed if necessary.

APPLICATION OF MEDICATIONS TO THE SKIN

The medications are either in a grease foundation such as lanoline, or as a lotion with water or glycerine added.

Ointments can be used by direct application to the skin. A thin film of the ointment is spread over the skin using a spatula, lint swabs or sometimes the fingers. The grease in the medication softens as it becomes warm on the skin. Excess ointment should be avoided; it cannot be absorbed, and is unpleasant. If the application is coloured, it may be advisable to cover the skin with thin cotton and a loose bandage to prevent staining linen.

Ointment remaining from a previous application is removed with arachis oil or soap and water before a fresh application is made.

Lotions, e.g. calamine may be applied with cotton wool swabs and left to dry. Frequent application is necessary.

Some lotions are applied by damping a large piece of cotton material such as muslin or lint, placing it over the skin and bandaging loosely over it. These applications are usually renewed when they have dried.

It is important that the medications are applied only to the area of skin prescribed for this treatment, and care is taken that no trickles of lotion or smears of ointment remain on other parts of the body.

Observations are made following the application for possible skin reaction such as reddening, swelling or a rash either over the area or surrounding it. Complaints of pain, discomfort and intense itching when the area is covered by a bandage should be investigated.

CHAPTER 30 | MOVEMENT

Muscles, Bones and Joints

Movement is brought about by the functioning of MUSCLE TISSUE the cells of which become shorter, i.e. contract, in response to a stimulus through a nerve fibre. When the stimulus stops the cells return to their original length. Not all the cells in a muscle contract at the same time, and some cells appear to be held in reserve. Like other cells, muscle cells need oxygen and food, and in extremely large quantities during physical exercise. Consequently during exercise the heart beats faster and the blood pressure in the arteries rises, so that the blood supply to the muscles is increased. When the muscle is subjected to excessive and continued stimulation, the contractions of the cells become less rapid and weaker so that eventually the muscle will not contract in response to stimulus. This is *muscle fatigue* and its treatment is *rest*. Normally, the muscles are never completely relaxed, but in a state of partial contraction. This *muscle tone* is important in preparing the body for swift action, protecting organs like bones, blood vessels and nerves, and is the basis of good posture.

General muscle action and muscle tone are improved by training in correct regular exercise either in one's work or recreation. Lying in bed or sitting in a relaxed position for long periods of time results in loss of muscle tone and efficiency.

FUNCTIONS OF MUSCLES (Fig. 23)
1. To enable the body to move.

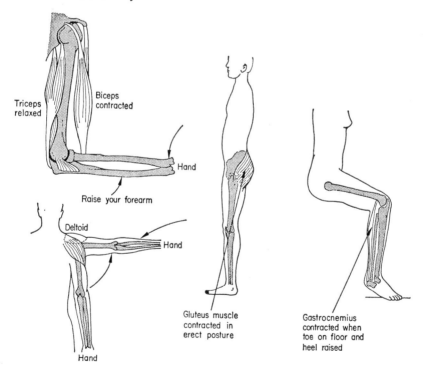

Figure 23. Movement—muscles, bones, joints.

2. During activity the muscles increase the flow of blood along the veins by pressing and squeezing them, and assist in the return of blood to the heart.
3. Muscles in tone maintain the body's correct posture.
4. They provide part of the warmth in the body; when the body is cold the muscles contract to produce heat (shivering).

The framework of the body is the SKELETON which is made up of rigid structures, the bones. These organs begin to develop before birth, though the long bones are not fully developed until physical maturity is complete at 21 years. Protein and calcium are necessary for proper development of bone, and so are important in the diet of pregnant women, women breast-feeding their infants, growing children and adolescents. Calcium does not become part of bone tissue unless vitamin D is in the diet or produced in the skin by the action of sunlight.

The surface of bone is hard and durable, but inside this compact layer is a spongy structure which contains red bone marrow. In the centre of the shaft of a long bone is a cavity in which fat is deposited (yellow bone marrow) (Fig. 24). Each bone has a blood supply and tiny openings can

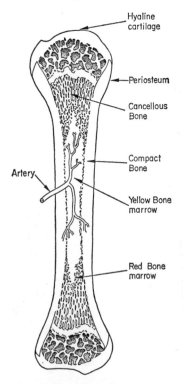

Figure 24. A long bone.

be seen in the surface of the bone through which arteries enter during life. In the body there are bones of varying sizes and shapes depending on their situation and function.

THE FUNCTIONS OF THE SKELETON

1. To provide, with the muscles, the means by which the body or parts of the body can move.
2. The protection of vital or delicate tissues and organs.
3. To produce, in the red bone marrow within the flat bones and at the ends of the long bones, the white blood cells.

The skeleton and muscles give shape to the body.

Usually the muscles end in *tendons* by which they are attached to the bones. *Ligaments* are strong bands of tissue which hold the bones together and prevent unwanted movement between them. Where the bones actually come into contact with each other are the *joints*, and these are characterised by varying degrees of movement determined by the fashion in which the joints are formed. Those where there is little or no movement have a thin layer of fibrous tissue between the bone surface and are therefore known as *fibrous joints* (Fig. 25), e.g. between the bones of the skull. *Cartilaginous joints* (Fig. 25) allow slight movement, e.g. where the ribs are joined to the breast-bone.

There is free movement at the *synovial joints* (Fig. 25), e.g. the knee, shoulder and hip. The bone surfaces concerned in these joints are covered with thin, smooth cartilage to ensure smooth movement without friction. Attached to these and forming a bag of fluid between the bone surfaces is the synovial membrane; in this way the joint is lubricated. A capsule of fibrous tissue encloses the joint and keeps the bone surfaces close together. Ligaments are outside the joint attached to the bones and these strengthen and stabilise the joint and prevent unwanted movement.

Bones and Muscles of the Head and Neck

The *skull* or cranium is box-shaped and formed from 8 bones, the fibrous joints between these (sutures) allowing no movement. As the basis for the forehead is the *frontal bone*, the two *parietal bones* are upper part of the cranium, and the *occipital bone* is posterior. These form the *vault of the skull* which covers and protects the brain. The remaining bones, with part of the frontal and occipital bones, are the *base of the skull* which supports the brain and accommodates the blood vessels and nerves passing to and from this vital organ. The frontal bone protects the eyes and within the temporal bones at either side of the head is the hearing apparatus.

The *bones of the face* are irregular in shape, and except for the lower jaw (mandible) are united by immovable joints. The cheek bones with the frontal bone protect the eyes. Teeth develop in the upper and lower jaws, 24 in the child, erupting from about 5 months onwards, and 32 in the adult.

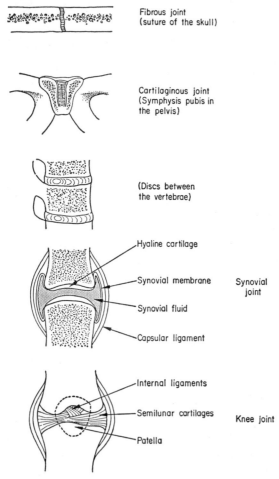

Fibrous joint
(suture of the skull)

Cartilaginous joint
(Symphysis pubis in
the pelvis)

(Discs between
the vertebrae)

Hyaline cartilage

Synovial membrane   Synovial
                           joint
Synovial fluid

Capsular ligament

Internal ligaments

Semilunar cartilages   Knee joint

Patella

Figure 25. Joints.

In the neck are the 7 cervical vertebrae of the spine. The upper two (atlas and axis) form a synovial joint which allows a side-to-side movement of the head, and the atlas supports the skull, at which joint 'nodding' can take place.

Muscles of *facial expressions* are small and attached to bone and skin. Those which surround the eyes are circular and when contracted 'screw up the eyes'. Similarly, contraction of the muscle round the mouth results in 'pursing of the lips'. Combinations of muscles in the eye-sockets control the movements of the eyeballs.

The lower jaw is attached to the skull by strong muscles, and the movements produced by these and other muscles of the face and mouth are made in biting and chewing (mastication) and in speaking. The *tongue* is a muscle attached to the lower jaw which pushes food between the teeth besides being necessary for speech. On either side of the neck are the *sterno mastoid muscles* and when these contract together the chin is brought down to the chest. The upper pointed part of the *trapezius* shoulder muscle is behind the neck.

The *spinal column* consists of 27 to 28 bones, the vertebrae. 7 cervical, 12 thoracic, 5 lumbar, 1 sacral, and 2 or 3 in the coccyx. They are intricate in shape to allow for the passage of the spinal cord through the centre of the spinal column. In this way it is protected from ordinary injury. Between the vertebrae are discs of cartilage which allow movement and form buffers between the bones. They prevent force or vibration travelling along the spine from the feet to the head as the body comes in contact with the ground after falling or jumping from a height as well as during the ordinary movements of walking or running. Ligaments and muscles join the vertebrae together and the result is a bony structure having great mobility combined with strength.

The muscles of the back include the *trapezius* muscles which draw the head and shoulders backwards and stabilise the shoulder girdle when weights are lifted. The latissimus dorsi pulls the arm backwards or down if it is raised, and the gluteal muscles which form the buttocks straighten the hip joint and/or move the leg outwards. Long, strong muscles of the back keep the spine erect.

Movements which are Possible in the Spinal Column

Flexion	— bending forwards
Extension	— bending backwards
Lateral movements	— side to side
Rotating movements	— twisting the trunk
Circumduction	— swaying in a circular movement while facing forward

The THORAX is a cavity enclosed within walls of bone and muscle. Posteriorly is part of the spine, the twelve dorsal vertebrae, in a curve which accommodates the lungs and heart. To the spine are attached by

I

movable joints twelve pairs of ribs which join the breastbone (sternum) at the front to form a cage. To make some movement possible as the lungs expand during breathing, the ribs are joined to the sternum by strips of cartilage, a tissue not so rigid as bone. Between the ribs are muscles which, as they contract, cause the ribs to be raised upwards and outwards, and the chest expands in circumference. The base of the thorax is a circular dome-shaped muscle, the *diaphragm*, attached to the lower spine, ribs and the tip of the sternum. In contraction it flattens and increases the chest cavity from top to bottom, and inspiration takes place. The mediastinum is a space between the breastbone and the spine in which are lodged the heart, aorta, venae cavae, the oesophagus, lymph vessels and nodes.

Outside the rib cage in front of the chest are two *pectoralis* muscles which bring the upper limbs towards the front of the body.

Surmounting the chest and supporting the upper limbs is the *shoulder girdle*. This is formed from two clavicles (collar bones) and the two scapulae (shoulder blades), the clavicles' point of fixation being the sternum. Between the shoulder blades is a gap and this means the shoulders are extremely mobile. Strong muscles are attached to the shoulder girdle. The skeleton of THE UPPER LIMB is composed of the humerus in the arm, the radius (above the thumb) and the ulna (above the little finger) in the forearm, the 8 carpal (wrist) bones, and the bones of the hand of which there are five metacarpals in the hand, 3 phalanges in each finger and 2 in the thumb.

The head of the humerus articulates within the socket of the scapula in a synovial joint, which has very full movement. Above the shoulder joint is a large muscle, the *deltoid*, and when this contracts the arm is raised.

The *biceps* flexes the elbow and is used in turning the palm of the hand upwards. The *triceps* works in the opposite direction to the biceps and extends the elbow; they act in conjunction with each other to produce a precise movement. Another flexor of the elbow is the brachialis and flexion at the elbow is a strong movement.

Flexors and extensors of the forearm and hand are in frequent use; their tendons are surrounded by sheaths containing a little fluid as lubrication.

Below the thorax and separated from it by the diaphragm is the ABDOMEN. This is a box-like cavity enclosed by muscles and supported posteriorly by the lumbar spine. In front is the strong muscle, the *rectus abdominis*, attached to the sternum and the pubic bones and in the centre line of which is the umbilicus. Between the rectus and the lumbar spine are the *abdominal muscles* with fibres passing in three different directions and forming a support for the abdominal organs (like a corset). The roof of the box is the diaphragm, the floor is the *pelvic diaphragm* through which passes the anal canal at the end of the alimentary tract and which supports the pelvic organs. These muscles are normally in good tone but this lessens as one grows older. They contract when standing upright, in rotatory movements of the trunk, and are necessary to breathing and lifting weights,. These muscles are used in micturition, defaecation and in a woman during childbirth. The pelvic diaphragm is a funnel-shaped muscle attached to the pelvic girdle. This firm, bony structure is formed from the two innominate bones of the hips and the sacrum at the base of the spine. It protects and supports the organs of the pelvis, the bladder, the rectum and the reproductive organs, and it forms attachment for the lower limbs in synovial joints with some free movements, but also a great deal of stability when the body is standing, walking, running, etc.

The bones of the lower limb are the femur in the thigh, the tibia and fibula in the leg, the seven tarsal (ankle) bones, five metatarsals in the foot and fourteen phalanges in the toes.

In the thigh the muscles are long and in most instances can produce movement at both hip and knee. The gluteal muscles (buttock) are hip extensors as well as being extensors of the spine. *Quadriceps extensor* muscles straighten the knee and they can flex the hip. They are anterior to the thigh and in their lower tendon is the knee-cap (patella). Acting in the opposite manner are the *hamstrings* posterior in the thigh, which flex the knee and straighten and stabilise the hip joint. In the calf is the *gastrocnemius*; when the muscle contracts, the knee flexes and the ankle joint is extended. It is used in walking on tip-toe and is attached to the heel by a strong tendon. There are flexors and extensors of the ankle joint, and muscles and ligaments in the foot.

The hands and feet have great importance in that they are the link or contact between the individual and his environment. They are highly developed in man and capable of small, precise, complicated movements like writing, and using instruments and tools, and are capable of great strength in grasping objects and lifting weights. When the hands are absent or without function the feet can be educated to perform activities like writing and painting. Smooth, easy movement in walking even on comparatively rough ground depends on the sensory nerve endings of touch and pressure and the muscles in the feet.

The nerve supply to the muscles is the means by which these organs are stimulated to contract and produce movement. The motor (or movement) pathway begins in the top of the brain. From a cell there stimulus can pass along a nerve fibre to the spinal cord. Here the stimulus is transferred to another motor cell and from there nerve fibres in a spinal nerve

to a muscle which then contracts. So for movement to take place in a
normal manner three organs participate:

 (i) muscles;
 (ii) their nerve supply;
 (iii) bones, and between these the synovial joints.

If one of these is damaged, then normal movement ceases.

Incorporated in the tissues round a joint are many nerve endings of
pressure. In this way the brain becomes aware of the movements taking
place at the joint.

The Purposes of Movement

To provide the body with some means by which it may
 1. fulfil its basic needs, e.g. obtaining food and shelter, and the
avoidance of pain and discomfort;
 2. protect itself and others in emergency by fight or flight;
 3. perform daily activities of eating, dressing, travelling to work,
communicating with others;
 4. carry out various forms of physical work and recreation;
 5. demonstrate self-expression, e.g. in adventure, construction,
creativeness, pursuit of knowledge.

Then one may reflect that for *thinking* no movement is required.

Joints, Muscles, the Skeleton in Health

DIET. As bone is a cellular tissue, protein is essential for its growth and
development. *Calcium* salts deposited in the cells determine bone rigidity,
but vitamin D is necessary for the calcium salts to act in this way. As
growth continues at various rates from before birth to physical maturity
the groups of people who need more protein and calcium than is contained in an average diet are infants, children, adolescents, pregnant
women and those feeding their babies.

Vitamin D is produced in the body by the action of the sun's rays on
the skin and is also obtained from the diet. When there is little sunlight
and the daily diet is likely to lack vitamin, then it is given in cod or
halibut liver oil or vitamin preparations. Deficiency of vitamin D in
infants causes rickets. In this disease the bones are softer than normal,
they bend and deformities occur. This is prevented by adequate amounts
of vitamin D and calcium in the diet, e.g. in full cream milk. Babies
with very dark skins do not absorb the sun's rays which are weak in
England, and may suffer this deficiency.

EXERCISE. The pull of the muscles on the bone shapes the bone in its early growth. In the same way the cervical and lumbar curves of the spine are formed, the first as the infant raises his head and the second as he begins to sit up. The actual growth of long bones is encouraged by exercise, i.e. use of muscles. When, through disease, muscles are inactive in childhood the bones affected do not grow and deformity or disability results. When muscles are not used at all, they become soft and then wasting occurs. The limb becomes very thin, with the bones more prominent.

RELAXATION of muscle is useful when it alternates with exercise to avoid fatigue.

Protection Against Injury
The methods depend on the situation.
(i) Special clothing, e.g.: steel-toed shoes, crash-helmets.
(ii) Machinery guards in factories.
(iii) Safety belts or harnesses in moving vehicles or machinery.

Protection Against Infection
Bone is infected only when the skin is broken, and infection is avoided by prevention of skin wounds and the proper treatment of wounds when they occur. Strict hygiene is maintained in emergency care of wounds. Later the removal of damaged tissue is performed under anaesthesia and the wound sutured. Small wounds are sealed with adhesive dressings after treatment.

Bones, Joints and Muscles in Disease

An adequate well-balanced diet prevents loss of weight and consequent exposure of the body prominences to pressure. Prolonged bed rest and no movement may result in bed-sores or the formation of stones in the kidney. These are reasons why the ill patient's position is changed two-hourly. The physiotherapist supervises bed-exercises, and as soon as possible, the patient sits out of bed and becomes mobile.

The muscles of an unconscious patient are relaxed and do not protect the underlying structures such as blood vessels and nerves. To avoid damage in these the limbs are placed in as near to the normal position as possible and no equipment is allowed to press on the limbs, e.g. a hard pillow under the thigh. Relaxed muscles can also become stretched and later the patient has difficulty in contracting the muscle. This can happen when the patient lies on his back and the bed-clothes press on his feet. He will have 'drop foot' and walking will be delayed when he recovers from his illness. To prevent drop-foot:
(i) the bed-clothes are loose over the patient's feet, and preferably a cradle is placed over his legs and feet;

(ii) he exercises his ankles at frequent intervals or the joints are put through a full range of movements by the nurse;

(iii) if exercise is impossible, a padded board is placed across the bed for his feet to rest against;

(iv) a back splint to fit the leg may be made from plastic material. This is bandaged on at night and removed in the daytime.

(v) adequate nourishing diet prevents wasting of muscle.

Changing the patient's position, exercises, sitting the patient in a chair, ambulation, occupational and diversional therapy all contribute to preventing stiffness of the patient's joints. This is not so likely to occur in the young patient but is common in the elderly who lie or sit in one position for long periods of time.

Symptoms and Signs in the Locomotor System

MUSCLE

Disease is rare in MUSCLE TISSUE and changes in its function are usually the result of disorders in the nerves, spinal cord and/or motor area of the brain, or inadequate blood supply to the muscles.

1. *Weakness of muscles*, e.g. the grasp of one hand being appreciably less than the other, or difficulty in sitting or standing upright without assistance. This usually indicates incomplete damage to nerves, e.g. neuritis and some varieties of spinal cord disease.

2. *Flaccid paralysis of muscle*, in which the muscle is soft and has no tone. Movement is totally or partially absent. This is usually due to complete damage to nerves.

3. *Spastic paralysis*. The muscle is in increased tone and contracted, so the limbs are drawn up with the joints flexed. There may be associated pain. It is usually due to damage to the spinal cord or brain.

4. *Convulsions* are forcible contractions of skeletal muscles which the patient cannot control. They are distressing and exhausting. This symptom originates in the brain.

5. *Muscle spasms* are contractions of small groups of muscles, e.g. in the face. More forceful spasms frequently indicate the onset of *tetany*, spasmodic contraction of muscle associated with lack of parathyroid hormone. This hormone controls the amount of calcium in the blood and also affects muscle contraction.

Severe muscle spasms occur in *tetanus*, which is due to infection of a wound by tetanus bacilli, micro-organisms which normally live in the soil.

6. *Pain* in muscle, when due to acute lack of oxygen because of some failure in the blood circulatory system, is usually localised and severe.

7. *Atrophy of muscles* is muscle wasting. The muscles become reduced in thickness, and as a result the body is thinner and the bones more prominent.

BONE

Symptoms and signs concerned with BONES include:

1. *Deformity,* i.e. a difference in shape or position from the normal or natural, in rickets and other diseases, or when a bone is broken.

2. *Loss of function,* e.g. a weight-bearing bone cannot bear weight when it is broken.

3. *Abnormal movement* in which the bone has lost its rigidity through fracture and the parts of the bone can move independently of each other.

4. *Pain,* which is severe in fractures and infections of bone.

5. *Swelling,* i.e. increase in tissue fluid, accompanies fractures and infection of bone.

6. *Enlargement* of the bone as with growths or when a bone is joining after fracture.

In addition to these a nurse may notice in some fractures *crepitus,* i.e. grating of the bone surfaces. It causes pain.

JOINTS

Symptoms and signs in diseases of the JOINTS:

1. *Stiffness:* the joint allows movement with some difficulty.

2. *Immobility:* there is no movement at the joint.

3. *Pain* is severe in (a) dislocation, (b) inflammatory conditions like rheumatoid arthritis or (c) infective conditions.

4. *Swelling* is a common symptom of sprains and dislocations.

5. Sometimes the joint shows *enlargement* as in rheumatic disorders.

6. *Deformity* results from previous injury or inflammation.

Clinical investigation is made by radiography when an X-ray film of a part of the body is made by skilled personnel (radiographers) using highly technical equipment. The bones being more dense than other tissues are opaque to X-rays and abnormalities can be detected in the films.

When the patient is in bed and too ill to be moved from the bed or even from the ward, a portable X-ray machine can be brought to the ward and the radiographer X-rays the patient with assistance from the nurses in moving the patient.

Preparation for X-ray examination. Rugs and blankets are necessary if there is likely to be some delay while the X-ray equipment is made ready for use, and if the patient is to remain in the department while the films are developed. Should the patient be very ill, a nurse stays with him. Dense materials like metal are completely opaque to X-rays and might cover a bone defect which would then be undetected. To prevent this, safety pins, buttons, and pieces of equipment are removed from the area to be photographed. Wool dressings appear as a shadow on the film and the radiologist usually prefers these to be removed and a single layer of gauze used if needed; this will be replaced by a complete dressing afterwards. The nurse may be required to maintain a limb in the correct position during this procedure.

The ability of the muscle to respond to nerve stimulation is tested by the physiotherapist, who applies a pad to the skin through which a very small-strength current can pass to the muscle.

Observations

The patient's general activity is noted, and to some extent this is difficult to assess as the nurse has not known the patient previously. Relatives can assist by giving information of his normal capabilities and ways in which these have altered during the course of his illness. During treatment and nursing care the nurse observes increasing or decreasing ability in ordinary activities, like pulling on stockings or slippers, tying shoe-laces, putting on a coat, and standing or walking. Decreasing ability is due usually to increasing stiffness or pain in joints. Awkward movements of which the patient may not be aware, and complaints of fatigue in one part of the body, due to pain or immobility (or fear of them) in other parts of the body, are also important. During treatment for a disability, a patient is taught how to make compensatory movements which the nurse will observe while he is in hospital. Examples of these are the swinging-out of the lower limb when walking with a caliper, which is an immobilising aid used following fracture of a femur, or when the knee joint is completely fixed. This movement compensates for the loss of knee flexion.

The patient with an anxious temperament or who lacks, for some reason, determination and perseverance may show less activity generally than the person who is optimistic, energetic and responsive.

Special range of movement is noted more precisely, sometimes by recording the angle through which a bone will pass in movement at the joint. Pushing, pulling and lifting can be measured by weights and pulleys by the physiotherapist. A small metal instrument is used in testing hand grasp; on hand pressure an indicator moves showing measurement in pounds per square inch.

Swelling, blue or white colour, pins and needles, numbness, and the *absence of a pulse beat* have already been mentioned.

It may be useful to measure the *length of a limb* to assess shortening of bone, or the *circumference of a limb* which is decreased in muscle wasting.

Pyrexia occurs in infections, e.g. osteomyelitis (inflammation of the bone tissue beneath the periosteum), and is also associated with some general rheumatic disorders.

During treatment for conditions in which the patient is immobilised or where the treatment itself curtails the patient's activity the nurse inspects the areas of *skin exposed to pressure* a least twice a day. Pressure sores result from the weight of the body on the bed or from equipment such as bandages or splints.

Friction also can cause reddening of the skin, abrasions and ulcers. Treatment of these is difficult and every suitable method of prevention is used, but observation is necessary in the first place of any situation in which pressure may be exerted on the surface of the body.

Observation of the Patient's Response to Treatment
In several orthopaedic conditions the treatment necessitates weeks or months confined to bed. Cure or relief may follow a series of operations when surgery may be performed in stages. The nurse–patient relationship is of special importance in the recovery of these 'long-stay' patients, and the nurse should be quick to observe signs of impatience, loss of confidence and anxiety regarding his condition, and nostalgia for his home environment and his work. These matters are rarely entered in a written report but spoken confidentially to the sister who will suggest means by which the patient may be given help and assurance. On the other hand, difficulties lie ahead if the patient becomes too dependent on the hospital staff and begins to lose his own initiative, or if his separation from a responsible and demanding, even competitive, life outside the hospital leads him to become restless or undisciplined in behaviour in the hospital ward. Sympathetic observations can quickly be followed by the provision of incentive or means of energy outlet as the situation demands. In hospital where these patients are treated the ward routine is geared not only to the physical needs of the patient but to his mental and emotional need also.

I*

Medical and Surgical Conditions in the Locomotor System

Congenital abnormalities are the result of inherited characteristics or may occur in the foetus while it is in the uterus, or during birth.

Examples of these abnormalities which are present after birth include:

Double thumbs, additional fingers, absence of fingers, absence of upper limbs, and fingers and parts of the hand attached to the trunk.

Torticollis or 'wryneck' in which the sterno-mastoid muscle between head and sternum on one side is shorter than the other causing the chin to be drawn downwards and towards the opposite side.

Talipes or 'club-foot' when the foot is drawn inwards and the heel is off the ground. There are different varieties of this abnormality.

Cleft palate. The hard palate is formed from two bones which unite in the roof of the mouth before birth. Occasionally one bone does not develop and the bony mouth roof is incomplete, i.e. it is cleft. Frequently this abnormality is accompanied by hare lip and the operations to correct it by plastic surgery are performed in a Children's Hospital.

Congenital dislocation of the hip in one or both hips is discovered during routine examination of the newborn infant. There is shortening of the limb. It is due to defective formation of the hip-socket, and treatment should begin as early as possible.

ABNORMALITIES in the shape of the skeleton occur in some cases as the result of injury or disease.

Examples:

Shortening of a limb is a complication of anterior poliomyelitis in a child, and this disease is prevented now by immunisation. This deformity is nowadays more commonly due to injury.

Rickets is a disease due to deficiency of vitamin D. The diet normally contains this fat-soluble vitamin in butter, margarine and fish oils, and it is produced also by the action of the sun on natural oils in the skin. It has become uncommon, as the standard of diet and living conditions has improved. Children who do not absorb fats easily need vitamin D supplement to prevent rickets. In this disease calcium salts are not laid down in the framework of the tissue, which causes the bones to be less rigid than normal and later they become distorted.

Hallux valgus is a deformity of the big toe which is aggravated by the wearing of high-heeled narrow-toed shoes or stockings which are too short or tight between toe and heel. The great toe is turned inwards under the other toes as the joint at its base becomes angulative. Pressure and friction from footwear result in a painful swollen joint known as a 'bunion'. It is treated by surgery.

ACUTE OSTEOMYELITIS. This infection of bone by staphylococci and occasionally streptococci which have already caused boils and abscesses in the body, or which have entered the bone through a wound in the skin as in compound fracture. The patient is usually a child who is very ill with raised temperature, and acute pain in the limb at the site of infection. The surgeon requests X-ray after his examination of the limb. Surgery is performed to drain the abscess and the limb is immobilised in a plaster of paris splint. Following examination of the pus and determination of the most effective antibiotic, this is administered as prescribed. As the patient is feverish, he is consequently dehydrated and requires adequate fluid intake, about $2\frac{1}{2}$ to 3 litres each day. Frequent sponging of the skin removes sweat and is comforting to the patient. Gentle moving of the patient prevents unnecessary pain.

SEPTIC ARTHRITIS. This is inflammation of a joint due to infection either carried in the blood from another part of the body, or due to injury, e.g. kneeling on a sharp object. There is pain and swelling in the joint. The surgeon removes pus by aspirating through a needle or by incision, the limb is immobilised in a plaster of paris splint, and he prescribes the appropriate antibiotic which the nurse administers, and which may also be injected into the joint cavity.

TUBERCULOUS INFECTION OF JOINTS is uncommon nowadays due to the pasteurisation of milk, immunisation by B.C.G. vaccine, modern treatment of tuberculosis and improved standards of living. It is a chronic infection, with pain and stiffness in the joint. Treatment is by a combination of streptomycin, para-aminosalicylic acid and iso-nicotinic acid hydrazide and surgery. The affected joint is immobilised in a plaster of paris splint, while the patient remains in bed. After intensive treatment, infected tissue is removed in operation, and a course of exercises begins.

SCIATICA is pain in the back of the thigh and the calf, which is severe when the limb is raised as the patient lies flat on a couch. This inflammation of the sciatic nerve may be due to the displacement of an intravertebral disc or cartilage and treatment is by rest in bed, skin traction on the lower limb to relieve pressure on the nerve by the displaced disc, or a corset support.

OSTEO-ARTHRITIS is wearing out of the ends of the bones within a joint. The articulating surfaces deteriorate and there is pain on movement. It affects weight-bearing joints usually, e.g. the hip or knee, and those affected are middle-aged or elderly. To maintain movement at the hip the surgeon may consider removal of the head of the femur, replacing it by a prosthesis which rotates in the hip socket without friction. To ensure the weight-bearing function at the knee joint, he may consider making the joint permanently stiff, an operation known as 'arthrodesis'. The patient in either situation is nursed in bed for a few days after operation and then sits in a chair with his leg raised. Exercises are important to improve muscle, bone and joint movement, and these are followed by rehabilitation. An overweight patient is encouraged to reduce his food intake of sugar and starches, and become as mobile and independent as possible.

RHEUMATOID ARTHRITIS is a disease more common in women than in men, and which begins at 40 to 50 years of age. The patient is ill with a raised temperature and feels weak and tired. Her joints are swollen and painful but improve on rest. Later she loses weight and becomes anaemic. If the condition continues, adhesions may replace the inflammatory changes in the joints, and if this takes place while the joint is in an unsatisfactory position, e.g. the wrist in flexion, there is residual disability.

In mild cases the patient has more rest than usual and is instructed not to overuse affected joints. Aspirin relieves pain. She is encouraged to continue with her usual interests.

Rest in bed for a few weeks is necessary when the illness is more severe. Painful joints in the lower limbs are protected by a bed-cradle and the feet are supported by a padded footboard. A fixed position in bed is discouraged and she lies flat alternately on her back or face downwards some time during the day. A severely affected joint is supported at rest and in the correct position by a plaster of paris or plastic splint applied to the patient's limb for correct fit.

Pain is relieved by analgesics, one of which is aspirin. The joints improve with the administration of prednisone, a synthetic preparation of cortisone, although this treatment is not always considered suitable. Heat is beneficial and applied by a heat lamp or electric pad. The patient may find it difficult to sleep and measures to relieve pain are of value. Diet is nutritious, containing protein and vitamins. An overweight woman will be given less sugar and starches in her food.

Rehabilitation of patients with arthritis. The patient goes to the toilet and sits out of bed as soon as pyrexia has disappeared, later becoming ambulant when this is possible, with walking aids to assist her. She will probably have difficulty in dressing herself and needs sufficient time and perhaps instruction on the best methods in managing this and other personal activities. The physiotherapist encourages simple, gentle movements in joints *not* acutely inflamed and later instructs and supervises her in exercises to maintain muscle, bone and joint movement and to improve her confidence in general outside activities which may include crossing busy roads and walking up and down stairs. In an occupational therapy department she may be shown aids for walking, dressing, eating,

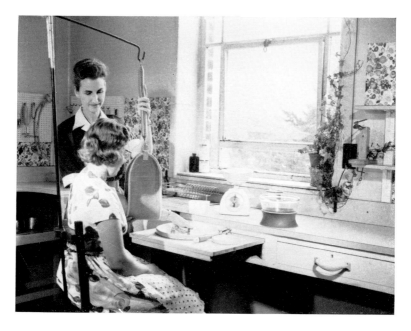

Figure 26. Rehabilitation in a kitchen (by courtesy of the Board of Governors, Queen Elizabeth Hospital, United Birmingham Hospitals).

writing, which will enable her to work in her own home and be as independent as possible (Fig. 26).

In the hospital ward the nurse attends to those needs of the patient which she cannot accomplish herself, e.g. bathing, cutting up her food, and fitting splints for supports. She gives the patient continual encouragement and most often when the patient appears slow and becomes impatient. The patient's garments should be loose and easy to fasten, the beds low so that she can sit with her feet firmly on the ground while she dresses, the floor safe for walking and the toilets and washbasins convenient to use. Occupations such as simple knitting or embroidery can be enjoyable as well as beneficial, and visits from relatives and friends stimulate and encourage the patient.

Injuries

SPRAINS

A *sprain* is a partial tear of a ligament guarding a joint when that joint is put under a stress which is too severe for the muscle to bear. Nerve endings are plentiful near a joint, which means that *pain* on injury is sharp and severe. There is damage to tissue; fluid leaks out from the cells and tissue spaces and collects under the skin as localised *swelling*. An X-ray may be necessary to exclude fracture.

The most common sites of sprains are the ankles, wrists and fingers or thumbs. In the wrist, however, a sprain is very often a fracture of a wrist bone and in the knee the cartilage may often be torn. Pain at the time of injury may be so severe the patient feels faint and it is arranged for him to sit or lie down. Should he actually become unconscious, he is laid flat and not disturbed for a few minutes, by which time he will have recovered from this effect of pain. The limb with the affected joint is placed in the natural anatomical position. *To prevent swelling*, a cold application is applied as soon as possible after injury. In a first-aid situation this may be a handkerchief lightly wrung out in cold water from a stream and wrapped round the joint, or by bathing the joint in running cold water. At home or in hospital, the foot or hand is supported in a raised position on a waterproof towel. A single layer of cotton material is placed around the limb and kept moist by spraying with cold water at intervals, for about an hour. As the water evaporates heat is withdrawn from the skin beneath the damp material.

Splints are used to support sprained fingers and prevent pain. If the ankle is sprained it should not be weight-bearing for a few hours but exercise of other joints is encouraged. Then normal activity is resumed as soon as possible so that *stiffness* is prevented. This third complication of sprains is due to the protein content of the tissue fluid which leaked during injury coagulating round the joint and pre-disposing to the formation of fibrous tissue. When some stiffness remains exercise should not be delayed and can be carried out most easily with the limb immersed in warm water.

DISLOCATIONS

In these injuries, the ends of the bones which articulate in a joint are no longer in their usual place, and have been described in ordinary terms as 'the bones are put out of joint'. The points most commonly dislocated are the shoulder, elbow, fingers and hip. This type of injury is usually associated with the unexpected accident, because normally the muscles surrounding the joint contract sufficiently firmly to protect the joint from displacement.

Pain occurs quickly, though not absolutely immediately; its severity can produce primary shock and the patient may collapse. Relief is by reduction of the dislocation, i.e. the ends of the bones are returned to their normal position. In some cases reduction takes place spontaneously when slight traction (pulling) is applied to the limb, particularly in the immediate painless period. More force may be necessary by manipulation, but if this treatment is carried out immediately no anaesthetic is needed. If, however, some time has elapsed since the accident occurred the patient is X-rayed and then has a general anaesthetic before the reduction is performed. After the manipulation the limb is immobilised in a splint, and observation of the extremity made carefully and frequently; the doctor may request the administration of analgesics when pain persists during the 24 hours following the treatment.

The *complications of joint dislocation* are damage to neighbouring structures, blood vessels, nerves or nerve tissue. When the doctor diagnoses a complication, the patient may be prepared for operation and open reduction is performed. After surgery, observation of the extremities is important, also prevention of infection.

Dislocation of the cervical spine. This injury usually follows falling in an awkward position, e.g. falling downstairs or on the games field, or after diving into a swimming bath. The first-aider may find that the person is paralysed below the site of injury, i.e. the neck, and cannot move his limbs, neither has his skin any sense of touch. The patient is not moved unless absolutely necessary until a doctor arrives (*see* First Aid), and the first-aider stays with him, sitting on the ground by the patient to reassure him. In hospital the method of reduction is by traction. Weights are attached to a cord which is secured to the head by a metal or leather device. The weights pull against the weight of the body, separating the cervical vertebrae and then bringing them into their normal position in line with each other. This takes some time, and in the meantime the nurse gives the patient the care necessary for a physically helpless individual.

Dislocation of hip is of two varieties:

(1) *Congenital*, in new-born babies where the socket is inadequately formed.

(2) *Traumatic*, where the head of the femur (the ball) is pushed out of the socket. The sciatic nerve is commonly damaged, causing partial paralysis and loss of sensation in the leg.

This dislocation is a very painful one, and a deep anaesthetic is always required to reduce the dislocation. The patient is not allowed to put weight on the affected leg for 6 weeks after injury.

Fractures

A fracture is a break in the bone and patients usually prefer this term to 'broken bones or limbs'. Degree of actual tissue damage varies considerably; some fractures are trivial, for example at the tip of the finger, but those which involve extensive bone damage or injury to skin and internal organs may be serious.

Most fractures are caused by injury, a few by disease. In the former the force may be directly applied to the bone by some hard object, as occurs when a blow is delivered or in a crush injury or fall. Indirect force can be the result of, e.g. a sudden forcible twist when the stress on the bone is sufficient to cause a fracture. Bones are predisposed to fracture in disease when they become softer as in Paget's disease and in malignant conditions when the normal tissue is replaced by tumour growth. In senescence (old age) the tissues are extremely brittle and can fracture with very little force having been exerted.

TYPES OF FRACTURES (Fig. 27) p. 260

A *greenstick fracture* is one in which the bone is not completely broken but bends at the site of injury. It occurs in growing children when the bone is not yet a rigid structure.

Several fragments of bone where the blow occurred give rise to the description of '*comminuted fracture*'.

In a *complicated fracture* structures other than bone are damaged, such as blood vessels, nerves, lungs, spinal cord, brain, or spleen.

A *compound* or *open fracture* is one in which the skin is torn by the injured bone, which protrudes through the wound. This type of fracture may also be due to a foreign body entering through the skin and damag-

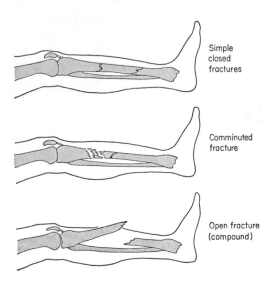

Simple
closed
fractures

Comminuted
fracture

Open fracture
(compound)

Figure 27. Fractures.

ing the bone, as in a bullet wound or in a head injury resulting from the impact between the patient's head and the road surface in an accident. There is a grave risk of infection in this kind of fracture.

A piece of bone is pressed down on the brain in a *depressed fracture* of skull.

SYMPTOMS AND SIGNS OF FRACTURES

Pain is localised and at the time of injury is likely to be severe. Shock due to the trauma, particularly in fractures of long bones like the femur and tibia, is aggravated by continued pain. Any movement at the joints above or below the fracture causes increase in acute pain. The part of the body affected may be in an *unnatural position*, for example, a fracture of the neck of the left femur will cause the left lower limb to be rotated outwards and shortened.

Unnatural mobility is most likely to occur in the limbs, the hand or foot being movable through a greater range than normal unless secured to a splint or held firmly in traction. When pain becomes severe the muscles in the locality of the fracture contract round the broken bone and decrease movement at the actual fracture to prevent excessive pain. Often this muscle 'splinting' is sufficient to cause the broken ends of the bone to overlap, causing the limb to be shorter than normal. This deformity is corrected during treatment by limb traction.

Loss of some function, though often not all of it, follows some fractures. For example, if the femur, a weight-bearing bone, is injured the patient cannot stand on the leg, and when the lower jaw is broken the patient cannot chew or speak properly. A patient with a crushed vertebra, however, may walk into the Accident/Emergency department. Swelling and bruising may follow the injury later.

Diagnosis of fractures is by clinical examination and X-rays.

Principles of Treatment

In the first-aid situation, a suspected fracture is immobilised in as near a natural position as possible. It is useful when applying temporary splints to secure the joints above and below the fracture. During transport an injured limb with possible fractures is immobilised to prevent pain and facilitate moving the patient. The Thomas's splint was devised for this purpose. The patient needs reassurance from the time of the injury; he should be moved as little as possible and gentle efficient methods of lifting him are necessary. Analgesics may be required to relieve severe pain at the scene of accident and are administered by the medical officer or specially appointed person. In the Casualty department or Trauma Unit his injuries are assessed and X-ray examination made. Severe pain is relieved by analgesics and acute complications such as haemorrhage are dealt with. An open wound (compound fracture) is cleaned thoroughly and dead tissue removed while the patient is anaesthetised in the operating theatre. The wound is then closed. A course of antibiotic therapy is usually prescribed.

The treatment for most fractures is then in three stages.

1. REDUCTION OF THE FRACTURE, i.e. bringing the broken ends of the bone together into a satisfactory position for healing.

The methods used are:

    (a) *Manipulation* by the surgeon.

    (b) *Traction*, i.e. by pulling on the lower part of the limb. Weights are then attached to the limb, or the lower part of the limb is secured to a splint by cords which are tightened each day, in order to maintain the good position.

(c) *Open reduction* in which a wound is made during surgical operation and the fracture is reduced by the surgeon through the wound, which is then closed. A metal plate is often applied in such an operation.

2. IMMOBILISATION when the bones are fixed in their satisfactory position. The most common method is by *plaster of paris splints* but a variety of *other splints* are also used. In some cases the surgeon operates and applies *internal fixation*, usually by nails (Fig. 28) in the medullary cavity

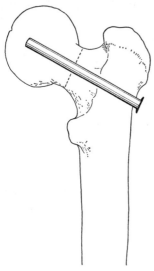

Figure 28. Smith Peterson nail.

of bone bridging the fracture, or by metal pins through the neck of the femur when a fracture occurs here as is frequent in elderly women. Metal plates and screws are also used. This part of the treatment is necessary while the bone heals (in about 6 to 12 weeks) although plates and screws are permanent and facilitate early ambulation.

3. Although the fracture, and probably the joints above and below it, are immobilised, it is essential that the remainder of the limb and the body should be as mobile as possible, and EXERCISES are an important part of the patient's treatment. These are arranged immediately he has recovered from the injury itself, and continue when he is confined to bed. This programme and occupational therapy prevents stiffness of the joints and loss of muscle tone besides making a contribution to his general health.

Complications of Fractures

Traumatic shock is severe particularly in fractures of long bones like the femur. It is aggravated by prolonged pain, haemorrhage, exposure to difficult weather conditions following accident and acute infections like influenzal pneumonia. In shock the general vitality of the body is lowered and the blood pressure falls and the pulse rate rises. If the pressure of blood to the kidneys become greatly decreased, these organs cease to function and the patient has acute renal failure. The nurse observes and reports the output of urine. When this is abnormally low and the water, urea and electrolyte balance in the blood is disturbed, the patient is treated by haemodialysis.

Mental confusion, particularly at night, is common in elderly patients, those with pyrexia and men who are accustomed to taking alcohol. The former need reassurance and should not be left alone for long periods of time. Cooling the feverish patient with sponges, a cold compress on the head and iced fruit drinks will help him to be more restful. The person who is accustomed to some alcohol each day becomes distressed when this is stopped, and his condition will improve when ale or beer is included in his diet.

Sepsis is a danger in compound fracture. The wound is cleaned then sutured in surgical operation and antibiotics are prescribed. Injections of tetanus toxoid and penicillin prevent possible tetanus infection from the wound.

Non-union or mal-union, i.e. union of the fracture in an unsatisfactory position, are possible later complications.

Injuries of the Face and Head

FACIAL INJURIES. These may be slight or severe. In either case pain and oedema are common, and eating and speaking can be difficult. There is also a measure of internal anxiety, for most people dislike wounds and scars which alter their outward appearance. For this reason the patient becomes quickly depressed. The small bones of the face may show comminuted fractures, the frontal bone simple fracture, or the lower jaw may be fractured and displaced. The eyes are usually well protected by the frontal and cheek bones, but teeth are often involved. The skin is not always damaged when there are fractures, but may be lacerated with no other injuries. Treatment in the more severe cases is carried out by a team of doctors including a plastic surgeon and dental surgeon, depending on the type of injuries.

SCALP WOUNDS may be complicated and careful examination is necessary to exclude complication. The nurse may be requested to shave part of the scalp to enable the examination to be carried out. The patient's permission is obtained. Temporary bleeding serves to clean the wound of dirt but may continue, in which case a pressure pad is bandaged over the area until the wound is sutured.

Infection of the wound is prevented by: removal of any foreign bodies present, e.g. grit or hair; trimming the edges of the skin in an irregular wound; cleaning the wound with an antiseptic; and suture of the wound. This operation is performed by the surgeon under local anaesthetic. Sometimes no anaesthetic is needed for simple suture as the scalp is not particularly sensitive to pain. Sutures are removed a week later.

HEAD INJURIES. The patient may not lose consciousness at the time of injury. It is important to remember that quite severe injuries of the head and skull can occur without loss of consciousness. This is usually the situation when there has been no rotating movement of the head during the incident. Examples are: the entry of penetrating foreign bodies, e.g. a bullet, without damage to the major blood vessels; a fractured skull when the head has been struck by a hard ball; or a heavy object falling on top of the head. It is obviously very necessary for the surgeon to examine the head closely. X-ray may be requested.

The nurse observes the general condition of the patient but reports particularly on levels of consciousness.

CONCUSSION. Sudden movement of the brain within the skull, particularly a rotatory movement as when the head hits the ground, or a moving object comes with force against the head, causes temporary unconsciousness. This is known as concussion. It may last only a few moments but the patient on being questioned later remembers nothing of the actual accident, and nothing of the events for a short time following the accident. Occasionally the state of unconsciousness remains for some days and even after recovery there is amnesia (loss of memory) from the time immediately before the injury until a short time afterwards.

OBSERVATIONS. It is necessary to report changes in the patient's general condition, and written records may be requested. Changes may indicate the development of some complication. See chart on opposite page.

Treatment and Nursing Care of Patient with Head Injuries

The patient may have suffered skull fractures with possible brain damage such as bruises or lacerations at the time of injury and will be deeply unconscious. The general nursing care is primarily that for an unconscious patient. The maintenance of an efficient AIR-WAY is necessary, by nursing the patient in the lateral position or by the insertion of an endo-

Chart to Indicate Levels of Consciousness

Patient's Name   Age   Date   Time of admission

Levels of consciousness	Times
1. Normal conversation	
2. Drowsy, with confused conversation	
3. Will answer simple questions only	
4. Will answer only yes or no	
5. Responds to painful stimuli	
6. Unrousable by any means	

The nurse places √ opposite the observation she has made, the time being inserted at the top of the column.

These points may be helpful for the nurse to understand the levels:

1. The patient replies normally and sensibly, is rational and co-operative.

2. He gives the same answer to different questions. He does not talk sensibly and is irrational.

3. He answers questions: 'What is your name?' 'How old are you,' 'Where do you live?' but no questions more difficult.

4. He answers 'Yes' or 'No' to questions but cannot explain in more detail.

5. When he is disturbed during bed-making he moves his limbs vigorously.

6. He does not respond to any movement or nursing attention. The pupils do not constrict in a bright light.

N.B. If the patient's level of consciousness falls or the *pulse rate* varies following head injuries, the doctor is notified immediately.

tracheal or tracheostomy tube. Excess secretions in the upper respiratory tract are removed by suction apparatus through the tube.

WOUNDS. Shaving of the head enables the surgeon to make a thorough examination of wounds. Prevention of infection is important. Later, the growth of hair is encouraged by regular shampooing of the scalp and gentle massage with nut oil.

SURGERY may be necessary to clean and suture wounds, to remove penetrating foreign bodies and blood clots, or to deal with fractures of the skull.

Disturbance to the heat-regulating centre in the brain will result in *hyperpyrexia*, and the body temperature rises to more than 39°C. When the blood supply to the brain may be deficient as a result of intracranial haemorrhage, the oxygen need of the brain can be reduced by lowering the body temperature to 32°C. This hypothermia is produced by the application of COLD PACKS as described in reduction of temperature.

FLUID AND ELECTROLYTE BALANCE is assessed by means of blood samples and fluid balance charts. Intravenous infusion of electrolytes in solution may be in progress. These are carefully checked before administration and accurate fluid balance charts are necessary. Loss of weight occurs rapidly and nutrition is important to prevent this.

DIET is comprehensive, e.g. Complan, and arranged in two-hourly feeds through an intra-gastric tube. Adequate protein intake assists in preventing bed-sores.

His POSITION is changed frequently, every half-hour when he is deeply comatose and generally at two-hourly intervals day and night, to prevent bed-sores and broncho-pneumonia. A special bed or mattress to protect pressure areas may be useful.

MICTURITION. During deep coma, catheterisation of the urinary bladder with continual drainage of urine may be necessary but as the patient recovers consciousness he is encouraged to pass urine into a urinal. By this time he is more mobile and probably finds it easier to stand by the side of the bed while micturating.

RESTLESSNESS. As the patient recovers consciousness he will struggle when he is restrained, and perhaps become noisy and violent. To prevent this, the nurse learns to move him *slowly*, and if he is restless she leaves him alone. Kindness and thoughtfulness are essential. If he is noisy and restless for no apparent reason, he may have a full bladder or be in a wet bed. The surgeon may consider lumbar punctures in some instances to relieve severe headache. Sedative drugs are not prescribed for the mentally confused patient with head injuries, because signs of complications would not become apparent if the patient were sedated, and the urgent treatment needed for these would be delayed. As soon as the patient's physical condition improves he sits out of bed and then walks about the ward, but as his mental state may not yet be normal he does this under a nurse's supervision, so that he does not wander away from the ward. This early mobilisation prevents absorption of calcium from the skeleton, bed-sores, micturition and defaecation problems and reduces weight and muscle tone loss.

REHABILITATION. The patient in hospital becomes mobile as soon as possible. Some physical disability, e.g. paralysis, may remain. Mental disability continues in some cases, and the patient when he returns home is irritable with members of his family, and finds work difficult. He may complain of headaches for some time. Recovery may take several months and he needs tolerance from his relatives and his employers while he is at work, during this time.

Relatives and friends need support, advice and reassurance from medical and nursing staffs and also from social workers. A club for these ex-patients has been formed in one accident unit. Meetings are held in the unit and patients and relatives attend until the rehabilitation programme is complete.

Multiple Injuries

These are usually the result of accidents involving vehicles on the roads, railways or in the air; falls of masonry, coal, or heavy machinery; the collapse of trenches or buildings; or where the person concerned has fallen from a height. The patient is not moved until a doctor has made a preliminary assessment of his condition or skilled personnel arrive to transport him by ambulance to a hospital or injuries unit. Emergency measures are in progress en route: visible haemorrhages are arrested, pain is relieved by analgesics, blood transfusion is in progress, temporary sterile dressings are applied to wounds and an efficient air-way is maintained. On arrival in hospital a second more detailed examination and assessment are made by the medical staff, and treatment includes a resuscitation programme and surgery for internal injuries and fractures. Occasionally the treatment of one injury takes precedence when this is urgent and other wounds receive full treatment later.

The bed prepared for this patient has a firm base. Bed accessories may be necessary to prevent pressure of bed-clothes upon the limbs. Oxygen apparatus is by the bed-side. Detailed observations will be required from the nurses throughout the day regarding the patient's wounds, level of consciousness, pulse, fluid output, etc. The patient's basic needs receive attention as with any helpless patient but special problems are lifting the patient who may have several fractures; and preventing pressure sores, broncho-pneumonia and weight loss. Eight members of staff may be necessary to act as a team under a leader in moving the patient, and in some cases a lifting machine is very useful. To operate this, canvas strips are placed beneath the patient's shoulders, waist, pelvis, thighs and legs, and fastened round rollers above the patient. The rollers can be raised by moving the appropriate handle.

This patient's relatives will need special consideration. Their visits are necessarily short, but contact can be made by telephone or hand message during the critical phase of the illness.

Amputations

These are performed following injuries involving a limb, e.g. crushed hand or foot, or to remove a limb the extremity of which has become gangrenous.

Gangrene is caused by:
   (a) injury which is complicated by damage to blood vessels;
   (b) infection by the organism of gas-gangrene—*clostridium Welchii*;
   (c) diabetes mellitus;
   (d) a disease of the arteries, such as severe arterio-sclerosis in the elderly.

There may be loss of a limb during an accident; this is a traumatic amputation and the surgeon usually refashions the stump during operation so that it is a more suitable shape for the attachment of an artificial limb later.

The possibility and significance of amputation are explained to the patient before the operation and his consent is obtained by the surgeon. The availability of an artificial limb (prosthesis) is also impressed on him as his rehabilitation for general activity and work will begin immediately following the operation. Loss of an upper limb, particularly the right if the person is right-handed, is a greater disability than loss of a lower limb, though a great deal depends on the occupation and adaptability of the patient. Amputation of a finger can be tolerated more easily than loss of the thumb.

A possible, though rare complication of operation is haemorrhage. The nurse observes the patient for pallor and would note a fast pulse with a rising rate. The wound dressing would be visible. Should bleeding occur, lay the patient flat and apply digital pressure over the pressure point nearer to the heart and seek assistance quickly. A tourniquet is kept near to hand and the assistant applies it over the towel around the stump with all speed (in about 90 seconds). The surgeon will attend to the wound in the operating theatre. Otherwise the tourniquet is released every 15 minutes and if bleeding begins again, is re-applied. The use of a tourniquet is avoided if at all possible.

Pressure bandages are applied to the wound to prevent oedema and to produce a cone-shaped stump which will fit into the artificial limb without friction or pressure. In a mid-thigh amputation the bandage includes a hip spica so that excessive flexion does not occur at the hip joint (Fig. 29). Similarly, the knee joint is maintained in an extended position rather than flexed. As soon as possible the patient sits out of bed and becomes ambulant with walking aids if he has had a lower limb removed. Then a rehabilitation programme begins with special strengthening exercises, including instruction in the use of the equipment and practice in

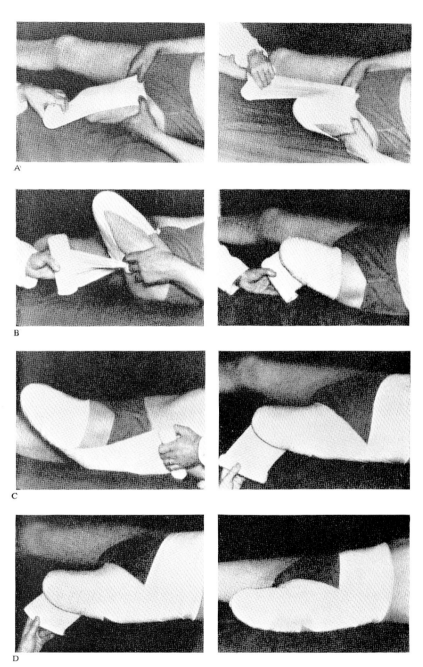

Figure 29. Stump bandage (from *Rehabilitation following Amputation*, Ministry of Health)

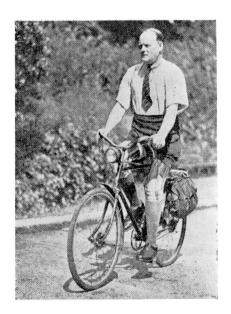

Figure 30. Cycling with two below-knee leg amputations (from *Hints on the Use of an Artificial Limb*, Ministry of Health).

wearing the prosthesis (Fig. 30). Artificial arms are made to have special attachments for various kinds of activity, either personal, like eating, or connected with work, as in operating a machine. Each article is made by craftsmen for the person for whom it is prescribed and the standard of work is extremely high. Throughout the programme the patient needs encouragement and praise for the progress he achieves.

A problem which may arise following traumatic amputation in an accident is that the patient may not be aware when he recovers consciousness that he has in actual fact lost a limb. As soon as he is sensible the surgeon or ward sister explains the situation to him. This is *not* the duty of the nurse but she should appreciate the procedure to prevent accidental knowledge of the injury.

Artificial limbs are being devised for children who are born without an arm or both arms or hands. The movements of the manipulating parts are operated from a small machine.

Preparation for the Application of a Plaster of Paris Splint

These splints are applied in a *special plaster room* when this is available. The floor is terrazzo and easy to clean. The person applying the plaster bandages wears a plastic apron to protect the clothing, and *sometimes rubber gloves* as frequent washing of the hands to remove plaster is harmful to the skin. Occasionally *orthopaedic cotton wool or stockinet* lines the splint and special equipment may be incorporated in it, e.g. *a walking heel on a leg plaster.* The splint itself is made from *plaster bandages* which are stiff muslin strips impregnated with plaster of paris powder, and rolled loosely into bandages. Usually these are bought ready for use as 'Cellona' or 'Gypsona' bandages. The width is selected as suitable to the part of the body to be treated, e.g. 3 inches for the forearm and 4 to 6 inches for the trunk, together with large dressing scissors for cutting them when necessary. *A large bowl of water* is prepared warm, to be just comfortable to the hand. Cold water retards setting, hot water makes setting more rapid but is uncomfortable for the patient, as a newly applied plaster becomes very hot. The water will be changed frequently or the bandages will not soak properly, and *sufficient tepid water is made available.*

Application of these splints may take some time, and the patient is made as comfortable as possible. The room is warm and the body not exposed more than necessary. The limb to be immobilised usually needs support such as a hand or foot prop, and the nurse may be requested to raise some part of the body into a suitable position, under the sister's direction.

The doctor or sister applying the plaster of paris splint takes a bandage from the supply close to his or her hand, and holds it under the water for 5 to 10 seconds until air bubbles cease to rise. Excess water is squeezed out lightly, and the bandage is applied in the skilled manner essential to the efficiency of this treatment, the principle of which is to immobilise a fracture, but allow mobility to the remainder of the limb.

SPECIAL CARE WHILE THE PLASTER IS DRYING. The patient remains in bed or on a couch, or sits in a chair after the application of the plaster. The splinted limb or trunk lies on something reasonably soft or it will dent. In a foot plaster the heel rests on a pillow or is unsupported until the plaster is dry. Absolute drying takes about 48 hours, but 3 days is much more reliable. When holding a wet plaster, the weight is taken on the *palm* of the hand not the finger-tips; if these are pressed into the plaster, pressure sores beneath the splint can occur. If the splint extends from foot to thigh, and the knee is slightly flexed, most of the weight is taken with the hand behind the knee, for lifting the limb by the foot will crack the plaster at the knee.

ARM PLASTERS. The nurse will observe that the splint has been applied so that it finishes above the metacarpal joint to allow full movement of the fingers, and during application the index finger and thumb are helped into position so that they can touch each other in the pincer movement so important in the use of our hands.

FOOT PLASTERS. Usually the foot is at right angles to the leg and the ankle in mid position between inversion and eversion. Either the plaster extends to the division of the toes or covers the toes completely, except for the tips, depending on the site of injury. The knee is often in slight flexion.

The swelling which accompanies a FRACTURE is quite severe for the first 24–48 hours, and an *incomplete plaster* is used in the first immobilisation so that the limb is not constricted. These are non-weight-bearing. The next day, or occasionally a little later, the incomplete plaster is enclosed with plaster bandages to become a complete plaster.

The patient returns to the ward or he goes home. In the latter instance, clear instructions are given personally by the surgeon or sister. It may be considered an additional advantage for these to be printed on a leaflet which is given to the patient or his relatives. The important points to be made are that he should see a doctor immediately if pain worsens, or if fingers or toes become blue or cold or cease to function, and that he returns to hospital *within 24 hours of the application of a new plaster* for a doctor to examine him. In hospital, the rules are the same. The nurse does not ignore a complaint of pain however trivial it may appear to be, but informs the sister.

Splints

These are used to immobilise a limb.

1. PLASTER OF PARIS bandages (for details of application see p. 269).

2. THOMAS'S SPLINT is a metal splint with a padded ring at one end which fits into the groin. The padding is of felt covered by kid. At the other end the metal is bent to form a notch. This is useful for securing the limb to the splint, and the splint and limb can be steadied during transport by fastening a cord round this notch and the end of the stretcher. Strips of calico six inches wide are placed round the metal sides of the splint to form a sling for the limb. The strips are fastened to the outer aspect by strong safety pins and sometimes bulldog clips. When the limb is placed on the splint, two-thirds of it should be above the level of the splint. If the slings are tighter the limb will tend to roll; if the slings are slacker the limb will rest on the metal of the splint and there will be pressure on the skin. The heel projects beyond the slings; pressure sores behind the heel are avoided by lightly bandaging a thin piece of sponge rubber round the ankle and heel. The patient is encouraged to exercise his foot and ankle to maintain the circulation of blood to the skin.

There are accessories which may be added to the splint, for example a foot piece against which the foot can press as an exercise.

When the splint has been used by a patient, the felt and kid are removed, and the splint is well washed and repadded before being used by another patient. The splint-maker attached to the hospital staff includes this job in his work.

The Thomas's splint is used:
    (a) to immobilise the lower limb during transport after injury;
    (b) as part of fixed traction to reduce a fracture of femur or tibia;
    (c) sometimes to support the lower limb while sliding traction is in progress.

3. BRAUN'S SPLINT. Slings to support the limb are necessary on this type of splint. The leg is supported with the knee and hip partly flexed. It is used when there are fractures in the leg and also just above the knee. It can be combined with traction.

4. Splints are made from PLASTIC MATERIALS moulded to the part of the body to be supported or immobilised. These splints are strong and light in weight but quite expensive and their making requires skill. They are useful for patients who need a splint for neck or trunk but who take part in normal activity. Leather straps can be fastened to them for easy application and removal.

5. METAL SPLINTS (aluminium) are occasionally used for hand or

finger injuries particularly when a dressing is applied over the hand or finger or while there is a great deal of swelling. They are padded with white wool or sponge rubber and a bandage.

6. WOODEN SPLINTS are convenient in an emergency or as a temporary method of immobilisation, following fractures or dislocations. A back splint is used to support the leg and foot, and possibly the lower thigh. This type of splint may be applied to immobilise the elbow during blood transfusion, when the patient is inclined to be restless.

For temporary use, the splint is covered by clean white wool or one-inch sponge rubber, and covered by a roller or tube gauze cotton bandage. The edges and ends of the splints must be well covered or there may be risk of pressure sores from contact with the skin. The splint is applied to the limb and secured by a calico or stretch bandage. After use the padding is removed and discarded, the sponge rubber and splint are washed well and can be boiled for five minutes.

Points to be observed when splints are used:

(a) Padding covers the splint edges and ends and is even in thickness.

(b) The splint is bandaged so that it does not move from its correct position. Bandages securing it are not too tight or too loose; they are inspected two or three times a day.

(c) Friction and pressure are prevented as far as possible. Circulation in the skin and dryness of the area are important.

(d) Complaints of pain from the patient are investigated immediately.

Reduction of Fracture by Traction

When a long bone breaks, the broken ends of the bone tend to overlap. This tendency is increased when the muscles round the fracture contract in an effort to prevent movement and consequent pain. If the bone heals while the broken ends lie over each other, the limb will be shorter than normal. This will be a disability, particularly in walking.

To bring the broken ends of the bone opposite each other so that healing takes place with the bone in a satisfactory position, the lower part of the limb is pulled away from the body. Pulling is TRACTION (as in tractor, or traction engine), and the limb is extended (lengthened) by traction.

THE METHODS OF TRACTION

The lower part of the limb may be pulled by fixing to it special orthopaedic Elastoplast to which a metal weight is fixed by a cord. This is SKIN TRACTION because the Elastoplast is applied to the skin. Alternatively a sterile metal pin or wire is inserted through the heel bone or the upper end of the tibia or lower end of the femur, depending on the place of fracture. To the pin or wire is fixed a horse-shoe-shaped metal plate with a weight fixed to it by a cord. This is SKELETAL TRACTION, and the procedure is performed in the operating theatre under anaesthesia. The *weight* is one or more metal discs like cookery scale weights but with a section cut from the centre. They are placed over a metal rod on a metal base. A small lever holds the weights in position so that they do not slide off. Sometimes a can of lead shot is used. The surgeon decides on the amount of weight to be used.

In both cases the weight is suspended over a pulley which is part of metal frame or bar attached to the bed. The effect of the 'pull' of the metal weight against the weight of the patient's body is increased by raising the foot of the bed on blocks or an elevator.

Because the weight cord slides over the pulley, the method is known as *sliding traction.*

Preparation for Sliding Skin Traction for Lower Limb Fracture
The limb is measured with a tape measure. A Thomas's splint is not necessary for this type of traction but is often used to support the fractured limb. A splint of suitable length and size is chosen. Calico slings are applied fastened with safety pins and possibly bulldog clips.

Hair is shaved from the skin to which the adhesive strips will be applied. If necessary the skin is washed and dried. Tincture of benzoin compound is applied to the skin which has been shaved and allowed to dry; this is antiseptic and appears to assist with application and later removal of the orthopaedic Elastoplast. The ankles and skin behind the heel are protected by orthopaedic felt or wool or thin sponge rubber secured by a bandage.

The orthopaedic Elastoplast stretches widthways and not lengthways. It is usually four inches wide and pink in colour. If the patient's skin is sensitive to Elastoplast, Ventafoam may be used. This is fixed to the skin by crêpe bandages.

The orthopaedic Elastoplast is applied to the inner and outer surfaces of the limb in two pieces. The ends of these extend about five inches beyond the foot. Here they are stitched to make neat, firm tongues which are secured by metal buckles to a piece of wood approximately 3 inches by $2\frac{1}{2}$ inches with a hole in the centre. This is called a spreader. A piece of window cord is threaded through the hole with a large knot on the foot side. The cord passes over a pulley fixed to a Balkan frame over the bed or a simple extended bar screwed to the bottom of the bed. The weight is attached to the cord so that it hangs free from the bed. It is released slowly and gently to avoid causing the patient pain and discomfort. The weight must not rest on any part of the bed frame or be lifted on to the bed as then the traction would be inefficient and possibly painful. Skin traction sets are now available.

SLIDING SKELETAL TRACTION is used in *fractures or dislocations of the neck*. The metal pins are inserted into the skull and attached to a curved metal bar with a weight suspended from it. The head of the bed is raised, the patient lies flat and his feet must NOT rest on a footboard or the effect of traction will be lessened. This patient is probably paralysed in all four limbs and needs sympathetic, skilled nursing care.

SLIDING SKIN TRACTION may be used in the treatment of *vertebral disc lesion* (causing sciatica). It is applied to both legs. The patient lies flat, the bottom of the bed is raised, and his head must not rest on the head of the bed. Thomas's splints are not used. This treatment relieves the patient's pain but it may be a little time before he is accustomed to this unfamiliar position.

Preparation for Fixed Skin Traction
In this procedure *orthopaedic Elastoplast* is applied to the skin and the limb is fixed to the Thomas's splint. Preparation for the procedure is similar to that already explained.

Strips of *lampwick* are sewn to the ends of the orthopaedic Elastoplast using strong thread. The Thomas's splint is applied over the limb; it is important it should fit correctly as the splint ring will be in close contact with the groin. The two pieces of lampwick are tied round the notch at the end of the splint. The tendency of the limb to twist outwards is corrected by taking the lampwick round the metal side of the splint first.

A piece of wood like a pencil may be slipped between the pieces of lampwick and twisted to shorten the distance between foot and notch, thus pulling out, i.e. applying traction to, the limb. The ward sister may do this on instruction from the surgeon.

To prevent the heel resting on the bed the splint is raised by a block placed beneath it, or it is supported by a cord from the Balkan beam.

Nursing Care of a Patient on Traction

If the fracture is in the lower limb, the patient is nursed in a divided bed with a flannelette sheet next to him. The injured limb is exposed.

GENERAL MOVEMENT AND EXERCISES prevent pressure sores, pneumonia and apathy in addition to being an essential part of the surgical treatment of fracture. Every assistance is given to the patient to become active and independent. He washes and shaves himself, uses a hand grip suspended from a pole at the top of the bed to raise his body during bed-making and while a bed-pan is placed beneath him. He flexes and extends his ankles and toes every hour during the day, sometimes being reminded to do so by the nurse. She can assess progress when he presses his foot against a foot-piece or her hand.

Hands and fingers also need exercise to prevent stiffness, particularly when the patient's occupation includes some manual skill. Occupational therapy of a suitable type, e.g. marquetry, provides not only physical activity but mental interest and helps the patient to release tensions which develop when a healthy energetic person is confined to bed. Some forms of clerical work may be considered. In a district where angling is a popular pastime some patients can be found making flies, floats, etc.

Pressure areas are inspected daily. These are likely to be:

The *skin beneath the splint ring*, particularly if the patient is sweating or there is some incontinence in a female patient. In this case a female urinal left in position may be considered. The nurse presses the skin beneath the ring gently away from the ring to relieve the pressure each time she inspects the area. Should any barrier cream be necessary, a smear only of anhydrous lanoline is smoothed over the area. As in all treatment of pressure areas the skin is kept clean and dry.

The *skin behind the heel* can become damaged with little or no pain, and observation is important. The splint sling should not have rolled at the edge, the heel may need some protection and the ankle and foot are exercised.

Buttocks and sacral area may be exposed to pressure, friction and dampness. It has been known for some patients to raise themselves on their elbows which have thus become reddened.

A nutritious *diet* in three good meals a day can usually be taken by the patient without difficulty. Protein and Vitamin C are important when injuries have been severe.

The patient may have problems with defaecation and micturition at first. Glycerine suppositories and an aperient may be necessary the day after the treatment begins. Then sufficient fluid and roughage (fruit and vegetables) in the diet will assist in continuing a daily habit. A special plastic receptacle for collection of urine may be needed by the elderly female patient who passes small amounts of urine often.

Mental confusion, particularly at night, is a complication experienced by some elderly patients admitted to hospital in emergency or those accustomed to taking alcohol each day.

Severe confusion may cause the patient to become very restless, and the traction worries him. The doctor may prescribe a tranquilliser temporarily until the patient settles down.

Pain is reduced or removed completely by the application of traction. Analgesics are rarely necessary and as soon as the patient settles down in hospital he usually sleeps well.

Progress of the patient is assessed by clinical examination and X-rays. Traction may be continued for six weeks, longer if necessary. The patient's limb is protected when he gets up by a caliper which is like a Thomas's splint but the metal rods fit into holes made in the heel of the shoes. He learns to dress and moves about assisted by a walking aid or elbow crutches. He becomes more confident until he can go about the hospital and eventually into the busy thoroughfares of the town.

Outline of the Treatment and Care of the Patient with Paralysis following Spinal Injury involving the Spinal Cord

PARAPLEGIA is paralysis below the place of injury or disease, most often waist level. The lower limbs are paralysed and the bladder and rectum do not function properly.

MONOPLEGIA is paralysis of one limb.

QUADRIPLEGIA is paralysis of four limbs. The spinal cord has been damaged at neck level.

Causes of paraplegia are: *spinal injury* following a road accident, falls of coal or rock, falling from a height, and penetrating bullet wounds. Other causes are spinal tumour and disease of the spine, such as tuberculosis.

The injury is either fracture or dislocation of the spine. Dislocation is usually at cervical level. Fractures are most likely at lower dorsal or lumbar level. The effects of injury include loss of sensation as well as loss of movement, and the patient is unaware of articles touching or burning the skin, and does not know the position of his lower limbs unless he can see them.

At the time of injury the patient is not moved by an inexperienced person. He will probably be lying flat on the ground. Send everyone away except someone who knows him and those who can help when the doctor arrives. His friend or relative, the first-aider or the nurse should kneel on the ground by his side; a person lying on the ground is confused and distressed by people standing round him and looking down on him. If possible his lower limbs are placed in as normal a position as can be managed without moving his trunk, and he is covered by a rug or blanket. His friend or relative can be near to comfort him.

The doctor makes a brief assessment and the patient will be removed to the nearest hospital or injuries unit.

During transport and on admission he lies flat with thin pillows placed beneath the neck and the waist to maintain the normal curves of the spine. There may be a small pillow under the knees and the feet are protected and supported. If his arms are paralysed they are folded across his waist. A bed made up of pillows on a firm base may be used.

During the next few days, a detailed assessment of his injury is made including X-ray photographs, muscle and skin tests. Where there is severe involvement of the spinal cord the patient will probably be transferred to a spinal injuries unit. While the assessment takes place the patient is beginning his mental and emotional adjustments, and his family are faced with the necessity for these too. It is important *never* to assume that he may become completely helpless. Immediately the extent of injury is recognised and it is known which groups of muscles retain activity a programme is devised by which the patient is trained to use these muscles as much as possible in a variety of activities. Some patients can eventually walk using walking aids, others with greater injury become mobile in wheel-chairs, and may be able to drive a disabled person's car. When the previous occupation cannot be resumed, the patient is trained for other more suitable work. Women receive instruction on house cleaning and how to manage their cooking, etc. Hobbies and recreations too are encouraged, and groups of patients in the unit at Stoke Mandeville have formed clubs, including archery, at which they have competed in other countries.

Nursing care of the patient with paraplegia includes the same nursing care as for all patients. *In lifting the patient*, the body is moved 'in one piece' so that the spine is not rotated. A lifting sheet under the pelvis is useful and 3 people are required to move him. *His position is changed* frequently, e.g. every one, two, or four hours. The *pressure areas are protected* by nursing him on a special bed such as one padded by pillows but on a firm base. Limbs are also protected from pressure and injury, but in positions which prevent stretching of muscles.

Nutrition is by a varied diet containing protein foods, roughage, vitamins and minerals so that he does not become thin or overweight. Adequate fluid is essential and it is convenient if he can have some means of taking drinks whenever he feels like it, and is not dependent on other people giving them to him.

Constipation is relieved by roughage in the diet and sometimes by a mild aperient. Regular manual removal of faeces may be necessary. In *retention or incontinence of urine*, catheterisation is avoided if possible. The bladder is re-educated to regain its muscle tone by special methods of drainage, when this can be done. The degrees of incapacity vary from patient to patient.

Throughout the treatment and nursing care the patient needs reassur-

K

ance and encouragement from others, and confidence in the staff and himself. His relatives too, join in helping him and are themselves given confidence and guidance in readiness for the time when the patient rejoins the family circle.

CHAPTER 31 | THE CARDIO-VASCULAR SYSTEM

The Blood

In order to carry out their functions, the body tissues require oxygen and foodstuffs, and these are transported to them in a liquid known as BLOOD. This vital fluid is contained within a system of tubes called BLOOD VESSELS. (When the blood escapes from a cut or diseased blood-vessel, *haemorrhage* is said to have taken place.) In life, the blood flows continually through the blood-vessels so that tissue cells are replenished with oxygen and foodstuffs, and the waste products which result from all living processes are removed. This movement of blood is maintained by the *heart*, which acts like a pump.

Blood is a sticky fluid, red in colour, which tastes salty and has a characteristic smell. It amounts to about one-fifteenth of the body weight in an adult, i.e. about $5\frac{1}{2}$ litres in a man, $4\frac{1}{2}$ litres in a woman. The red colour is given by large numbers of tiny RED BLOOD CELLS. These are produced in red bone marrow and contain a material called haemoglobin which itself contains iron obtained from the diet. They carry oxygen around the body, and the blood leaving the lungs contains large amounts of oxygen and is bright red in colour (Fig. 31). When it returns to the lungs, there is very little oxygen attached to the red cell haemoglobin, but during respiration oxygen from the air is again absorbed into the red cells. These cells live about 120 days and are then destroyed in the spleen, so it is necessary for more to be produced continually in the red bone marrow.

In the blood also are the WHITE CELLS, which are pale in colour. They are fewer in number and larger in size than the red cells and are of two kinds which differ both in appearance and, slightly, in function, but both protect the body in inflammation and infection. Most of the cells are formed in the red bone marrow, and during infection are produced in large numbers. They are needed to rid the body of disease-producing bacteria, together with the remains of cells which have been damaged or destroyed.

In addition to red and white cells there is a number of extremely small particles named PLATELETS which are important in the clotting of blood when it escapes from a blood vessel; a clot of blood frequently seals the hole in the vessel and prevents further bleeding. There is an unusual condition called haemophilia in which blood does not clot easily, so that trivial injuries such as cuts in shaving or tooth extraction become a hazard.

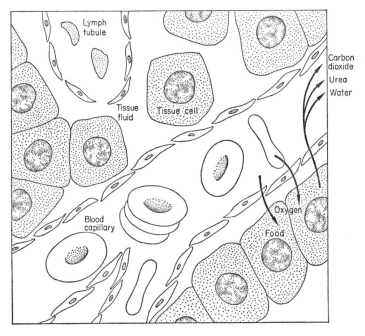

Figure 31. Tissue cells, tissue fluid and blood supply.

The blood cells flow in a straw-coloured sticky and slightly alkaline liquid called PLASMA. The stickiness is due to plasma proteins which prevent it from leaking out through the vessel walls.

As in all fluids in the body, the plasma contains a certain amount of sodium chloride (common salt). Foodstuffs necessary for the different cells in the body are transported in the plasma liquid.

As the blood flows round the body it takes waste products, carbon dioxide and urea from the tissues and transports these to the kidneys, lungs and skin to be excreted.

The blood plasma contains *hormones* produced by the endocrine organs, and *antibodies* which are formed in certain body tissues. Heat is distributed round the body by the circulating blood.

The Blood Vessels

Blood with its oxygen and nutrients comes close to all the cells in the body by flowing through very small tubes called CAPILLARIES. The walls of these are only one cell thick and allow substances in solution to pass through into the tissue fluid which surrounds the tissue cells, and from there into the cells themselves. Waste products pass in the opposite direction and are being continually removed as they are produced.

So that this process of supply and removal can continue, capillaries penetrate all the tissues of the body. Organs which are concerned with controlling amounts of nutrients in the blood (the liver is one) or remove waste from the blood (kidneys) or are capable of great activity (skeletal muscles), are well furnished with capillaries and consequently appear red in colour.

Blood travels to the capillaries in the tissues through small arteries called *arterioles*. These are branches of main vessels named *arteries*. The largest artery in the body is the *aorta* leaving the *heart*, the organ which pumps the blood to the capillaries in the tissues. After circulating through the capillaries the blood returns to the heart by *veins* (Fig. 32).

ARTERIOLES are able to narrow (constrict) or widen (dilate). These actions are organised from the brain and control the amount of blood passing into an organ. For example, when the arterioles in the skin dilate, blood flows into the skin and it becomes flushed and warm. If, however, they are constricted the skin is pale and cool.

The pressure of blood in the *arteries* is high. Therefore if an artery is cut the blood will escape in a jet. It will also be seen to spurt with each heart beat. The AORTA passes from the heart through the chest, behind the diaphragm and into the abdomen, where arteries branch from it, and eventually it divides into vessels entering the pelvis and lower limbs.

The flow of blood returning to the heart is maintained by *valves* in the VEINS and by the action of muscles which squeeze the vessels as the body is exercised.

THE PULMONARY (LUNGS) CIRCULATION

Blood, from which oxygen has been taken up by tissue cells needing it, returns to the heart, which pumps it round the lungs. In these organs, blood in capillaries surrounds the tiny air sacs. As the lungs inflate during breathing, oxygen passes from the air sacs into the blood and carbon dioxide passes from the blood into the air sacs. The oxygenated blood returns to the heart to be pumped round the body.

The PORTAL CIRCULATION includes veins from the stomach, intestines and spleen which join to form the portal vein entering the liver. It is in this way that nutrients and some other substances which have been absorbed in the alimentary tract pass to the liver. Those needed immediately for tissue cell activity are released into blood which leaves the liver and returns to the heart for general circulation.

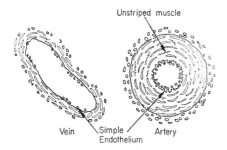

Figure 32. Vein and artery cut across.

The blood vessels are named to identify them and most of the descriptions come from the bones near which they are situated. All the arteries and most of the veins are well protected by bones and muscles, but the superficial veins lie beneath the skin. They are therefore exposed to injury and, not having the full support of the muscles, may in some people become stretched and widened. This condition is known as varicose veins.

The HEART (Fig. 33) is a cone-shaped organ, the size of a closed fist, and situated in the chest a little to the left of mid-line. It is formed from special muscle issue called the myocardium and is surrounded by a double bag of membrane, the pericardium, between the layers of which is a small amount of fluid to prevent friction when the heart muscle contracts during heart beats. There are four chambers in the heart, the left atrium, left ventricle, right atrium and right ventricle. These *atria* have thin muscular walls, and the two *ventricle*s have thick powerful walls. The chambers are lined with a thin smooth tissue called endocardium over which blood can flow easily without clotting. The left side of the heart is separated from the right by a wall, the septum. Between each atrium and ventricle is a valve which prevents blood from flowing backwards when the heart muscle contracts, and there is another valve at the outlet of each ventricle.

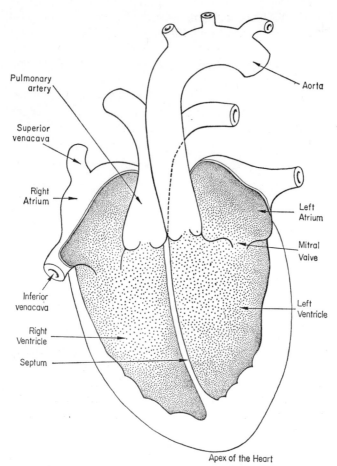

Figure 33. The heart.

Blood Vessels Entering the Heart

Into the right atrium—superior and inferior venae cavae containing de-oxygenated blood from head, trunk and limbs.

Into the left atrium—four pulmonary veins containing oxygenated blood from the lungs.

Blood Vessels Leaving the Heart

From the right ventricle—pulmonary artery with deoxygenated blood flowing to the lungs.

From the left ventricle—aorta with oxygenated blood which will flow to the head, trunk and limbs.

The heart muscle receives its own oxygen and nutrition from the two coronary arteries which come from the aorta. Its nerve supply is adjusted so that its muscle contracts and relaxes rhythmically. In the average adult at rest this is about 60 to 70 times per minute. The contractions are known as heartbeats and can be felt on the anterior chest wall to the left of the sternum between the ribs. The contraction of the left ventricle forces blood along the arteries and the pressure of blood at each heartbeat can be felt where arteries are near the surface of the body as at the wrist, and this is where the *pulse rate* can be counted.

By means of the nerve supply from the brain the speed of the contractions can be increased when demands are made on the body, e.g. in an emergency, and the heart works to a greater capacity as a pump so that certain parts of the body, like the muscles and brain, receive more blood. When the heartbeat increases in rate, the relaxation periods are shortened in comparison with the contraction. This means that a long, continuous period of increased heart rate can sometimes place the heart muscle under stress as in prolonged fever. Like other muscles, the heart improves in efficiency with properly organised exercise, and a slow pulse rate is common amongst athletes.

The Cardio-Vascular System

1. *In Health*
The heart is a muscle, and, like voluntary muscles, improves in tone and efficiency when exercised regularly by physical training or activity.

Changes take place in the size of blood vessels with the needs of organs, dilating in the muscles during exercise and in the stomach and small intestine during digestion, and so on.

The arterioles in the skin change size with temperature, narrowing in cold surroundings to prevent heat loss and dilating to get rid of heat when the environment becomes hot.

Nervous control of blood vessels is shown by pallor in fear and worry, blushing with embarrassment, etc.

2. *In Disease*
When blood is lost in haemorrhage, the loss is made up by increased production of red and white cells, and fluid is replaced. Transfusion is necessary if haemorrhage is severe.

Plasma is lost from the skin in burns, and is made up if necessary by plasma infusions.

Electrolytes in varying proportions may be required to replace loss in sweating or diarrhoea.

(There are compensatory mechanisms for all these happenings and special treatment is not always necessary.)

Common Symptoms and Signs in Diseases of the Blood

1. *Colour.* In lack of blood or haemoglobin the patient's skin and conjunctiva are pale. When there is an excess of red cells the skin is bluish red.

2. *Breathing.* Haemoglobin deficiency means less oxygen is available for the body tissues and the patient breathes rapidly and complains of being short of breath. Severe haemorrhage causes the patient to have *air-hunger* for he needs oxygen urgently.

3. Weakness and tiredness.

4. Swelling of the feet.

5. Purpura (bleeding into the skin, appears like bruising). Haemorrhages from mucous membranes.

Clinical Investigations Concerned with Blood

Blood Count. By special techniques the number of erythrocytes (red cells,) leucocytes (white cells) and platelets can be counted, and are expressed as a number per cubic millimetre of blood. The proportion of each type of white cell can also be counted, and this is called a differential white cell count. Immature erythrocytes, called reticulocytes, can also be counted.

Haemoglobin can be assessed by examination of a drop of blood from the lobe of the ear. The normal is taken as being 100 per cent.

Blood Groups. In blood there are factors which are responsible for different blood groups, and these factors are known as A or B. Some people have A factor, some have B factor, some both factors (Group AB), and others have none (Group O). The plasma of blood from individuals in one blood group will sometimes cause red cells of another blood group to clump together. Should this occur in the bloodstream it would be dangerous, as these clumps could act like clots of blood. For this reason the patient's red cells are compared with the serum (plasma without its fibrin) of blood from four people of the different blood groups A, B, AB, and O. An examination of the results will show the blood groups to which the patient belongs.

Group O is most common, and as the cells have no reacting factor this blood can be donated to almost all other people. People of group AB blood have a non-reactive plasma and therefore can receive blood from most people.

Group A and Group B blood react with each other, and a patient with

Group A blood is not given blood in transfusion from a Group B donor, and vice versa.

There is another blood factor, the Rhesus factor, which may be present (Rh, positive) or absent (Rh negative). There are more Rh positive (Rh$^+$) group people than Rh negative (Rh$^-$) group people.

In hospital, the blood from donors which is most frequently used is Group O Rh$^+$.

The clotting time of blood is assessed when the patient has been prescribed anti-coagulant drugs for treatment of thrombosis, and for patients who bleed abnormally easily, e.g. haemophiliacs.

Marrow Puncture is performed when the physician requests the examination of bone marrow, the blood-forming organ, to assess the activity of the tissue and whether the cells being produced are normal. A needle is inserted through the skin over the sternum into the bone cavity, and a small amount of marrow is withdrawn in the shaft of the needle. Asepsis is necessary. Examinations of blood and marrow are made in the haematology laboratory.

Blood sugar urea and electrolyte examinations are carried out in the biochemical laboratory. Ten millilitres of blood is obtained by the doctor from the patient's vein, injected into a bottle or jar containing potassium citrate or fluoride, a substance which will prevent the blood from clotting. The bottle or jar is shaken well immediately to mix the blood with the substance.

Conditions and Diseases Concerned with Blood

SEVERE HAEMORRHAGE. Rapid loss of blood produces symptoms of thirst, increasing weakness and fainting. The patient is pale and restless with air-hunger. His pulse is rapid and full in volume but if the bleeding continues the rate increases, the volume becomes weak. He may collapse and become unconscious. Sometimes the restlessness develops into mental confusion as the brain becomes anoxic (lacks oxygen). The bleeding may be visible, for example from wounds in external injuries or as vomit from a peptic ulcer (haematemesis). In cases such as a ruptured spleen in injury, or ruptured uterine tube following ectopic gestation, the haemorrhage is internal and recognition of the signs and symptoms is important. The principles of treatment are to stop the bleeding and to replace the lost blood by transfusion.

ANAEMIA is lack of blood but refers mainly to lack of red blood cells (erythrocytes). The patient is pale, and this loss of colour extends to the conjunctiva. In *anaemia of long duration* he is breathless, listless, complains of fatigue and has slight oedema of ankles.

K*

Anaemia is due to:

1. *Loss of blood.* Epistaxis, bleeding from haemorrhoids, and in menorrhagia when the menstrual loss is heavy. A minor degree of bleeding over a long period of time can have serious consequences.

The blood count and haemoglobin are estimated, and blood groups determined as blood transfusion may be required. Measures are taken to deal with the cause of haemorrhage. Later iron medicines are prescribed to replace that which has been lost.

2. *Iron deficiency* is the result of chronic haemorrhage, deficiency in the diet or non-absorption of iron from the intestinal tract. It is treated by dealing with the cause when this is possible and the administration of medicines such as ferrous sulphate or ferrous gluconate tablets by mouth. When absorption of iron is inadequate or the iron deficiency is acute the physician may prescribe an intra-muscular preparation (e.g. Imferon) which is injected into the gluteal muscle of the buttock, or he injects an intravenous preparation (e.g. Ferrivenin).

This patient needs a nutritious well-balanced diet.

3. *Pernicious anaemia* caused by the failure of the stomach wall to absorb vitamin B12 from the diet. This vitamin is required for the production of blood cells by the bone marrow, and its deficiency is responsible for a reduced number of red cells in the blood.

Treatment is by intramuscular injections of vitamin B12 either as the pure substance or in the form of liver extract injections. The injections must be continued every few weeks throughout life and the patient attends a clinic for blood count and supervision of his progress.

4. *Failure in the blood-forming organ, the bone marrow.* The cause for this is often unknown. Occasionally it occurs as a toxic reaction to certain drugs such as sulphonamides, chloramphenicol and thiouracil, and may result from excessive exposure to radio-active materials or X-rays. This condition is known as *aplastic anaemia,* and it is relieved by blood transfusions. As the leucocytes are also involved, nurses prevent infection as far as possible by cleanliness and aseptic techniques when attending to the patient, and antibiotic therapy is frequently prescribed.

LEUKAEMIA is a disease in which there is an abnormal production of white blood cells. This overgrowth of white cells prevents a normal production of red cells and the patient has symptoms of anaemia. The platelets also are affected and there is bleeding into the skin, producing purpura which appears like bruising.

There are three chief types:

1. *Acute myeloid leukaemia.* The bone marrow is affected. This disease is like an acute infection with pyrexia, bleeding in the mouth, purpura and intense pallor. It is a serious illness and patients are either children or

young people. Basic nursing care performed with great gentleness is required. The patient's mouth is treated as often as is necessary, perhaps half-hourly, but with soft wool swabs moistened with water and a mild antiseptic such as glycothymoline, or irrigation of the mouth using a syringe may be more suitable. The diet is soft and non-irritating to the mouth, avoiding added salt. Clear fluids are usually preferred to milk. The patient is mentally alert and appreciates frequent visitors for short sessions.

The patient may be nursed in a side ward (reverse isolation) as he has very little resistance to infection.

2. *Chronic lymphatic leukaemia* is a chronic disease of older people, usually men, in which the lymph glands are enlarged.

3. *Chronic myeloid leukaemia.*

Cytotoxic drugs which slow down white blood cell production are used in treating these diseases. Blood transfusions relieve the anaemia and antibiotics prevent infection. Deep X-ray therapy reduces the enlargement of glands in lymphatic leukaemia.

Common Symptoms and Signs in Diseases of the Blood Vessels

Pain in the legs during walking occurs when the arteries to the lower limbs are narrowed, so that the blood supply, and therefore oxygen, is reduced in the leg muscles.

Numbness may occur if the blood supply to the extremities is poor. The colour of the limbs may become *white* if the arterial supply is restricted, and *blue* when the venus return is impaired.

The skin may be *cold.*

When valves in superficial veins become inadequate they distend and are visible in the leg as varicose veins.

Clinical Investigations

Arteries can be X-rayed by first injecting into them a substance opaque to X-rays which will outline the arteries. This is an *arteriogram* and the film shows blockage, dilation or abnormal position of arteries.

Diseases and Conditions of Blood Vessels

An EMBOLUS is a blood clot moving in the circulation which blocks an artery at a point where the artery divides into smaller vessels, e.g. in a cerebral artery, a branch of the pulmonary artery, the lower end of the aorta, or the femoral or popliteal arteries.

This may arise from a clot of blood forming in the heart in mitral stenosis or in bacterial endocarditis or from a clot of blood forming in the veins of the leg.

A PULMONARY EMBOLUS sometimes occurs about ten days after operation. A sudden acute pain in the chest causes the patient to be very distressed; he is pale and has difficulty in breathing, and sometimes has an acute urge to defaecate. In a severe attack the patient collapses and does not survive more than a few moments. In less serious instances the patient has a sudden pain in the chest and coughs, and often has blood-stained sputum. He becomes pale and breathless. The nurse disturbs him as little as possible, sends for his doctor and administers oxygen.

CEREBRAL EMBOLISM (blockage of a cerebral artery by an embolus) results in hemiplegia, i.e. paralysis on one side of the body. This is called in simple terms 'a stroke', and in severe cases the patient becomes unconscious; in other cases he may be aware of his surroundings and disability but is unable to explain them as there is disturbance of speech.

EMBOLISM IN THE FEMORAL OR POPLITEAL ARTERY causes the foot to become cold and numb. On inspection the limb below the blocked artery is white. The ward sister is informed *at once* and surgery (embolectomy) may be urgently necessary.

A THROMBOSIS is a clot of blood stationary in a blood vessel which occurs in the cerebral and coronary arteries, and in deep veins of the lower limbs.

Deep-vein thrombosis in the calf or thigh is a complication of bed rest when the patient lies in one position. It is predisposed by pressure on the veins through relaxed muscles when hard pillows are placed under the calves or thigh, and by infection and its general effects of toxaemia. The patient complains of pains in the muscle, the limb is stiff and slightly oedematous with a bluish colour. In treatment the limb is immobilised on a thin, soft pillow for a few weeks and protected by a cradle. Infection is controlled by antibiotics, and anticoagulant drugs may be prescribed. Recovery of the patient from illness or operation is delayed. Measures to prevent this complication include getting the patient to walk as soon as possible after operation. If the patient cannot walk in the ward, he has exercises in bed, often supervised by the physiotherapist but performed at frequent intervals during the day. The position of a helpless patient is changed at least every two hours.

Sitting in a chair so that the edge of the seat presses against the lower thighs for two or three hours can also predispose this condition in a woman who is short in stature. It may be advisable to place a pillow behind the patient's sacrum and a stool beneath her feet, and to encourage her to move and walk in the ward every twenty to thirty minutes.

VARICOSE VEINS. The valves in superficial veins of the lower limbs sometimes become inadequate and the veins distend. The patient complains of itching of the skin over the vein and pain in the limb after standing for some time. They are unsightly when visible. When injured there can be severe bleeding, and slight damage may lead to varicose ulcers which are painful and difficult to heal. In mild cases an elastic stocking or support hose or crêpe bandage gives relief. Resting with the limb raised for a time during the day is helpful.

Treatment is by an injection into the vein to cause an aseptic thrombosis and consequent thickening of the vessel walls, or by operation. Either the vein is ligatured near the groin or the whole vein is stripped out. In these cases other veins take on the passage of blood previously sustained by the ligatured or removed vein. A crêpe bandage to provide firm support is applied to the limb before the patient gets out of bed, beginning at the foot but omitting the heel and finishing just above the knee.

GRAFTS OR REPAIRS ON MAJOR BLOOD VESSELS are operations to overcome a block or weakness in the vessel. Blocks are due to an embolus, and weakness in an artery is the result of a dilation (aneurysm) of the vessel.

Observations of lower limbs after operation include:
noting the colour of the foot, and whether the feet are cold; should the feet become white, blue or cold or the pulse cannot be felt, the nurse reports this to the ward sister *without delay* as the surgeon will wish to be informed.

As in all operations, nutrition, prevention of infection and pressure sores are essential parts of the patient's general treatment.

Common Symptoms and Signs in Diseases of the Heart

The *arterial pulse* is usually observed in the radial artery at the wrist below the thumb. The rate, volume and regularity are noted and give an indication of the heart efficiency and activity. The pulse rate is faster than normal in some heart diseases, in fevers and in excitement. An extremely low pulse rate, e.g. 30 per minute, is a sign observed in 'heart block'.

When the patient is in a state of collapse and no pulse can be felt 'cardiac arrest' has occurred. (The heart has stopped.) This is an emergency situation.

The rhythm of normal pulse is regular, but in a few healthy people there are extra beats. One cause of irregularity in the pulse rhythm is *atrial fibrillation*, when the walls of the atria twitch erratically and frequently instead of having regular efficient contractions. The impulses reaching the ventricles through the Bundle of His are ineffective and do not always occur when the ventricle contains blood. The output of blood from the heart becomes inadequate.

There are changes in *blood pressure* in heart disease, and high blood pressure may also cause heart disease. The patient is *cyanosed* and breathless when the cardiac condition affects the pulmonary circulation.

Pain is not always a feature but some patients complain of sub-sternal pain, which they sometimes regard as indigestion. Angina pectoris is a gripping pain in the chest, which may radiate down the left arm. It occurs when the patient is active, ceasing when he is at rest.

In chronic heart failure the patient's general circulation is inefficient and he develops *oedema*, fluid in the tissues, which gravitates to the lowest part of the body. The *urine* output has decreased.

Exercise intolerance is observed by the patient and his relatives. There may be *mental confusion* at night.

Clinical Investigations

X-ray of the chest reveals any abnormal position or size of the heart and major blood vessels.

Electric impulses produced by heart muscle as it contracts can be picked up and conducted by leads (cables) from the patient to an electrical machine which translates the impulses into a graph drawn on paper. This is an *electrocardiograph* which indicates to the physician the activity of heart muscle during the cardiac cycle.

Diseases of the Heart

Acute rheumatism, or rheumatic fever, is an allergic reaction of the body to streptococcal infection such as a sore throat. It occurs usually in children and is becoming less common since streptococcal infections are now more easily controlled. The joints are swollen and painful, the pain moving from joint to joint, and the child is feverish with a high temperature, sweating and general malaise. It is thought that in some children the symptoms may be so slight that the disease is not recognised. The heart tissues may become inflamed causing endocarditis, myocarditis or pericarditis. In some cases there are severe symptoms, e.g. acute dyspnoea and chest pain in pericarditis. Because of the likelihood that the heart may be affected the patient is nursed at rest in a comfortable semi-recumbent position and dissuaded from general activity. Sponging of the skin relieves the discomfort of fever and the joints are kept warm and free from weight and pressure of bedclothes. A cradle is placed over the feet, the nurse flexes and extends the patient's ankle when changing his position at frequent intervals. Fluid intake is increased to 3,000 millilitres a day. The acute condition responds to salicylates and the physician prescribes penicillin to deal with causative infection. The patient is nursed in bed until his temperature, pulse and electrocardiograph are satisfactory.

It is usually decided that penicillin therapy shall continue indefinitely so that he has protection against further infection.

Chorea is another manifestation of the reaction to streptococcal infection but this affects the child's nervous system and he has uncontrolled jerky movements with fever. It has been known as 'St Vitus' Dance' and is uncommon at the present time. As he is continually restless the child's skin is exposed to friction.

HYPERTENSION means a raised blood pressure. It can be due to the increased resistance in the blood vessels in arterio-sclerosis (hardening of the arteries), a change which takes place in the arteries of some older people. Occasionally it occurs in a severe form in a young person. Hypotensive drugs are prescribed by the physician to relieve the condition and avoid complications, and the patient should lead a quiet life, for the blood pressure rises in emotional crises.

ATHEROMA is a condition in which the tissue lining the arteries degenerates and fatty deposits appear as patches on the endothelium, causing narrowing of the artery. When this condition occurs in the coronary arteries there is poor access of blood to the heart muscle, and this may be inadequate for its increased activity in general exercise. Muscle deprived of oxygen produces pain and in physical effort the patient experiences an acute pain in his chest radiating down the left arm. This is *Angina pectoris*. He is distressed, then stands still and rests, and the pain is relieved.

Dissolving tablets of glycerine trinitrite under the tongue relieves the pain by dilating the arteries, the coronary arteries in particular.

Atheroma may predispose to clot formation in a coronary artery (coronary thrombosis) and this will block an artery supplying the heart muscle with oxygen. Heart function is seriously disturbed and the patient collapses with severe pain in the chest. He is pale and sweating and the condition may be very quickly fatal. He should be disturbed as little as possible, lying on the ground with a coat or rug beneath his head and covered by another until a doctor or ambulance men arrive. He is lifted carefully into bed at home or taken to hospital. Treatment is usually by rest in bed with a minimum of activity until his heart activity improves, then graduated exercises are arranged. Pain at the time of collapse is relieved by analgesics, e.g. morphia, and sedation by barbiturates may be necessary for the patient to obtain adequate rest; these drugs are prescribed by the physician who has examined the patient. Oxygen is administered by nasal spectacles at 4 litres per minute or by a plastic mask at 6 litres per minute. The blood pressure may be very low at the time of admission and stimulants are prescribed.

Anti-coagulant therapy is used in some cases to prevent further blood clotting.

The patient is discharged from hospital in 4 to 6 weeks and advised to stop smoking (which accelerates heart activity), assume fewer responsibilities with their attendant stresses and strains, take more physical exercise and lose weight when this is above average.

This condition is becoming increasingly more common in men over the age of forty-five and is occurring now in younger age groups.

CONGESTIVE HEART FAILURE is failure of the muscle on the right side of the heart which results in congestion of the tissues from which the veins return blood to the right atrium.

The nurse will observe in this patient *oedema* which is easily detected in the ankles and feet when he has been standing, and in the sacral area as he lies in bed. The abdomen may be enlarged with an increase of fluid in the peritoneal cavity and this is *ascites*. *Urine* is decreased in amount and contains albumin, indicating congestion of the kidneys. The patient loses his appetite, complains of indigestion and nausea, and is constipated. As the condition progresses and the lungs become congested he becomes cyanosed and is breathless, sometimes unable to breathe unless he is sitting up in bed or in a chair (orthopnoea). During the night he may be confused.

In the treatment of this patient, the physician investigates the cause of the heart failure and appropriate measures are prescribed, such as drugs to reduce the effects of thyrotoxicosis or hypertension should either of these conditions be discovered.

General Nursing Care. The patient finds sitting up in bed well supported by back rest and pillows most comfortable for breathing. In orthopnoea he leans forward on a bed-table, his arms on a pillow. Oedematous feet are supported on a thin, soft pillow and protected from the weight of bed-clothes by a cradle. A water pillow or sponge rubber cushion is placed beneath the oedematous sacral area. Patients with cardiac failure and oedema do not tolerate cold well. Draughts are avoided and a thin, warm flannelette sheet or cellular blanket covers the feet and can be tucked closely round his body. A loose cardigan or bedjacket protects the shoulders while the patient is sitting up in a cool room or ward and is more easily removed than a vest beneath the pyjamas or nightdress.

The nurse relieves the patient of all activities causing effort. She washes and feeds him, a colleague assists her in lifting the patient when making the bed or placing a bed-pan beneath him. Sedation is necessary on some occasions.

A weight-reducing diet is introduced with less sugar and starchy food, as these cause indigestion, and meals are small in bulk to prevent embarrassment of the heart by a distended stomach.

Digitalis is frequently prescribed by the physician, the action of the drug being to slow down and strengthen the heartbeat. The nurse observes the pulse rate, and when this falls to below 60 a minute the doctor is consulted before the drug is administered.

Oxygen is administered through Ventura mask (28% oxygen), when there are pulmonary complications causing dyspnoea.

The patient in hospital may be worried, even distressed, in the unfamiliar surroundings. He feels extremely ill and during the night can be anxious and afraid. The nurse attends to him frequently and is available when required. If he finds bed-rest difficult to tolerate (at home, where he has already been ill, he has probably been dressed and assisted into a room to be with other members of his family except when extremely ill), it may be considered satisfactory for him to be lifted out of bed into a chair for a few hours a day. Frequently the patient finds using the commode less exhausting than a bed-pan in bed; and the bed-sheets can be changed while he is out of bed.

Reduction of oedema is by *restriction of salt intake*, none being added to the diet. To improve the flavour of the food a synthetic salt can be used.

The physician prescribes diuretics such as Mersalyl by intra-muscular injection or Chlorthiazide by mouth, and the nurse measures the urine output. Assessment of improvement is made by weighing the patient once or twice a week at the same time each day.

When the oedema persists or is severe the physician may consider the insertion of Southey's tubes in the legs to drain the fluid. In ascites he introduces a cannula into the peritoneal cavity under local anaesthetic to remove the excess fluid and relieve the patient's discomfort.

Convalescence is slow, and the patient's physical activities and responsibilities need to be reduced. This is difficult for those whose lives have included these in good measure, and they sometimes need help in adjusting to a quieter life.

LEFT-SIDED HEART FAILURE is due to hypertension. The patient has a cough with sputum, sometimes blood-stained. He is distressed at night by attacks of acute dyspnoea. This is *cardiac asthma*. The patient finds sitting in a chair more comfortable than lying down in bed and appreciates some ventilation from an open window. In hospital, he leans forward on a bed-table, and the nurse remains with him while the attack is in progress. This condition may eventually become complicated by right-side failure.

PULMONARY CARDIAC FAILURE is heart failure associated with long-standing lung disease, e.g. chronic bronchitis or emphysema. The lung condition is treated and the patient requires the nursing care given to those with congestive heart failure.

OPERATIONS ON THE HEART

These are performed in the treatment of the following conditions.

1. Congenital Heart Conditions

Openings in the heart septum which normally close at birth occasionally remain open. Blood is able to pass from the left to the right side of the heart. Consequently the amount of blood passing through the lungs is greater than normal and the heart enlarges to pump this extra amount of blood.

In surgery these defects (holes) are closed either by sewing the edges together or by sewing in a patch of plastic cloth. The heart is exposed by opening the chest (thoracotomy) and its action is taken over by a heart and lung machine which collects the blood from the large veins, oxygenates it, and returns it to the patient's arteries.

Some children are blue and the commonest cause of this is *Fallot's tetralogy* in which there are four defects of different types. Patients are breathless, blue and often have clubbing of the fingers. They frequently squat on exertion and sometimes have fainting attacks. An operation is performed to correct the defects.

2. Heart Defects which Occur Later in Life

MITRAL STENOSIS is the result of inflammation of the valves in rheumatic fever. The flow of blood from the lungs is obstructed and lung congestion follows. In surgical treatment thoracotomy is performed and the surgeon dilates the opening of the valve with his finger or an instrument so that blood can flow through more easily.

When a valve in the heart is diseased and the opening enlarges, the heart's pumping action becomes less efficient. The surgeon is often able to replace the diseased valve with an artificial type which is now available.

Operations are performed while the patient is at normal temperature or in hypothermia. His temperature will be 35°C when he returns to the ward.

Preparation for operation is careful and detailed. After an advanced operation the patient is nursed in a recovery ward or intensive care unit.

Preparation for and Care of the Patient during the Introduction of Fluid and Blood into the Cardio-vascular System

ADMINISTRATION OF FLUID BY THE INTRAVENOUS METHOD

The technique is sometimes known as intravenous infusion (infusion means 'the *pouring* of something into').

The occasions when intravenous infusion is used as treatment are as follows:

1. The administration of water in severe dehydration. A prescribed amount of sodium chloride is included.

2. The administration of electrolytes, sodium or potassium, when there is a deficiency of either of these in the blood.

3. The replacement of fluid lost from the circulation during or following surgical operation.

4. The replacement of fluid lost from the circulation in shock due to injuries, burns or surgery.

5. The continuous slow administration of drugs into the blood stream. *Fluids* which are introduced into the body by intravenous infusion are:

Water containing *sodium chloride* in prescribed amounts, usually 0·18% or 0·9%. The latter is sometimes referred to as 'normal saline'. 0·18% sodium chloride in water is called one-fifth normal saline.

Potassium is prescribed in varying amounts according to the patient's blood analysis, and is carefully and accurately prepared in the dispensary as a sterile solution for slow intravenous administration.

Simple food is in the form of dextrose 5% in water, to which is added 0·18% or 0·9% sodium chloride.

Dextran is an example of a solution in which particles of a special substance are suspended in water. These particles are too large to escape from the capillaries through the tiny spaces between the epithelial cells, and therefore assist in keeping the blood inside the blood circulatory system. This solution is administered in prevention or treatment of shock, preventing a dangerously low blood pressure which would interfere with the flow of blood through vital organs like the brain and kidneys.

Plasma is separated from the cells in human blood from donors, and dried by a heat process so that only the solid part of the plasma remains. This is composed largely of plasma proteins. It is collected under aseptic conditions into a sterile bottle which is sealed. Immediately before the intravenous infusion is commenced the seal is broken, the cap is removed from the bottle and special distilled water is added. The water is as pure as it is possible to make any water, so that it is safe to 'pour into' the blood stream. The dried plasma and distilled water are mixed thoroughly. The solution is ready for administration.

Nor-Adrenalin is a drug which is added by the doctor to sodium chloride and water solution for intravenous administration sometimes as treatment in shock.

EQUIPMENT for intravenous infusion includes:

>   Basic dressing trolley.
>
>   Antiseptic lotion for cleansing the skin.
>
>   Sterile 2-millilitre syringe and needle with local anaesthetic, e.g. procaine hydrochloride 2%.
>
>   Blood pressure machine.
>
>   Sterile intravenous set.
>
>   Sterile intravenous needle or cannula, e.g. Guest cannula.
>
>   Tubing clip to regulate flow of fluid.
>
>   Covered splint or protected pillow to support or immobilise the arm or foot if necessary.
>
>   Adhesive tape to secure the needle to the skin.
>
>   Bottle clip by which to suspend the bottle of fluid from an intravenous stand.
>
>   Bottle of prescribed fluid, usually 500 millilitres. Fluid is checked by noting that the names on the label and the prescription signed by the medical practitioner are identical. Fluid balance chart on which to record the amount on the Intake Column.

PREPARATION OF PATIENT

The doctor or nurse explains that he is going to have some fluid through a needle in his arm (or foot), that the fluid will take some time to go through and he may need to lie quietly for that time. He will have a prick in his arm before it begins, and then he will not feel anything. It may be advisable to offer a urinal or bed-pan before the procedure begins.

When the needle or cannula is to be inserted into the arm and may be in position for some time, the nurse will no doubt consider it sensible to remove the pyjama sleeve from that limb, as it is not possible to remove the jacket after the apparatus is set up. (Occasionally bed-gowns which have tapes along the shoulder and sleeve are provided, so that the garment can be removed easily.) The same problem may arise with pyjama trousers, when the site of infusion is a vein in the foot. The limb is kept warm by a small flannelette sheet light in weight, which can be replaced by a clean one at least once a day. It is dangerous to place a hot-water bottle near to the limb, as burns can easily occur. Usually the doctor chooses the site with regard for the suitability of the vein. Injuries, operations and skin conditions may exclude certain areas which would otherwise be suitable. Should there be no special reason for choosing a certain site, the nurse should ask the patient whether he is right- or left-handed. Then the more useful upper limb can be kept free for manipulating drinking-cups, spoons, handkerchief tissue, urinal, etc.

Splints are covered by clean white wool and sponge rubber, tube gauze bandage, or are specially prepared with a waterproof covering. They are only necessary when the patient is restless. Fixed at the elbow by bandage or adhesive tape, a splint tends to keep the joint too straight and stiff, and the needle is not accommodated easily. When a pillow is used beneath the arm or leg it is protected by a waterproof cover beneath its clean cotton cover, as there may be a little bleeding. A cradle will be required to raise the bed-clothes from the leg.

The procedure is carried out by the doctor with the assistance of the nurse. It is helpful if the nurse attends to the patient and observes any change in his condition, reporting this to the doctor as it arises. She places equipment so that it is easily available to the doctor. They both check the fluid to be administered with the prescription form. If the fluid is turbid or has a sediment it is not used but returned to the pharmacy.

The sites used for intravenous infusion are:
Suitable vein at the elbow.
Suitable vein on the back of the hand or above the wrist.
Suitable vein above the foot or ankle.
It is an aseptic procedure, and the main steps now are these:
The nurse arranges the blood pressure machine in position above the site for infusion.
The doctor washes and dries his hands, assembles the equipment, cleans the area, administers local anaesthetic.
The nurse inflates the cuff on the patient's limb to about 100 millimetres on the doctor's instruction.
The doctor inserts the needle or cannula.
The nurse deflates the cuff.
The doctor releases the tubing clip so that the fluid flows from the bottle and then he regulates the flow.
The needle and tubing may be secured to the limb by adhesive tape.
Before leaving the patient, his general condition is noted.

Supervision of the Patient during Intravenous Infusion
The general nursing care of the patient continues with the addition of any particular treatment. It is possible for some patients after operation to

walk in the ward with the cannula in the hand or arm and the intravenous bottle supported in a metal carrier, but usually the patient is nursed in bed. As far as possible any restlessness is prevented by attending to the patient's basic needs—to pass urine, to relieve thirst, pyrexia, pain, excessive heat or cold. When prevention or treatment of restlessness is difficult, the limb is secured by a splint or a loosely applied clove-hitch bandage attached to the side of the bed.

The limb is visible, an arm being supported on top of the bed-clothes, whilst a foot is viewed through the open-ended bed when the cradle is in position.

Tension on the needle is avoided by allowing the tubing some freedom. A loop of tubing can be fastened to the sheet by a safety pin. No kinking of the tubing must be allowed to occur. Care is taken when making the patient's bed, or changing his position, that the tubing is not dragged as this may move the needle.

The flow of fluid is noted at frequent intervals. It is regulated according to the doctor's instructions by opening or closing the clip, and is measured either by the drops per minute through the drip-chamber usually 15 to 40, depending on the reason for the infusion), or the time for 1 bottle, i.e. 500 millilitres in 8 hours. It is important that the patient has the correct amount given in the stated time at a continuous rate, otherwise his fluid and electrotype balance will be disturbed. A State Registered Nurse is notified when the bottle is emptied to $1\frac{1}{2}$ inches from the neck so that she may change the bottle if this has been requested. Inform her if the flow of fluid through the drip-chamber ceases.

OBSERVATIONS OF THE PATIENT

Any movement of the needle, swelling round the site of infusion, local inflammation or bleeding, and complaint of pain by the patient are reported to the ward sister or charge nurse. If the patient's breathing becomes more rapid with increased mucus secretion and an inclination to cough (i.e. he is 'chesty'), this is also reported. His general condition is again noted.

When drugs are being given to the patient in this way, it is necessary to observe their effect.

In some cases insertion of a needle or cannula directly into the vein is considered unsuitable. One reason for this is that the patient's blood pressure is low and the vein is collapsed. Then the doctor cuts down through the skin to the vein, which is carefully exposed. The vein is encircled by 2 ligatures using an aneurysm needle. The ligature farther from the heart is tied off. A small incision is made in the vein with a scalpel. Into this an intravenous cannula is inserted, and this may be supported in the vein by the second ligature. This procedure necessitates the making of a wound. A local anaesthetic is required, and an aseptic technique is employed. Splint covering and protective covering for the limbs should be quite clean. A sterile dressing is placed over the wound, and the nurse's hands are washed before attending to the dressing or cannula.

Extra Sterile Equipment for Cutting down to the Veins
    2 pair mosquito forceps (very fine artery forceps).
    1 pair suture scissors.
    1 scalpel or Bard Parker handle and blade.
    1 aneurysm needle.
    2 cutting edge needles, 1 straight and 1 curved.
    Ligatures and sutures, e.g. linen thread.
    Intravenous cannula.

CHANGING A BOTTLE OF FLUID DURING CONTINUOUS INTRAVENOUS INFUSION is performed by the doctor or a State Registered Nurse. The nurse in training, however, may be asked to check the fresh bottle with the prescription signed by a doctor, and witness the commencement of its administration to the patient. The points to bear in mind are:

1. The correct fluid is presented for administration. See page 297.

2. No air is allowed to enter the apparatus during the procedure, as this would interfere with blood circulation.

3. Aseptic technique is necessary.

If the intravenous infusion stops, the sister or nurse in charge of the ward is informed at once. Is the bottle empty? It is useful to check immediately whether the needle has moved from the vein in which case sister will close the tubing clip. The nurse makes sure that the tubing is not kinked, and that it is not trapped beneath the patient's body or some bed equipment. She does not interfere with any part of the intravenous apparatus unless she has been so instructed.

Taking down intravenous infusion apparatus is carried out by the doctor, though the ward sister or staff nurse may sometimes remove it on the instructions of the doctor when there has been simple insertion of a needle. If there has been an incision to expose the vein the doctor will remove the cannula, ligature the vein and close the skin with a suture. For this procedure he needs sterile dressings and forceps, cutting needle and nylon suture for the skin, and suture scissors. A bandage, strapping or collodion will seal the wound.

Any signs of local inflammation such as pain, redness and swelling within the next 24 hours are reported. The total amount of fluid administered is entered on the fluid balance chart.

If a vein has been ligatured at the end of this procedure, the blood which would normally flow through this vein now passes along smaller veins alongside. These enlarge to some extent to take the extra load. A vein which has been incised can rarely be used again at the same point, and this is one reason why the care of the patient who is having intravenous infusion is important, as there may be only a limited number of suitable sites in the patient for this method of treatment.

Intravenous Infusion in Infants and Children
The veins are very small and the needles used are extremely fine. Sometimes the site chosen in an infant is a scalp vein. The needle is secured by a rubber strap round the wrist or ankle, or by collodion. As the child may find the procedure unpleasant, a sedative may be ordered by the doctor to be given before the treatment commences.

The regulation of the amount of fluid administered to infants particularly is of the greatest importance. Water and electrolytes are in very small amounts compared with those in the adult body and even a slight alteration in balance can produce rapid and intense effects. Definite amounts may be ordered to be given in each hour. To provide for greater accuracy, a reservoir to hold, for example, 100 millilitres is sometimes fixed above the drip-chamber. This is filled from the bottle above at each hour. During the hour this fluid flows through the drip-chamber into the vein.

Infants and children have amazing powers of adaptation to situations in illness as well as in health, but during lengthy treatments of this kind they need quiet and soothing comfort. When a child cannot move easily, the nurse speaks to him with her face towards him, so that he can focus without effort. When she leaves him his favourite toy is placed where he can see it.

Blood Transfusion

The REASONS for which blood is transfused:
1. To replace blood loss resulting from injury, disease (such as peptic ulcer, haemorrhoids) uterine bleeding following childbirth, or surgical operations.
2. To treat anaemia (lack of blood).
3. To provide extra blood for the machine which pumps blood round the patient's body during major heart surgery. This is extracorporeal circulation (circulation from outside the body).
4. To replace the blood of a few newly born infants. These are the Rhesus positive babies of Rhesus negative mothers. Rhesus negative blood is used.

When the doctor decides the patient needs blood transfusion he with-draws a sample of blood from a vein. The laboratory technician discovers from this the patient's blood group, Blood is received from the blood transfusion centre as required by the hospital. The most common type being Group O Rhesus positive. Each bottle has a large label showing the blood group of its content, and information regarding storage, etc. There is also a space for the patient's name, ward and number when the blood is reserved. Attached to the bottle is a small screw-cap bottle con-taining a few millilitres of the same blood. The technician adds a few drops of this to a few drops of the patient's blood on a glass slide, and looks at the result under the microscope. This is cross-matching—when the donor's blood is satisfactory there is no clumping of red cells. In this case the blood is reserved for the patient, and his name, etc., is written on the label. The bottle is now stored in a refrigerator at 4°C to 6°C where it is accessible to ward staffs.

Sometimes the blood is collected into a polythene bag (or pack). This is lighter in weight and more convenient for transport and storage.

There are two types of pre-sterilised intravenous sets in common use:

(a) for use with *bottles of blood*. The apparatus includes an air-entry tube. As blood leaves the bottle, air enters the bottle to replace it;

(b) for use with *packs of blood*. There is *no* air-entry tube in this set. As blood leaves the pack the polythene bag collapses. The short tube in the apparatus is included for the administration of drugs.

In an emergency the patient's blood is cross-matched immediately with a donor Group O blood, and the patient's blood groups are assessed later. It is useful if people who know their blood groups carry a card to show this.

When urgent treatment is required and blood from the Blood Trans-fusion Service is not available, the doctor may consider transfusing a relative's blood after cross-matching. Most hospitals have 500 mls blood which is suitable to transfuse any patient in extreme emergency. Jehovah's witnesses refuse blood transfusion treatment on religious grounds.

Equipment

This is the same as that for intravenous infusion of fluid, and the patient is prepared in the same way, but it is explained to him that blood is to be transfused. Some new patients feel that this treatment is carried out only in extremely serious and urgent situations, and need assurance that it is frequently used to raise the general physical condition by improving the blood. If they have lost blood, they usually accept that recovery is speeded by blood replacement.

The bottle of blood is brought to the ward only a short time before it is required. It is not placed where there is extra heat, but is allowed to come to room temperature.

Checking of Blood

This precaution is carried out by a doctor or State Registered Nurse. A second reliable person (this would be a nurse in training) witnesses the checking of the details:

1. The full name and age on the bottle label is the same as that of the patient to be transfused.

2. The registration or laboratory number on the bottle label is the same as that of the patient to be transfused.

3. The blood is transfused to the patient whose full name is on the bottle label.

Nurses may find it helpful to notice a patient's blood group, as this aids in checking also. It is as well to bear in mind that the patient may be transferred from one ward to another as this could cause confusion.

If the patient is unconscious or for some other reason cannot give his full name, this may be found on a wrist identification band and on his charts on the bed or locker.

The PROCEDURE is the same as for intravenous infusion. The transfusion may begin with a sterile normal saline solution 0·9%, this bottle being replaced by the bottle of blood which has been checked. The rate of flow is from 20 to 40 drops a minute. Occasionally, for example after or during severe haemorrhage which cannot be stopped immediately, the rate may be very fast indeed. Regulation of rate is on the instructions of the doctor.

OBSERVATIONS OF THE PATIENT are also the same as for intravenous infusion, with the addition of rise in temperature, rigors (shivering attacks), jaundice, skin rash, twitchings, pain in the limb where the cannula or needle is introduced or in the lower back or chest, or haematuria. Any of these signs are reported at once.

OBSERVATIONS OF THE APPARATUS. When the bottle is nearly empty it is reported. The rate is regulated correctly. The tubing is handled carefully, and no tension is put on the needle. Should the flow of blood stop, the sister or nurse in charge is informed.

When the transfusion is completed, the bottle is usually returned to the laboratory *unwashed*. This is in case further examination of that particular blood is required.

The patient may be interested to know who donated the blood he received, as he often feels he would like to express his gratitude personally. This is not possible as the names of donors are not disclosed with their donated blood. Donors in this country give blood as an offering, without payment, to any person who needs blood transfusion through the Blood Transfusion Service. The gratitude of the patient is to all donors who have this consideration for others less fortunate than themselves.

The cost to the National Health Service financed by the taxpayer is considerable. Because of this, bottles of blood are stored and used under precise instructions. In this way no blood is ever wasted.

The Lymphatic System

In the tissue spaces surrounding the body's cells are tiny tubules which join to form thin-walled tubes leaving the organs as lymphatic vessels. It is thought that plasma proteins which escape from the capillaries into the tissue fluid are removed through these tubules. If plasma proteins were allowed to accumulate in that tissue fluid, water would flow from the capillaries into the tissue spaces, causing oedema.

LYMPH is the name given to the fluid as it passes along the lymphatic vessels. Its flow through the body is made possible by the large number of valves in the thin-walled lymphatic vessels and the squeezing effect of skeletal muscles in action. Lymph vessels accompany the deep and superficial veins. They enter LYMPH NODES (Fig. 34) which are small organs found in groups at the base of the neck, in the axillae, groins, and deep in the chest and abdomen. Larger vessels from the nodes join to form two main vessels which enter the blood circulation at the base of the neck.

The lymphatic system is one of the means by which the body protects itself from harmful material produced during inflammatory changes. As the result of infection lymph flows through the tubules together with the remains of dead tissue and white blood cells, and possibly a number of bacteria. In the compartments of the lymph nodes are large white cells which ingest the unwanted material as the lymph flows by them. In this way all harmful substances have been removed by the time the lymph enters the blood circulation.

Lymph nodes also produce *lymphocytes*, one type of white blood cell.

In the lining of the small intestine is another group of lymph tubules into which fats are absorbed from food digested in the alimentary tract. These tubules join with the other lymph vessels in the system.

To summarise, lymph contains:
 1. Fluid from tissue spaces.
 2. Substances to be removed from tissue spaces:
    (a) plasma proteins escaped from the capillaries;
    (b) cell debris and micro-organisms in infection.
 3. Fats absorbed from the small intestine.
 4. Lymphocytes.

If lymph drainage from a part of the body is interfered with in injury or disease, oedema occurs in that area.

Carcinoma is a disease which can spread to various parts of the body through the lymphatic system.

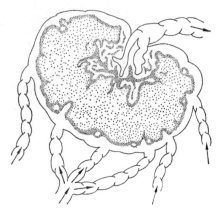

Figure 34. Lymph node (gland).

CHAPTER 32 | RESPIRATION AND THE RESPIRATORY TRACT

Respiration is the act of breathing. During respiration air is drawn or sucked into the lungs from the atmosphere surrounding the body; this is *inspiration*. Then air is pushed out from the lungs; this is *expiration*. The act of breathing takes place in a healthy adult between 16 and 20 times a minute, and is under the control of the medulla which is part of the brain. The moving of air into and out of the lungs is called *pulmonary ventilation*. This movement increases in exercise, and decreases when a patient lies very still, for example after major surgery or during unconsciousness or when he experiences pain on breathing.

The Organs of Respiration

The LUNGS are two organs in the chest. They are cone-shaped with the upper point at the level of the first rib and the lower border or base resting on the diaphragm, which is the circular muscle separating the chest (or thorax) from the abdomen. In life the lungs are pink owing to the blood circulating in a large number of lung capillaries, but if the person lives for many years in a dust-laden atmosphere, as in a city, or a coal mine, the lungs appear dark. They are spongy in texture because of the air-spaces in them. Entering each lung are two vessels, one is an air-tube (or *bronchus*) which is the end of the open air-passage from the nose and throat, and the other is a branch of the pulmonary artery from the heart, which contains deoxygenated blood.

The bronchus divides like the branches of a tree into tiny tubes or *bronchioles*. At the end of each of these is an air-space (alveolus). The air-spaces (alveoli) are surrounded by capillaries, through which blood flows on its way from the branch of the pulmonary artery to the two pulmonary veins in each lung.

Throughout the lung tissue there is elastic tissue and it is *this* tissue which enables the lungs to enlarge and collapse as inspiration and expiration take place.

Each lung is surrounded except where vessels enter and leave the organ by a double serous membrane, the pleura, in the same way as a fist pushed into an inflated balloon becomes surrounded by the balloon. Between the two layers of pleura is a small amount of serous fluid, just enough to allow the lung to expand and deflate in the chest without friction or discomfort.

The Act of Respiration

The small amount of carbon dioxide dissolved in the blood, which is normally present, stimulates the respiratory centre in the medulla and impulses pass along two nerves called the two phrenic nerves to the diaphragm. Then the muscle (which, when relaxed, is dome-shaped) contracts and flattens, thus enlarging the chest cavity from top to bottom. At the same time, the muscles between the ribs contract and the ribs rise upwards and outwards so that the chest cavity is also enlarged from side to side and front to back. On measuring round the chest before and after a very deep inspiration it will be found that it enlarges by 2 to 3 inches in circumference. The pleura is drawn out with the chest wall and the lung tissue stretches with the pleura. The alveoli become larger and to fill the resulting increased space in them air is drawn in through the open air-passages (Fig. 35).

The impulse ceases, the muscles relax, the chest cavity becomes smaller, the air-spaces collapse and air is pushed out through the open air-passages. This is called expiration.

As the air is drawn into the lungs, it enters through the nose and through the mouth when the latter is open. The nose, formed from bone and cartilage, is covered with skin and lined with numerous membranes

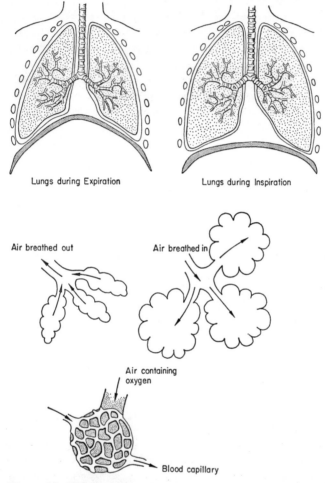

Lungs during Expiration

Lungs during Inspiration

Air breathed out

Air breathed in

Air containing oxygen

Blood capillary

Figure 35. Respiration in the lungs.

which warm and moisten the air on its way to the lungs. It is divided into two nostrils by the septum. There are hairs in the nose which prevent dust and other particles from entering the lungs. The endings of the nerve of smell are in the roof of the nose.

The air passes through the nose into the *pharynx* which is a tube formed from unstriped muscle. The adenoids are found here; these assist the body in preventing some respiratory infection. In childhood they sometimes grow large and partially block the upper part of the pharynx, causing difficulty in breathing through the nose. Then the child breathes through the mouth. As the child grows older the adenoids usually shrink in size.

It is not usual to breathe through the mouth in ordinary activity, but, for example, swimmers learn to take very large amounts of air into the lungs quickly by drawing in air through mouth and nose at the same time. A patient who is unable to breathe easily or efficiently will also breathe in through his nose and mouth and the latter will become very dry and uncomfortable if not treated frequently.

From the pharynx, air is drawn in through the *larynx* which is made up of cartilages, one of which is the thyroid cartilage (Adam's apple). This is the narrowest part of the upper respiratory tract and inhaled foreign bodies may obstruct the air-passages at this level. Below the larynx is the *trachea* in the lower part of the neck and entering the chest. This part of the tube is kept open by U-shaped sections of cartilage joined together by unstriped muscle. It divides into the two *bronchi*, each entering one lung.

In expiration, as the air is pushed out of the lungs, it passes through the larynx and can cause the two vocal cords there to vibrate, thus producing a sound. The sound becomes speech by the use of the lips, teeth, tongue and cheeks. The vocal cords are moved by contracting and relaxing tiny muscles and when these are close together the sound has a high pitch, and when separated a low pitch.

Physiology of Respiration

The purpose of breathing is to take a supply of oxygen into the lungs and so to the blood and at the same time to remove the carbon dioxide given off by the blood.

When respiration is disturbed or difficult the person always becomes anxious and distressed. He becomes blue (cyanosed) as the blood in the body is not becoming oxygenated when it passes through the lungs. It is necessary for the cause of the difficult breathing to be removed or for the patient to be given some aid.

When respiration is impossible, the patient is cyanosed and he quickly becomes unconscious. Relief is necessary at once, as the nervous system especially is extremely sensitive to a lack of oxygen. Causes of difficulty or cessation in breathing:

1. Lack of air round the individual—the air may have been replaced by water (drowning) or harmful gases or smoke.

2. Obstruction of the upper respiratory tract by
   (a) foreign bodies, e.g. dentures, food;
   (b) swelling which follows the swallowing of acids or alkalies causing burns of the throat, or bee or wasp stings of the throat;
   (c) some material covering mouth and nose, e.g. a pillow or soft plastic bag.
3. Injury to throat.
4. Open chest wound with fractured ribs and air in the pleural space preventing expansion of the lungs. Fractured ribs. Pneumothorax.
5. Disease or accident causing inability to contract the diaphragm, e.g. poliomyelitis, electric shock.
6. Inhalation of vomit or respiratory secretions.
7. When a patient has very weak heart function, his breathing becomes difficult. In deep coma also the patient cannot cough and normal respiratory secretions tend to collect in the lungs.

Interchange of Gases in the Lungs and Body Tissues

While the air is in the expanded lungs, oxygen is absorbed into the blood capillaries where it combines with the haemoglobin of the red blood cell to form oxyhaemoglobin, and the blood becomes bright red. The oxygenated blood returns to the heart through two pulmonary veins from each lung, and is pumped round the body. The various tissues, which require oxygen in order to carry out their functions, take up oxygen from the blood as it passes by them in the capillaries. At the same time, the tissues give up carbon dioxide, which is a waste product from their cell activity and this is absorbed into the plasma. The blood is bluish red.

The blood returning to the heart therefore has little oxygen with its haemoglobin and a large amount of carbon dioxide in the plasma. As the blood is pumped through the lungs, the haemoglobin again absorbs oxygen from the air in the expanded lungs (i.e. during inspiration) becoming oxyhaemoglobin, and the carbon dioxide passes from the capillary plasma into the air-spaces, and is secreted from the body in expiration.

Under ordinary conditions air which is breathed in contains a small amount of carbon dioxide, together with some oxygen and a larger amount of unimportant gas (nitrogen). It may also contain dust and bacteria. Some of the latter are possibly disease-producing organisms like tubercle bacilli or the influenza germ and then the patient becomes ill, though frequently his body defences resist the organisms. The air which is breathed out contains four times as much carbon dioxide and only three-quarters the amount of oxygen.

Maintenance of Health in the Respiratory System

Pulmonary ventilation improves by GENERAL EXERCISE and BREATHING EXERCISES. The former includes the normal active duties of work, also walking, gardening, games and physical recreation. In breathing exercises it is useful to expand the whole lung instead of only part of it, and this is practised when people are trained, e.g.: in swimming and singing, but also it can be achieved in simple daily breathing exercises.

POSTURE is the position of the body. If this be erect and well balanced with ease, either when sitting, standing, walking or in the performance of physical skills, then efficient respiratory function is expected together with absence of fatigue. It is an advantage to health if the air which is breathed in is free from dust, harmful particles and gases, and disease-producing bacteria as well as containing adequate oxygen. This supply is maintained by efficient ventilation. In industrial areas, local authorities make every effort to reduce the amount of smoke by controlling the production and discharge of smoke. In a smokeless zone, householders and industrial firms are required not to use any fuel which will produce smoke. The reduction of smoke also results in less fog (fog plus smoke means 'smog'). 'Smog' aggravates chronic inflammatory diseases of the chest, e.g. chronic bronchitis, and its effects can be severe. In occupations where dust or fine particles pass into the air, these may be trapped by a fine water or oil spray and be carried away by a drainage pipe. Harmful fumes are sometimes produced in industry and these are drawn out by extractory fans through a metal flue to a safe and convenient place. Special masks are worn by workers in some occupations to prevent inhalation of disadvantageous substances.

The inhalation of cigarette smoke as by heavy habitual smokers, i.e. over 15 cigarettes a day, is harmful to lung tissue. There can be no civil regulations regarding this aspect of health, but health education is arranged especially for young people to encourage them to protect their healthy lungs.

Maintenance of Respiratory Function in Disease

Breathing exercise, posture and ventilation are important in assisting towards satisfactory respiratory function and in preventing complications during illness. For example:
   (a) after surgery on one lung it is important that the healthy lung should expand efficiently;
   (b) in poliomyelitis (inflammation of parts of the spinal cord) some groups of muscles become paralysed, and the physiotherapist will

L

ensure the correct *posture* of the body, otherwise the strong muscles will overact and the chest cage may become deformed. The lack of adequate room ventilation increases the risk of respiratory infections and the patient feels less well generally; ventilating a ward is part of the day's routine. When the patient suffers from oxygen lack (this may happen in a haemorrhage, partial obstruction of the respiratory tract, heart and lung diseases, and gas poisonings) then it is necessary to administer oxygen to the patient.

OXYGEN ADMINISTRATION

The gas is obtained from cylinders which can be recognised by the white-painted top. On the head of this cylinder a porter fixes a pressure gauge on which dials show the amount of oxygen in the cylinder, and the rate at which it flows out when the appropriate tap is turned on. The gas passes through pressure tubing which will not kink easily to a plastic *oxygen mask* which fits over the patient's nose and mouth. It is light in weight and fairly comfortable besides being inexpensive so that it can be discarded after use. Sometimes it is more convenient to use a *nasal catheter* than a mask, and this is lubricated and passed about 2 to 3 inches backwards into the nostril. A piece of adhesive tape is necessary to keep it in position. Plastic nasal tubes with ear-pieces attached are light in weight and comfortable.

If the oxygen is required to be moistened then it may be passed through a humidifier, a bottle containing water, which may also measure the rate of flow. An atomiser may be available. Oxygen may also be passed through a medication fluid according to the doctor's prescription. The rate of flow through a plastic mask is 4 to 6 litres per minute. The rate of flow through a nasal catheter is 2 to 4 litres per minute.

Note: the patient does not breathe pure oxygen but a mixture of air and oxygen through the mask or air *round* the catheter together with oxygen through the catheter. Breathing pure oxygen will interfere with the act of breathing.

Oxygen Tent

This may be hospital equipment or hired from a firm. Instructions for use are issued with the equipment or are included in the Nursing Procedure manual. Servicing is necessary at intervals, e.g. after each time of use, and when a fault is suspected. The tent covers the bed or half the bed including the patient's head, shoulders and arms. It is made of plastic material which is transparent, is supported by metal rods and the lower edge tucks underneath the mattress. Oxygen enters from large cylinders outside the tent or from a piped supply. The temperature inside the tent will rise, and is uncomfortable for a patient above 21°C to 24°C (as registered on a thermometer inside the tent) so the oxygen entering passes over a cooling system, e.g. ice container, and becomes moistened at the same time. Warm expired air passes out from the tent through a small vent.

The patient can receive attention by the nurse inserting her hands through openings in the tent. It is necessary to observe the patient frequently for changes in colour, pulse rate and any signs of restlessness; also the equipment is inspected—oxygen cylinders, for example, are likely to become empty and need to be exchanged. The patient who is somewhat confused, as when he is feverish, may be frightened inside the tent and needs much reassurance and should not be left alone. His agitation may be due also to inadequate supply of oxygen or the temperature inside the tent becoming raised. Children particularly should be given a special introduction to the tent to prevent fear and apprehension and it is useful to allow them to sit inside one before the type of operation after which it will be a part of the essential treatment.

If the patient is an infant a 'croupette' may be used. This is a dome-shaped transparent case which fits over the infant or a smaller edition of the oxygen tent which fits over the cot.

Precaution during Oxygen Therapy
Burning will take place with great speed when oxygen is present in large quantities. For this reason no naked light is allowed near oxygen and oxygen apparatus, and a notice may be displayed 'No smoking' for patients and their visitors. It is unwise to allow a child in an oxygen tent to have toys which produce sparks, or adults to use wireless ear-phones or electric bells. Electrostatic materials, e.g. plastic mattresses and pillow covers on the bed, are avoided. No grease or oil is used on the pressure gauge. A reserve cylinder is on the ward, near the tent, ready to replace the cylinder in use when this becomes empty.

Artificial Respiration

When the patient cannot breathe (this is asphyxia) for one of the reasons mentioned on page 152, *artificial respiration* is carried out at once, and this is continued until medical aid arrives. Whichever method is used, first a finger is inserted into the mouth and foreign bodies (e.g. stones or weeds after drowning) or a denture are removed quickly and clothing round the neck and chest loosened. If the patient has been immersed in and inhaled water, the body is placed in prone position (face downwards) with the head lower than the chest if possible and turned to one side to allow the water to flow out of the lungs and stomach. It is advisable to begin resuscitation, i.e. mouth-to-mouth breathing, without delay.

MOUTH-TO-MOUTH BREATHING (Fig. 36). The patient lies on his back on a rigid surface like the ground or floor, with the head extended backwards slightly. The nurse kneels at his left side and compresses his nose with her right finger and thumb. She takes a fairly deep breath through her nose and mouth looking to the right above the patient's head, then places her open mouth over the patient's open mouth. If he is a child she may be able to place her mouth over *his mouth and nose*. And she breathes out into his mouth. Her left hand may lie lightly over his chest and she will feel the sternum (breastbone) rise as the lungs inflate. Then she raises

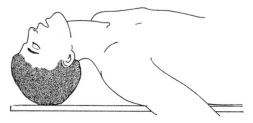

Figure 36. Position for mouth-to-mouth breathing.

her head, turns it to the right and breathes in again. *Gentle* breaths only are introduced into a child's lungs. The procedure is timed to take place 16 to 18 times a minute. The nurse takes care not to breathe *out* too much air otherwise she may become rather dizzy and breathe less often. In hospital wards and departments a Brook air-way or Ambu bag may be available and this is used in place of mouth-to-mouth resuscitation.

When breathing is extremely difficult or distressed, or the patient is deeply comatose, an artificial opening in the trachea may be necessary to save life, or be beneficial in relieving his symptoms. The patient takes in air more easily and in greater quantities. This operation is TRACHEOS-TOMY (Fig. 37), and the incision is made under local or general anaesthetic in the mid line low down in the neck. The surgeon inserts a silver, plastic or rubber tube, which is curved to fit into the trachea. The tube is secured by 2 tapes which are tied at the side/back of the neck by a *reef knot* and therefore cannot become accidentally untied. Immediately after the operation and during the next few days, secretions from the lungs may block the tube. These are removed as they accumulate by passing *sterile* whistle-tipped catheters to approximately 1 cm beyond the end of the tracheostomy tube (i.e. to the division of the trachea into the two bronchi) and attaching to it a low-pressure suction apparatus. The catheter is inserted and then withdrawn slowly so that suction takes place. The catheter is removed and another used when necessary. This is continued till the tube is clear. This procedure may be necessary every few minutes up to two-hourly. A supply of catheters is at hand and these must be sterile to prevent infection of the lungs, which could lead to broncho-pneumonia. Catheters are handled using forceps or sterile disposable gloves to prevent lung infection. The position of the tube in the trachea is maintained by tying the tapes attached to it round the neck. If the tube moves from the correct position the patient will become distressed and blue. It should be rapidly adjusted and the doctor informed.

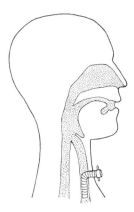

Figure 37. Tracheostomy tube in position.

The *silver tube* will be observed to consist of two parts: (a) the outer tube which is never removed by the nurse, (b) the inner tube which can be removed for cleaning with a fine bottle brush or ribbon gauze, after which it is boiled and then replaced.

The *rubber tube* may be surrounded by a rubber cuff which is inflated with air, e.g. 5 to 10 millilitres from a syringe. This ensures a secure fit of the tube within the trachea, and for this reason it is the most suitable for patients who have an excess of secretions in their pharynx, and those who need the assistance of a mechanical respirator. But to prevent *continuous* slight pressure from the inflated cuff on the lining of the trachea, the cuff is deflated at intervals, e.g. for 5 minutes every hour, and then re-inflated. Plastic tracheostomy tubes are used in some cases. These are sterilised by the manufacturer and arrive in sealed packets. They are discarded after use.

After this operation, the patient cannot use his voice, as the opening is below the larynx (voice-box), so a writing-pad and pencil are required at his bed-side, as well as a bell to summon the nurse. Later he learns to speak by placing a finger-tip over the tube opening.

If the tracheostomy is permanent, a small plastic tube may be kept in the opening, and is cleaned when necessary. If the larynx has been removed, the patient can be taught to speak again by a speech therapist.

An *endotracheal tube* is passed through the mouth or nose into the trachea. The procedure is called intubation and it is performed sometimes in resuscitation and the administration of an anaesthetic.

Observations

Various observations are necessary in conditions concerned with the respiratory tract.

RESPIRATIONS. In sleep or when resting, the *rate and depth* of breathing are less than in normal activity. They are increased during exercise and also in emotional states such as fear, excitement or distress. When the body reacts to infection, more oxygen is required and the respiration rate rises. In asthma and pneumonia, less air is exchanged during each respiration and the rate increases to compensate this. When the body vitality is lowered in shock, breathing is quick and shallow, but in ketosis the patient has air-hunger and the inspirations are long and deep.

Respiration rate and depth are influenced by some drugs. Stimulants, e.g. adrenalin and nikethamide, produce quicker and deeper respiration, but the patient breathes slowly after sedatives like barbiturates, and general anaesthetics.

Difficult or laboured breathing is observed as dyspnoea; the patient is distressed with a drawn expression and dilated nostrils. He becomes cyanosed. Following a number of forced expirations when CO_2 is expelled in excess, the blood level of CO_2 is lowered and respirations cease temporarily. This is a period of apnoea ($=$ no breathing) and it may be seen in a baby at the end of a bout of crying. Sometimes in advanced illness apnoea alternates with periods of deep breathing and this is known as *Cheyne-Stokes respiration*. A *cough* is a sudden explosive expiration produced as a reflex response to foreign material in the air-passages so that this is not inhaled into the lungs, or to rid the respiratory tract of excessive secretions of mucus or pus, or it is a voluntary action. During unconsciousness the cough reflex is absent and therefore no foreign material must be allowed to enter the air-passages. Before a general anaesthetic the patient's stomach is emptied either by starving him for four hours or by aspiration. No fluid or food is given to an unconscious patient, neither is the mouth cleaned using swabs which are not secured safely in *clip forceps*. When the mouth and throat are anaesthetised before an examination like bronchoscopy, the sensory stimulus for the cough reflex action is absent, so fluids to drink are not given to the patient until the mucous membrane recovers its ability to appreciate the presence of fluids etc.

In disease, the patient coughs to get rid of some excess material from the respiratory tract. In carcinoma of the bronchus, the malignant tumour cannot be expectorated so there is no relief from coughing, and the cough is harsh, dry and unproductive. Occasionally a small blood vessel is eroded and then the patient expectorates a little blood (*haemoptysis*). There is excessive mucous secretion in acute bronchitis and the sputum is frothy due to the air mixed with the mucus, which may be large in amount (like the discharge from the nose in the common cold). Should a secondary infection occur, then the sputum contains pus and is yellow as in chronic bronchitis. Coughing produces relief. In acute pneumonia, the the cough is dry and irritating; the sputum is small in amount and may be blood-stained, but in broncho-pneumonia, the production of sputum can be profuse, thick with mucus and pus, and an elderly or immobile patient has difficulty in expectorating it. This is a serious situation and is prevented by changing the patient's position at least two-hourly, encouraging chest movements (by physiotherapy), postural drainage and prevention or treatment of chest infection.

There may be no cough in early pulmonary tuberculosis, but the disease may be manifested by a sudden haemoptysis. Late in the untreated condition there is a purulent sputum which is highly infectious.

In bronchiectasis (dilated bronchioles which eventually become infected and allow pus to collect in them), and in lung abscess large amounts of purulent sputum are expectorated, especially when the patient moves about after lying still for some time. The pus is greenish yellow and offensive.

When reporting the characteristics of SPUTUM, the following points are made:

    (i) amount;
    (ii) appearance, e.g. mucoid, muco-purulent, purulent, blood-stained;
    (iii) time of expectoration;
    (iv) whether there is difficulty in expectoration.

The patient expectorates sputum into a waxed cardboard container with lid and it is disposed of by burning.

Clinical Investigations

When a specimen of sputum is required for bacteriological examination the patient is given a specimen jar with a screw cap the previous evening and the nurse explains that he should cough sputum into the jar as soon as he wakes up the following morning. He will expectorate most sputum at this time of the day. The jar is labelled and collected with the appropriate laboratory request form. A specimen of saliva only is of no value. Specimens from three consecutive mornings may be requested.

For X-RAY of the upper respiratory tract and/or chest the patient stands, or sits on a stool. If he is very ill, a portable X-ray machine is brought to the ward and he lies flat, being lifted carefully while the radiographer places the photographic plate beneath his chest, or he is supported in an upright position by the ward nurse who observes his condition and can deal with an emergency situation should this arise, e.g. collapse. He wears a cotton flannelette gown and *no* pins, buttons, brooches or medallions are allowed to remain in the X-ray field, as these may obscure an abnormality. Instructions to him to breathe in and out will be given by the radiographer. Later the plate is developed and the resulting X-ray is reported on by the radiologist and used by the physician in making a diagnosis or as an indication of progress. An X-ray of the chest may show abnormalities other than in the lungs, such as an enlarged heart or fractured ribs.

MASS RADIOGRAPHY is used for large numbers of healthy and apparently healthy people to have an X-ray of the chest. It is a method of exposing early disease before the individual experiences symptoms which would lead him to consult a doctor. Patients may also be referred by their family doctors direct to have their lungs checked radiographically.

BRONCHOGRAM is the X-ray film of the chest when a substance opaque to X-ray, iodised oil, e.g. 'neohydriol', has been introduced into the bronchi. The fluid is injected through a tube in the pharynx and trachea, or through a needle through the skin in the neck into the trachea with the patient in such a position that the dye will flow into the lobe to be investigated. The resulting film will show any dilations of the bronchioles. It may be necessary to empty the dilations if these be filled with pus, before the injection of the oil by postural draining.

BRONCHOSCOPY is a method of direct inspection of the trachea and bronchial tree by a hollow tube passed through the mouth and pharynx with illumination of the distal end. It is carried out under local or general anaesthetic and is used particularly for diagnosis of malignant growths of the bronchus (lung cancer) and for removing foreign bodies which have been inhaled and secretions that cannot be coughed up.

If under local anaesthetic the pharynx is anaesthetised, it is important that patients should not attempt to swallow fluid or food until this effect has worn off.

Sometimes a specimen of tissue is removed by long forceps through the bronchoscope and there may be some spitting of blood following this procedure. The patient should be observed carefully on return from the operating theatre to see that the amount of blood is not excessive. He should be encouraged to expectorate and his air-way should be kept free. The mouth is cleaned as required and his first drink should be of plain water to ensure that he can swallow safely.

CHEST ASPIRATION. This is a technique performed by the doctor to obtain fluid from the pleural cavity when a pleural effusion is suspected or it is necessary for the fluid to be examined in the laboratory. *Pleural effusion* occurs after pneumonia, in tuberculosis and carcinoma of the lung. It can be detected by X-ray of the chest and when extensive it causes breathlessness. If it is infected an abscess forms—empyaema. This is unusual since sulphonamides and antibiotics have cured pneumonia.

Aspiration is an aseptic procedure and the sterilisation of the equipment is important. During the preparation the patient sits up in bed with pillows to support his lower back, and leaning over a bed-table so that his ribs are separated as far as possible. He coughs now if he wishes before the procedure begins. The physician or surgeon cleans the skin on the affected side over the area where the fluid is suspected, and anaesthetises it. He introduces a chest exploration needle (which has a wide bore) between the ribs and withdraws fluid with a syringe. The patient is asked not to cough during the procedure and a cough linctus may be administered, immediately prior to the aspiration. Specimens of fluid are prepared for the laboratory.

An extensive effusion (up to 1 litre) necessitates more complicated equipment, either a large chest-needle with 2-way tap, 40-cc syringe, and rubber tubing leading into a measure or bottle which collects the fluid, or the Potain's equipment by which the fluid is drawn from the chest into a large bottle by a pump. The patient is usually ill and requires constant attention and observation by the nurse. Should he become pale and sweat appear on his face (often first on the upper lip), his skin becomes cold and his muscles lose their normal tone, the attention of the doctor is drawn to his condition. A stimulant is easily available, e.g. nikethamide 5 ml by hypodermic injection, if the doctor requests an immediate administration. The procedure is stopped and the patient placed almost flat in bed, unless he is dyspnoeic, kept quiet and as comfortable as possible until he recovers.

The patient is given sips of water or of cough linctus if he shows an inclination to cough towards the end of the procedure.

CHEST ASPIRATION is carried out when bleeding into the chest has

L*

occurred during injury (haemothorax) and also sometimes after lung operations, to remove fluid which collects there.

Diseases of the Respiratory Tract

The COMMON COLD is a virus infection of the upper respiratory tract (see diseases of the ear, nose and throat).

In BRONCHITIS, the bronchi are inflamed and when the disease is acute the patient is feverish with a temperature raised to 39°C and he expectorates mucoid, then muco-purulent sputum. He is nursed in bed and the doctor prescribes a cough expectorant medicine, and steam inhalations with added medications like tincture of Benzoin Compound to enable him to expectorate more easily.

This condition begins in the winter and tends to recur in following years usually between November and March. As it becomes CHRONIC, the patient coughs throughout the year, expectorating mucoid or purulent sputum with secondary infection of the respiratory tract. After repeated attacks it is probable that emphysema will develop. The lungs become distended and inelastic and increasingly inefficient so that shortness of breath is more persistent and crippling. After a time the heart too is affected (the condition of heart failure secondary to pulmonary disease is known as cor pulmonale) and signs of failure appear, with cyanosis, exercise intolerance and oedema of the feet and ankles.

Chronic bronchitis is associated with living in industrial areas where the air contains impurities such as sulphur, and is also damp; it is more common in the Midlands and North of England than in the South and East. This condition is aggravated by cigarette smoking and is more common in men than in women. It is a disabling disease affecting the patient from 45 years onwards, and is responsible for much loss of work time. Treatment includes expectorants, and antibiotics to deal with respiratory infection. Giving up cigarette smoking, and moving to a more suitable district in which to live when possible, are means by which progress of the illness may be halted.

PNEUMONIA is the result of a bacterial or occasionally virus infection of the lungs. ACUTE LOBAR PNEUMONIA is the type in which the infection is localised to one lobe of a lung. The patient has a raised temperature, is feverish and very ill, and may be delirious. Treatment includes rest in bed, nursing care and sulphonamides or antibiotics. These drugs cure the infection quickly and complications are unusual. The patient is nursed at home unless complications arise.

BRONCHO-PNEUMONIA is a widespread inflammatory condition affecting the bronchioles of the lungs. The alveoli become filled with the secretions from the lower respiratory tract, which are excessive as a result of the inflammatory process, and interchange of oxygen and carbon dioxide is difficult. The patient becomes cyanosed, appearing grey in colour and is dyspnoeic. His breathing is distressed and he is nursed supported in an upright position at complete rest. He is encouraged to cough and expectorants, with changes in position when possible, assist in this. Oxygen is administered continuously by nasal spectacles or plastic mask. Chemotherapy or antibiotics deal with the mixed infection in the lungs. The general comfort of the patient, intake of fluid and some nourishment and prevention of bed-sores are important.

Broncho-pneumonia can occur in older patients suffering from other diseases which necessitates them lying still in bed and also in patients who are unconscious for some time. Steps are taken to prevent this from happening by changing the patient's position every two hours, by suction using sterile catheters when the patient is unconscious, and by encouraging a conscious patient to breathe deeply and to cough if any sputum is present.

INFLUENZAL PNEUMONIA is an infectious acute manifestation of an epidemic disease. It has a very short onset and runs a rapid course but is serious in young people and the elderly. A vaccine is available but this is effective for only the current year as the type of organism varies from year to year.

STAPHYLOCOCCAL PNEUMONIA varies in its severity. The patients are often elderly and may have a similar infection in another part of the body. If the staphylococci are drug resistant, they are contained in the sputum and the patient in hospital may be isolated to prevent infection to other patients.

PLEURAL EFFUSION is a collection of fluid in the pleural cavity and is a complication of pneumonia. The fluid compresses the lung and the patient has quick, shallow respirations. His temperature remains above normal. The fluid is often absorbed by the tissues.

INJURIES include:
    (i) fractured ribs;
    (ii) open chest wounds.

Fractured ribs are painful but not serious unless the bone enters a lung, causing haemoptysis. If several ribs are broken, each in two places, so that the chest wall loses its stability, breathing is dangerously affected. The patient may have haemoptysis, or blood collects in the pleural cavity (haemothorax). In the latter case, blood is removed by the doctor using a machine which provides suction through a wide-bore needle inserted in the chest wall. Prevention of infection is important.

As an emergency procedure for open chest wounds, it is advisable to

seal off the wound immediately with dressings of a thick wad of clean
linen covered firmly by a piece of material like clean plastic and a firm
bandage or Elastoplast. This will prevent air from entering the chest,
allowing the lung to collapse. The mechanism of breathing as explained
on page 305, cannot proceed normally when the chest cage is incomplete
as in injury. Infection also is prevented by closing the wound.

PNEUMOTHORAX is air in the pleural cavity. This condition may occur
without warning for a reason not always known (spontaneous pneumothorax). The patient is acutely breathless. After X-ray of the chest, air is
aspirated from the chest and a tube inserted with under-water seal drainage. Pneumothorax occasionally complicates road injuries involving the
chest.

TUBERCULOSIS is a disease caused by tubercle bacilli. It may affect
many parts of the body. Pulmonary tuberculosis occurs when tubercle
bacilli have been inhaled and the body has diminished resistance to the
infection. The patient is young or old and may say he has lost weight at
the same time as complaining of fatigue. There may be a rise in temperature and X-ray examination shows changes in the lung such as infiltra-
tion in a cavity. If he coughs sputum, this is examined and the discovery
of tubercle bacilli seen under the microscope confirms the diagnosis.
Occasionally there is no sputum and the person seems reasonably fit and
energetic, but an X-ray photograph of the chest shows evidence of the
disease. This fact has been used in Mass-radiography methods to reveal
otherwise unsuspected cases in an early stage. In some instances the
individual is seen by his doctor when he coughs up blood (haemoptysis),
and tuberculosis is found to be the cause of this.

Medical treatment is by a combination of three drugs, streptomycin
(given by intra-muscular injection), para-aminosalicylic acid, known as
P.A.S., and isoniazid (I.N.A.H.), both given by mouth. The organism can
become resistant to any one of these drugs but this is less likely to happen when at least two are combined in administration. More drugs are
now available. Often treatment is desirable in hospital for domestic reasons and to minimise the chance of infecting others in the active stages.
Occasionally the lesion is localised or obstructed and the affected part
may be removed by partial resection of the lung. General treatment includes a nourishing, well-balanced diet and rest, combined with graduated exercise so as not to cause pyrexia or fatigue. During and after recovery the patient is seen by the doctor at intervals, and his chest is
X-rayed repeatedly.

Standards of food and housing, and habits of cleanliness are important
in the prevention of this disease. Industrial conditions too have improved.
When a diagnosis is made, investigations are carried out in the patient's

family or amongst school or work colleagues, to discover a possible un-recognised source of the disease and this person will be treated. Infection is spread by droplet infection and sputum must be disposed of with great care, preferably by collection in waxed cardboard containers which are burned. Infected crockery and cutlery should be boiled after use. Dis-posable handkerchiefs are preferred. In flats and houses where no fire is available a disinfectant is poured on to the sputum and it is flushed away in the lavatory. Patients rarely leave hospital with positive sputum, i.e. sputum which contains tubercle bacilli.

Many people in the population have reasonable resistance to the infec-tion, but to safeguard those who may become infected and who have not already required some resistance, immunisation is offered by a vaccine named B.C.G. (Bacillus Calmette Guerin). This contains bacilli treated so that they are not virulent and it is administered by injection or by skin application. It is important that young people between the ages of 13 and 20 years have this protection whenever possible as this is the age when they are most susceptible. The positive tuberculin test shows that a per-son has already had a primary infection. The reaction is positive when there is a raised red area on the forearm 48 hours after the injection, or skin application (Heaf test).

CANCER OF THE LUNG is a malignant growth usually arising in a bron-chus. The patient is generally over 45 years of age and it is more common in men than in women. Common symptoms include coughing, shortness of breath and a pain in the chest. There may be expectoration of some blood (haemoptysis). An attack of pneumonia may indicate its presence. X-ray examination is essential with the slightest suspicion so that an early diagnosis can be made. Heavy continued cigarette smoking predis-poses to carcinoma of the lung. Health education attempts to discourage this habit, particularly in young people who do not always realise its consequences.

Treatment is by resection of lung when the position of the growth makes it possible and the disease has not spread, or by radiotherapy.

BRONCHIAL ASTHMA is a condition in which the patient has difficulty in breathing due to spasmodic narrowing of the bronchioles. The asthmatic attack may be a response to the inhalations of some substance to which he is hypersensitive, i.e. allergic. These substances include pollens from grasses or flowers and dust from feathers or fur. Skin tests may show the causative substance, and then it may be avoided. A respiratory infection may precipitate attacks as also can psychological disturbances.

In an attack of bronchial asthma the patient breathes out with great effort and becomes extremely distressed. The bronchioles which are constructed from unstriped muscle are in spasm, giving rise to the symptoms. He needs reassurance and is helped by having a knowledgeable person near at hand. Treatment is by drugs which relax the bronchioles like adrenalin or aminophylline and oxygen. There are a number of treatments to prevent attacks and ensure a healthy condition of the respiratory tract which are arranged by general practitioners and the medical staff of out-patient clinics. Patients with complications or a continuous series of attacks (status asthmaticus) are admitted to hospital. In severe or prolonged attacks the steroid drugs (e.g. prednisolone) may be prescribed. These may produce side effects which would be observed and reported by the nurse should they appear.

CARBON MONOXIDE POISONING occurs following the inhalation of coal gas or motor car exhaust fumes. It may be accidental or self-administered and the patient quickly becomes unconscious. The skin is bright pink due to the combination of carbon monoxide and haemoglobin in the blood.

First-aid treatment is to turn off any gas taps, or switch off the car engine. It is dangerous to light matches. The patient is pulled quickly into the fresh air outside the room or garage. If he cannot be moved immediately, the windows and doors are opened wide.

The clothing is loosened round the neck, dentures, if present, are removed from the mouth and artificial respiration begun at once. Emergency number 999 (or whatever code is in use for emergency calls) is dialled as soon as possible as the patient needs hospital treatment urgently. This consists of oxygen therapy, stimulants and the general care of the unconscious patient.

PREPARATION OF PATIENTS FOR LUNG OPERATIONS is important and includes investigations of the unaffected lung for its efficiency and absence of infection. The co-operation of the patient and his relatives is essential as he is ill for 24 to 48 hours afterwards and his confidence is required. Antiseptic preparation of the skin is either indicated by the surgeon who will carry out the operation, or it is done in the operating theatre. The anaesthetist takes over the breathing of the patient during the operation with the respiratory and anaesthetic machine.

Following the operation the patient is encouraged to cough as soon as possible and at frequent intervals, e.g. hourly, to clear the respiratory passages of secretion and prevent blockage. The nurse supports him and places a hand firmly over his wound while he coughs. He is supported upright in bed but his position is changed slightly every two hours. He sits out of bed after 24 to 48 hours and becomes mobile quickly, even with drainage tubes. Breathing exercises are important throughout and attention is given to correct posture as the patient tends to incline the shoulders to the affected side. Rehabilitation is an essential part of postoperative care.

Under-water Drainage

The operations most frequently performed in a chest surgery unit are *Resection of the whole lung* (pneumonectomy) and *Resection of part of a lobe.* There is specialised post-operative care which includes the supervision of drainage from the pleural cavity by a tube through the chest wall.

The principle is to ensure that fluid collecting in the thorax after operation drains away while at the same time preventing air from entering the chest. This would collapse the lung, and prevent inflation of the organ with the possibility of the collapse becoming permanent. There is also a risk of pleural infection in an open chest drainage.

The drainage tube in the chest is connected to a length of tubing by a glass connection. The lower end of the tubing is attached to a long glass tube passing through a rubber bung into a large drainage bottle which stands in a tray or holder on the floor. A short glass tube allows air to enter and leave the bottle. Inside the bottle is water sufficient to cover the end of the long tube. The amount of fluid is measured periodically to indicate the quantity of drainage. The equipment is sterile when assembled. As the tubing is heavy and may drag on the chest drainage tube, a loop of tubing is fixed to the bed with a strong safety pin.

During drainage, the level of the water in the long glass tube is seen to rise and fall with every inspiration and expiration the patient makes. Fluid is also draining into the bottle. When the fluctuation of the water level ceases, the tubing is inspected to ensure that it is not kinked in any part. If the fluid draining from the chest is thick, it may have blocked the tube. In this case the drainage tube is clamped off with forceps, and the tubing and bottle are replaced. Should this be unsuccessful the blockage is in the drainage tube and the doctor will advise. Any leak in the tubing or a blockage in the exit air tube will prevent normal fluctuation of the water level. The rise and fall of fluid in the tube will also cease when, after partial resection of lung, the remaining lung tissue has re-expanded and filled the pleural cavity.

PRECAUTIONS are necessary in the management of the under-water drainage.

The bottle must *never* be lifted to the level of the patient's chest, or the water will flow into the chest. The occasions when this may happen are during the cleaning of the ward and during bed-making. If this type of drainage is infrequent in the ward, a large label may be attached to the bottle: 'Do not lift above 6 inches from the ground'. While the bed is being made and the patient's position is being changed, it may be necessary to move the bottle to the other side of the bed; then the tube is clamped off with forceps, the tubing disconnected and the bottle carried round the bed and re-connected. The clamp forcep is removed or the drainage will not continue.

The drainage bottle and tubing are replaced at intervals by a clean, sterile bottle and tubing, the necessary liquid having been poured into the bottle. Drainage fluid amount is assessed from the removed bottle by subtracting the original water from the total collection and the resulting figure is recorded on the chart.

A suction machine, e.g. Roberts suction motor, is used in some cases to encourage drainage from an intercostal tube. This is attached by tubing to the air exit tube in the rubber bung of the drainage bottle. If it is driven by electricity, and when the power is switched on, the negative pressure is regulated to 3 lb.

Nursing Procedures

INHALATIONS IN RESPIRATORY CONDITIONS

1. *Oxygen.* This has been explained earlier in the chapter.

2. *Air* may be administered from a cylinder by similar methods.

3. *Steam inhalations* are a useful treatment in acute bronchitis and infections of the upper respiratory tract when the mucous membrane is dry and sputum is difficult to expectorate. They are also important after tracheostomy to make the air inhaled moist and prevent crusting inside the trachea. Steam is administered in three ways:
   (a) using a Nelson's inhaler;
   (b) using a household jug or measure;
   (c) steam tent.

4. *Humidified air.*

(a) *Using a Nelson's Inhaler*
This is a china receptacle to hold 1 litre of fluid. The glass mouthpiece is covered by a piece of material to protect the patient's lips from the warm glass. 500 ml of boiling water is poured into the inhaler and the level does not reach the spout or there may be an overflow of hot water. By the time the inhaler is used, the temperature of the water will be about 92°C. The cork and mouthpiece are placed so that the spout faces away from the patient. A cover is placed round the inhaler, which is fixed securely in a bowl and given to the patient with instructions for him to breathe in through his mouth and out through his nose while the mouthpiece is in position. A sputum carton should be close at hand. The procedure lasts about 6 to 10 minutes and is comforting to the patient. It is unsuitable for patients who are unable to hold the equipment securely and co-operate, such as young children, elderly patients with disabilities, or patients who are restless or irrational.

(b) *Using a Household Jug or Measure*

The receptacle holds at least 1 litre of water and the most suitable type is the deep, narrow-top jug, which does not slip in the hands or become very hot. 300 ml. of boiling water is poured into the jug. A smooth towel is arranged so that it covers the rim completely. The jug may be more stable if it is placed in a suitably sized bowl. A wool or cellular cover keeps the jug warm. The patient is instructed to breathe in with his face over the jug, then raise his head and breathe out. The treatment lasts about 5 minutes while steam is rising from the water.

These inhalations can be administered 3 or 4 times a day. The patient may feel chilled if he moves into a cool atmosphere immediately afterwards and this should be avoided. Medications which are expectorants are frequently prescribed to be given with the steam inhalations, e.g. *tincture of Benzoin compound*, 1 fluid drachm (4 millilitres) or 3 *menthol crystals*. Either drug is added to the hot water immediately before taking it to the patient.

(c) *Steam Tent*

This is the method used when the patient is very young or helpless. Apparatus may be improvised by using screen frames and draping over these sheets to form a tent at the top of the bed with the front open (i.e. a half tent). Otherwise special frames and covers are made for use in the hospital wards. The steam enters from an electric steam kettle, capacity 1 to 2 litres, from which a long spout enters the tent behind the patient. A room thermometer hangs inside the tent away from the kettle spout, and the temperature should remain constant at 21°C to 24°C. If it tends to rise above this, the steam inflow is stopped temporarily. Too much heat with the water vapour in the air will cause the patient, especially a child, to become restless and uncomfortable.

In the steam tent, the patient's general care and treatment continues, and the nurse assists the patient to cough. It is suitable procedure to continue for a few days if the necessity arises. The patient's vision is restricted by the tent and the nurse should be with him frequently.

Care of the kettle is as for other electric equipment; the flex and plugs are checked before use, sand is available within the ward in case of fire from a wire fault, and the kettle is not allowed to boil dry.

(d) *Humidified air*, i.e. moistened air, is administered by an atomiser. There are various types of these. They are attached to oxygen or air cylinders or air is drawn into the machine.

(e) *Drugs* to be inhaled are sometimes administered through atomisers which change the liquid into a very fine spray. They are usually attached to oxygen cylinders.

Postural Drainage (Fig. 38)
The patient lies in such a position (or posture) that excess respiratory secretions and discharges will drain out of the affected part of a lung. It is a treatment used in bronchiectasis, and necessary before a broncho-gram, and as part of the pre-operative treatment in lobectomy and resec-tion of the lung.

It is wise if the patient does not have this treatment immediately fol-lowing a meal or he may vomit. The procedure is explained to the patient as his co-operation is necessary.

A sputum carton is available and following the procedure the amount of sputum is measured. It is usually carried out two or three times a day.

The physiotherapist may assist by 'clapping' the patient's back.

CHAPTER 33 | NUTRITION

To carry on their work, the tissues require food. The body accepts food through the mouth into the alimentary tract where most of it is digested and absorbed into the blood. This transports the simple foods to the tissues requiring them.

The provision of foods to the body is NUTRITION. The arrangement of foods into meals eaten by the individual is a DIET.

Certain types of food are necessary for the growth and health of the human body and these are classified as follows:

Proteins provide the body with material for growth and repair of tissue, some energy and replacement of gland secretions and juices. Meat, fish, cheese, eggs and milk are first-class proteins and some of these are necessary in the diet for health. Lentils, peas, beans and nuts are second-class proteins and are useful additions to the diet. Pregnant women, nurs-ing mothers, growing children and adolescents need extra protein.

Carbohydrates provide the body with calories (heat and energy).

Sugars are soluble in water and include cane sugar, glucose, milk sugar and fruit sugar. They are sweet and added to food make it more palat-able, but can easily be taken to excess.

Starches are insoluble in water. Potatoes, flour, cereals and bananas contain starches.

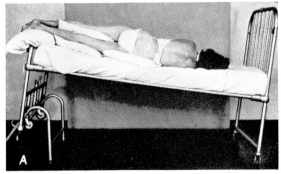

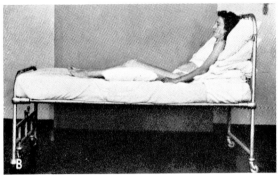

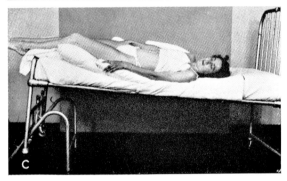

Figure 38. Postural drainage-positions.
A: left lateral and posterior lower segments;
B: upper segments of upper lobes;
C: right middle segments;

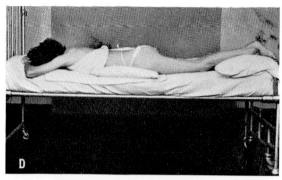

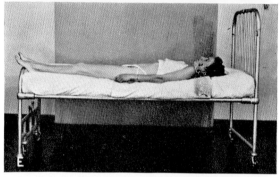

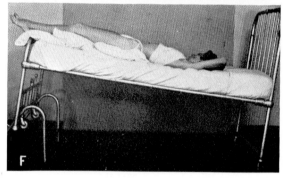

Postural drainage-positions. (continued).

D: upper segments of lower lobes;

E. anterior segments of both upper lobes;

F. anterior segments of both lower lobes.

(from D'ABREU. A.L. *A Practice of Surgery*,
Edward Arnold)

Excess carbohydrate is converted into fat and stored.

Fats provide the body with plenty of heat but are more difficult to digest than carbohydrates. They are therefore taken in smaller amounts. Fats remain longer in the gastro-intestinal tract and delay hunger.

Animal fats include fatty meat, fish such as herring and salmon, cream butter and fish oils. They contain useful vitamins.

Vegetable fats include olive oil, nut oils and margarine. Vitamins are often added to margarine.

Minerals. Sodium chloride (common salt) is essential for health. It is taken as a condiment and is in salted foods such as bacon and kippers.

Iron is in red meat and some vegetables. Liver is rich in iron.

Iodine is present in plant foods which grow near the sea, and in sea fish. In some countries (Britain is one) iodine is added to some table salts.

Calcium is present in hard water and in milk.

Vitamins are required in very small amounts but are necessary for the maintenance of health and the prevention of certain diseases.

Fat soluble vitamins A and D are found in fish oils and some animal fats.

Water-soluble vitamins B are present in yeast, unrefined cereals, some vegetables and liver.

Water-soluble vitamin C is in fresh fruit and vegetables. It is destroyed by prolonged exposure to sunlight and heat as in cooking.

Water is a constituent of the diet and is essential to life. The requirements of individuals vary greatly but an average amount is 2 litres a day.

Roughage has no food value but provides bulk in the intestine and so prevents constipation. The parts of the diet providing roughage are the fruits and vegetables, wholemeal flour, bread and cereals.

The most efficient method of introducing all foodstuffs into the diet is to provide as much variety as possible in the menu. The normal appetite as a rule controls amounts of food quite well. Each day the diet of an adult should contain approximately 70 grammes of protein by weight, the same amount of fat and four times as much carbohydrate. Proteins and fats (meat, fish, cheese and fats) are expensive. Carbohydrates (bread, potatoes and cereals) are cheaper. Fruit and vegetables are expensive in towns and cities.

The heat produced by food when it is made use of in the body is measured in *calories*. Proteins, carbohydrates and fats provide the body with calories, but fat gives more than the other foods.

A person undergoing average activity needs 2,500 to 3,000 calories each day. Manual workers and active children need more than an average amount. Inactive and elderly people require less.

FACTORS other than those in disease WHICH CONTROL DIETS are:

1. Availability of food. In countries where agriculture and fishing are difficult there is a lack of food. Failure of crops can cause famine.

2. Knowledge in adapting to new methods of producing food. *Education* in recognising foods, preparing and cooking them.

3. Availability of fresh water and fire (or other heating methods). Access to shops and food stores.

4. Finances. Family income, size of family, and the ability to budget well.

5. Racial and religious differences in diet.

6. Family eating habits.

7. Reactions to certain foods are unusual but may be encountered. A small number of infants and children (and possibly young adults) are allergic to milk. Shell fish can cause a rash or swelling in a few people.

A diet may be adequate and balanced in content, but to be eaten and enjoyed, some further points need consideration:

(i) Cleanliness of the cooking utensils, crockery and cutlery, the cook's hands and the food, will prevent gastro-intestinal infection.

(ii) The standard of cooking can vary very much.
The addition of flavourings or herbs makes the dish more interesting, and stimulates the appetite.

(iii) The meal should be served in an attractive manner. When combined with a pleasant environment this makes eating the food a pleasure. Quarrels and an atmosphere of noise and haste can interfere with appetite and should be avoided at meal-times. Eating a meal can be part of a festive occasion (dinner is an important part of the Christmas celebrations). Patients in hospital appreciate an occasional diversion and, where possible, they are given a birthday cake or their relatives are encouraged to bring some special gift to celebrate an anniversary.

Some people feel grateful for the food they receive, and may thank the hostess after the meal. The nurse may find amongst her patients a child who says Grace before his meals and she should uphold him in this family habit.

Conditions Resulting from Inadequate or Unbalanced Diet

STARVATION follows severe reduction in all foods. There is loss of weight and general weakness. When a person in this condition is re-introduced to food, the diet contains easily digestible but nourishing fluids given in small amounts. Complan and milk are useful (p. 231).

MALNUTRITION is the result of lack or deficiency in one or more types of food in the diet. There may be sufficient food in calorie value but the diet is not correctly balanced. Improvement takes place quickly when the foods previously omitted are included in the diet and are replaced by medicines in treatment. Malnutrition can be due to disease. The patient's weight may be satisfactory but he is not healthy, and children do not grow at the normal rate.

OBESITY or overweight is more common now than in previous years and causes some anxiety, particularly when it occurs in children, people who are middle-aged (45 to 60 years) and those who suffer from heart conditions. It is due to eating more than the body needs, and there appear to be a variety of reasons for either increased appetite or lack of exercise or the combination of both. Obesity is associated with some diseases like under-secretion of the thyroid gland.

Any underlying cause is treated when possible. The diet is reduced by omitting sugar and some starches (low-calorie diet). The patient is advised to avoid sweets and snacks between meals but encouraged to eat plenty of meat, fish, eggs and cheese, fruit and vegetables. He visits his medical practitioner or a special clinic periodically. Weight-watchers' clubs have been formed and are popular with women especially, who are over-weight and wish to reduce.

WATER DEFICIENCY is dehydration and this can be due to insufficient water in the diet.

VITAMIN DEFICIENCIES

Deficiency in vitamin A causes the conjunctiva, skin and tissue lining the body cavities to become dry and unhealthy. It also causes night-blindness.

Deficiency in the various B vitamins can cause a form of neuritis (inflammation of the nerves). There are two severe deficiency diseases but they are uncommon in this country. Lack of vitamin B_{12} causes pernicious anaemia.

Deficiency in vitamin C causes scurvy, in which disease there is bleeding from the gums. In an infant, bleeding into the ends of long bones causes intense pain. The patient is anaemic.

Deficiency in vitamin D causes rickets at eighteen to twenty-four months. The bones become soft and deformities occur which can become permanent.

In treating vitamin deficiencies, the patient's diet is investigated and then adjusted so that it includes all the necessary nutrients. Symptoms of the disease are relieved by vitamins given in the form of medicines.

MINERAL DEFICIENCIES

Lack of iron causes anaemia.

Lack of iodine causes an enlarged thyroid gland (goitre).

Lack of salts causes dehydration.

Occasionally the body is unable to absorb a certain foodstuff in the diet.

Failure to absorb fats in the small intestine is a symptom of coeliac disease. It is the result of an allergic reaction to wheat flour in the diet. The child is treated by giving him a wheat flour (gluten) free diet.

Failure to absorbe vitamin B_{12} from the diet is due to lack of certain activity in the stomach wall. The patient needs large amounts of the vitamin in the diet (in liver) or it is given by injections.

Special Diets in Illness

FLUID DIETS

Clear fluids. Water, fruit juices with glucose in water, weak tea, Bovril, clear soups.

Bland fluids are prepared from water thickened slightly with barley, arrowroot or corn flour. Blackcurrant or lemon juice is added for flavour.

Fluid diets containing sufficient nutrients, fluid and calories for patients with partial obstruction of throat or oesophagus, or who are being fed by a tube into the stomach. COMPLAN (Glaxo) is a complete food. One pound packet makes eight cupfuls and is sufficient for one adult for one day. If Complan is not available a fluid diet is prepared, for example:

2 pints milk

4 oz dried skimmed milk

2 eggs

$\frac{1}{4}$ pint cream

2 oz glucose

1 teaspoonful Marmite.

Vitamin concentrate is added. The juice of an orange or two tablespoons of blackcurrant juice is given in the feeds or in water as a separate food.

This mixture is not very pleasant to take by mouth.

Soups. An ordinary cream soup is made more nutritious by adding Casilan, beaten eggs or cream.

A machine is available (homogeniser) which can reduce solid food like meat and vegetables to a thick liquid. This can be sucked from a spoon by a patient who cannot open his mouth easily, or given through a tube after soup or gravy has been added to make it more liquid.

Casilan (Glaxo) contains mostly milk protein and can be added to milk, soups or water, $1\frac{1}{2}$ oz (4 heaped dessertspoons) to each pint.

GASTRIC DIETS are prescribed as part of treatment to reduce the general activity of the stomach. The main principles in the diet are:

1. Frequent *small* meals.
2. Foods which are difficult to digest or will irritate the stomach are avoided. These include fatty meat or fish, fried foods, pastry, sauces and pickles. Fruit and vegetables are sieved.

The patient is encouraged to have snacks of milky drinks and biscuits, and should not be more than three hours without food.

LOW-RESIDUE DIET is prescribed for patients with inflammation of the colon or diarrhoea or sometimes in the preparation of a patient for surgery. It is similar to a gastric diet in most cases (a few patients are allergic to milk and then a special diet is arranged). Foods which have a laxative action such as prunes and figs are avoided. Occasionally *no* fruit or vegetable is allowed.

GLUTEN-FREE DIET is ordered in the treatment of coeliac disease. No food containing wheat flour or rye (in crispbreads) is given. Corn flour, rice flour or wheat starch are used in baking and making gravies and sauces. Nescafé and tea may be used as drinks but not Horlicks or Ovaltine.

LOW-PROTEIN DIET gives the kidneys less work to do.

Not given in the diet are fish, meat, cheese and eggs. Milk, bread and biscuits are reduced.

Given in the diet are certain cereals (rice or rice crispies or corn flour), vegetables, salads, fruit, sugar and fats.

LOW-SALT diet helps to reduce oedema.

Not given in the diet are salt added at table or in cooking, kippers, bacon, ham, tinned meats and fish, pickles and sauces. Puddings, cakes and biscuits.

When the diet is strict, special bread and margarine are used and milk is left out.

HIGH-PROTEIN DIET repairs damaged tissue and replaces lost protein (as in burns). Double portions of meat, fish or eggs are served at three main meals a day. Three ounces of Casilan in a litre of milk are given each day. Milk is useful and is added in cooking and in milk drinks.

LOW-FAT DIET is ordered when jaundice is present.

Not given are cream, cheese, fried foods, pastry, biscuits, cakes; *very little* butter or margarine, and skimmed milk. One egg is allowed each day.

DIET TO REDUCE WEIGHT is ordered for obesity.

Not given in the diet are fried foods, sugar, sweets, pastry, puddings, thick soups, sauces. Bread, cakes, biscuits, milk, potatoes are reduced.

Given in the diet are average (or raised) amounts of lean meat, white fish, cheese, eggs, and all fruits and vegetables except potatoes. Moderate amounts of fats are given with plenty of *unsweetened* fluids, preferably between meals.

DIET IN DIABETES

The diet is sufficient to maintain the patient at his correct weight. There is no food he may *not* eat, but attention is paid to *carbohydrate in the diet*:

(i) Foods containing large amounts of carbohydrates are avoided (except in emergency). Sugar, sweets, cakes, sweet biscuits.

(ii) Foods containing carbohydrate are eaten in controlled amounts: bread, crispbreads, plain biscuits, cereals, porridge, potatoes, peas and beans, dried fruits, some fresh fruits (oranges, apples), milk, and Ovaltine.

(iii) Foods containing protein with some carbohydrate are allowed freely (unless the patient is overweight). Meat, fish, eggs, cheese, as well as fats may be eaten.

(iv) Foods containing little carbohydrate are allowed as often as the patient desires: most vegetables, sour fruits, Oxo, Bovril, clear soups, and all diabetic products such as diabetic jam, marmalade and chocolate.

DIET WITHOUT MILK in any form is part of the treatment in some cases of ulcerative colitis. A few infants cannot tolerate milk and a milk-free diet is devised for them also.

Naso-oesophageal Feeding

Feeding a patient may necessitate a tube being passed through the nose and oesophagus into the patient's stomach, so that he may be provided with food for adequate nutrition while he is unable to swallow.

This situation occurs:

1. In unconsciousness.

2. In paralysis of muscles used in swallowing, for example in tetanus.

3. In partial obstructions which may be due to stricture (narrowing), a complication of inflammation of the oesophagus.

4. Following major operations on the throat, such as laryngectomy.

5. In treatment of gastric ulcer when a continuous flow of milk into the stomach relieves the patient's discomfort.

6. When the mentally disturbed or confused patient refuses to take food.

This method of feeding the patient is a clean procedure. The equipment is clean and the nurse washes her hands before preparing the equipment and feed.

Two trays are required:
(a) for passing the tube;
(b) with the prepared feed.

EQUIPMENT

Naso-oesophageal tube. This is at least 60 cms long. (The nose and pharynx are about 20 cms and the oesophagus 25 cms in length in the average adult.)

Jacques's oesophageal tubes and Ryle's tubes are made of rubber. If the tube is soft and needs to be stiffened a little before passing it through the nose it can be placed in a bowl of ice for a few minutes. Plastic tubes such as the Levin's tube are received in a sterile pack.

Wooden applicators or nasal forceps with damp swabs attached are used to clean the nose if necessary.

Arachis oil. A few drops of this on a swab lubricates the tube to be passed through the nose.

A *2-millilitre syringe* and *blue litmus paper* are used to test if the end of the tube is in the stomach.

A small piece of *adhesive tape* is needed to secure the end of the tube to the patient's cheek.

A *small clean towel* protects the patient's clothing.

PROCEDURE is explained to the patient unless he is unconscious, and his co-operation is obtained. Some privacy is preferable. If possible the patient sits up in bed with a pillow in the curve of his back and his head bent slightly forward. The nostrils are cleaned when this is necessary so that the patient can breathe easily through the nostril not concerned in the procedure.

The nurse, who has washed her hands, lubricates the end of the tube with a *very small amount* of nut oil. The point of the tube is then passed in a *backward and downwards* direction along the floor of the nostril into the pharynx. (Note that the nose has curved turbinate bones on the outer walls of the nostrils—these are avoided by the backwards direction of the tube. The pharynx opens into the back of the nose. If the nurse introduces the tube upwards, it will irritate the mucous membrane and the patient will want to sneeze.)

It is helpful if the patient swallows as the tube enters the pharynx. The nurse passes the tube a little farther into the oesophagus as he completes the swallowing action. The muscle in the pharynx and beginning of the oesophagus is relaxed at that moment (Fig. 39).

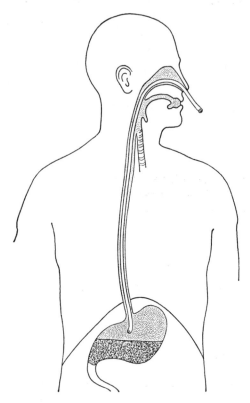

Figure 39. Naso-oesophageal tube in position.

As the air-passage joins the food-passage at the lower end of the pharynx, it is possible for the tube to enter the air-passage. This rarely happens in the conscious patient who is able to co-operate, but if by any chance this did take place he would cough and become blue, and there would be some respiratory distress. The nurse withdraws the tube at once as the patient would wish to expectorate.

It is obvious that although passing a naso-oesophageal tube in a conscious patient can be accomplished with little difficulty, it demands a great deal of skill when the patient is unconscious and then the procedure is usually carried out by the doctor, ward sister or experienced staff nurse.

As with the insertion of any tube into the body, it must be *introduced* gently though firmly, and never *pushed* through an opening (orifice). If there is any difficulty the nurse withdraws the tube and seeks advice; the tissues of the body are delicate and can be easily damaged. Two important points in this connection are:

(a) the nurse knows the simple anatomy of the part of the body with which she is dealing;

(b) ʋhe gains the co-operation of the patient.

Occasionally a patient prefers to pass the tube himself. There is no reason why he should not do this but it should be under supervision.

About 20 inches of the tube is introduced into the nose and oesophagus. Some fluid may be withdrawn and tested with blue litmus paper. If this turns red, the fluid is acid. As gastric juice is acid it is assumed that the end of the tube is in the stomach. The free end of the tube is attached to the patient's cheek with adhesive tape.

The total intake of food in one day is between 1200 and 1800 ml. There may be 9 or 10 two-hourly feeds of 120 ml or five feeds of 250 ml at four-hourly intervals. Two or three times during the day and between these feeds the patient receives diluted fruit juice, orange or blackcurrant, through the tube.

Preparation of the feed is similar to that for other meals. Tray and equipment are scrupulously clean. The presentation is as attractive as possible for the patient's pleasure in receiving food aids his digestion. The liquid food is in a kitchen measure and is warmed by placing it in a bowl of hot water. If the feed has been recently mixed with hot milk, the temperature is checked with a food thermometer. It should be at 38°C (100°F). The food is kept covered until it is given to the patient.

The food to be administered through the naso-oesophageal tube is liquid and nutritious. It can be:

(a) A mixture of milk, dried skimmed milk (4 tablespoons to 3 cups of milk), eggs, cream and glucose, thickened with flour. Minerals such as salt and iron medicine, as well as vitamins, are added. Casilan is a preparation of protein and can be added.

(b) Complan (Glaxo) of which a 1 lb packet makes 8 cupfuls. It is added to water.

The patient's diet cloth is placed in position. A funnel and tubing with glass connection are attached to the open end of the naso-oesophageal tube. About 30 ml of cooled boiled water are poured into the funnel. This prevents milk sticking to the sides of the tube like rinsing a saucepan before milk is put into it. The food is then given holding the funnel higher than the level of the patient's stomach. Then another ounce of boiled water is poured down the tube to remove as much of the milk as possible. The funnel and tubing are detached and cleaned thoroughly. If the food is regurgitated through the tube, the patient being restless or unconscious, the end of the tube is closed by a spigot.

The patient's mouth is cleaned after each feed as the natural cleansing action in chewing and producing more saliva is absent. The amount of food given would be recorded on a fluid balance chart.

When the nurse gives the patient his next feed, she checks that only the expected amount of tube is outside the patient's nose. If there is more than this, she requests the advice of a more experienced person before proceeding. It is possible that the end of the tube is no longer in the stomach, so that a little milk could flow from the end of the tube, into the air passages and cause infection in the lungs.

To remove a naso-oesophageal tube, the nurse asks the patient to swallow and draws out the tube section by section at the end of each swallowing action.

Oral-oesophageal Feeding

In this procedure the oesophageal tube is passed through the mouth, at the side of the tongue, to prevent retching. There are disadvantages. The tube easily moves out of position as the mouth is moist and the tongue mobile. Closing the mouth is impossible; this causes discomfort, and infection can occur. Speech is made difficult. It would be preferable to pass the tube each time the feed is administered.

Gastrostomy is an opening in the stomach made so that the patient's nutrition can be maintained when there is severe disease or injury of the oesophagus. A tube is inserted by the surgeon into the opening and it is closed with a spigot between feeds. Encircling the tube over the wound is a small dressing which is renewed as necessary.

The patient being fed in this way can usually be given an ordinary diet reduced to semi-liquid so that the food can pass through the tube. Meat is minced or fish pounded and gravy or a thin sauce added to this and the puréed or creamed vegetables. Milk puddings and custards are diluted with milk. The nurse can use her ingenuity in adapting and modifying the diet and presenting it attractively on a tray. It is best for the patient to have his meals at the same time as the other patients, for he will be hungry at that time. He needs some privacy. If he is able to administer his own feeds he can be shown how to do so. The method is the same as that used with a naso-oesophageal tube.

To encourage the flow of saliva which keeps the mouth in a healthy condition and to stimulate the digestive juices in the alimentary tract, he chews a little food as the meal is being given. This may be a piece of meat from the ordinary meal or a raw apple. He cannot swallow it but expectorates it into a bowl and this is removed with the tray at the end of the procedure.

Continuous milk infusion may be ordered, for example, for a patient with a gastric ulcer. The presence of milk in the stomach prevents pain. It is sometimes in use during the night so that the patient can sleep when very frequent feeds ordered as treatment would necessitate his being wakened each hour.

A naso-oesophageal tube is passed and a flask or glass reservoir is attached to this by tubing and glass connection. 150 millilitres of milk are poured into the flask each hour. A tubing gate clip controls the rate of flow. 15 millilitres of cool boiled water are poured through the tubing before each feed. The flask and tubing are removed from the naso-pharyngeal tube twice a day, cleaned thoroughly and sterilised. A plug of wool enclosed in muslin or gauze in the opening of a glass reservoir prevents dust from entering it as it hangs from a prop attached to the bed or locker.

As on all occasions when methods of artificial feeding are employed, the mouth requires regular and conscientious care. The patients respond to reassurance and simple explanations of the procedures. A high standard of cleanliness and knowledge of simple diets are essential.

CHAPTER 34 | THE ALIMENTARY TRACT

Tissue cells require foodstuffs in order to perform their functions. It is in the alimentary tract that food is taken into the body and broken down into simple substances which can be absorbed into the blood stream. As the blood circulates through the tissues, the nutrients which the cells require pass from the plasma into the cells where they can be used. Materials which have not been digested and absorbed are passed along the canal to be excreted as faeces.

The *alimentary tract* (Fig. 40) is a long muscular tube which begins at the mouth and ends at the anus.

The MOUTH is a cavity, the roof of which is called the hard palate. On the floor is the tongue, at the sides lie the molar teeth and cheeks and the incisor teeth and lips are at the front. The teeth are embedded in facial bones named the upper jaw (maxilla) and lower jaw (mandible). There are three *salivary glands* on each side of the face. One (the parotid) lies in front of the ear, one under the tongue (sub-linguinal) and the other (the submaxillary) lies in the neck immediately beneath the lower jaw. The pressure of food in the mouth and also the smell and taste stimulate the glands to produce *saliva* without which the food cannot be properly chewed or swallowed.

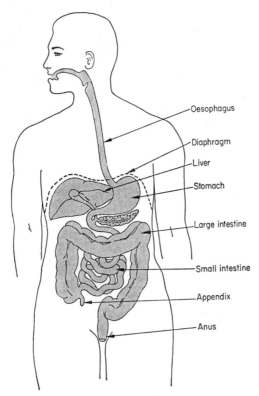

Figure 40. The alimentary tract.

Saliva has the following functions:
(1) It keeps the mouth moist and is slightly antiseptic in action.
(3 It is necessary for the taste of food to be appreciated.
(3) It is also necessary for speech.
(4) It contains a digestive substance, ptyalin, which changes cooked starches into sugars.
The front teeth (incisors) bite a portion from solid food and the tongue pushes it between the back teeth (molars). In chewing, the muscles of mastication contract, the jaws come together and the food is ground into a soft mass with the saliva.

Swallowing. The lips close and the soft mass is pushed by the tongue upwards against the hard palate and it passes backwards against the soft palate. This is a muscle structure joined to the hard palate and directs the food mass downwards into the *pharynx*, a cavity which lies behind the nose and mouth. It has muscle walls which on contraction move the food into the *oesophagus*. While swallowing takes place, a flap called the epiglottis falls across the opening which leads to the larynx (air-passage), and prevents choking. Chewing and swallowing are automatic actions, but under some voluntary control. From the oesophagus onwards, the contents of the alimentary tract move along the canal by peristaltic action.

Peristalsis is rhythmical contraction of circular and longitudinal muscle fibres in the walls of the tube so that wave-like movement takes place. The material inside the tube is squeezed along continuously. Normally the individual is quite unconscious of this movement.

The *oesophagus* is about 25 cms in length and passes through the chest, pierces the diaphragm and enters the stomach.

The STOMACH is a dilated portion of the alimentary tract situated beneath the diaphragm in the upper left abdomen. Its muscular wall has additional fibres which enable it to contract in several directions so that food within it can be churned up ino a semi-liquid consistency. At both ends of the stomach are ring-shaped muscles (sphincters) which close while food is being partly digested in the stomach (Fig. 41).

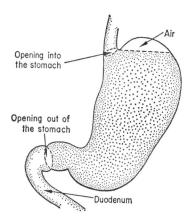

Figure 41. Stomach.

Glands in the wall of the stomach produce *gastric juice*. This is a fluid which is acid and contains digestive substances (rennin and pepsin) which change milk protein and other proteins into simpler substances.

Other cells in the stomach wall secrete a substance necessary for the absorption of vitamin B_{12}, which prevents pernicious anaemia.

DIGESTION IN THE STOMACH

(1) Churning of the food mixes it with the gastric juice and makes it more liquid.

(2) Proteins are changed into simpler substances called peptones.

When the process is over the pyloric sphincter at the exit of the stomach opens and the contents pass into the duodenum of the small intestine.

The *duodenum* is about 25 cms in length and lies fixed in front of the spine in the upper abdomen. It is C-shaped and the head of the pancreas fits into its curve. Ducts or tubes enter the duodenum carrying bile from the gall bladder and the pancreatic juice, and the food is mixed with these. By continuing peristaltic action, the contents of the tube move on into the *remainder of the small intestine*. This is about 20 feet in length and lies coiled in the centre of the abdomen. Further digestive juices are added from glands in the walls of the intestine.

DIGESTION IN THE SMALL INTESTINE

Bile emulsifies the fats in foods, making them more digestible.

Pancreatic juice contains:

  Lipase which changes fats into SIMPLE FATTY SUBSTANCES.

  Amylase which changes cooked starches into sugars.

  Trypsin which changes peptones (from proteins) into AMINO-ACIDS.

Intestinal juice contains:

  Maltese, inverbase and *lactase* which change all sugars into GLUCOSE.

  Erepsin which changes peptones into AMINO-ACIDS.

  Bile and *intestinal juice* are alkaline.

Absorption of foodstuffs in the Small Intestine

The lining of this part of the food canal is in the form of countless tiny projections called villi which contain blood capillaries and small lymph vessels. As the digested foodstuffs pass over the villi amino-acids and glucose are absorbed into the blood capillaries and are carried to the liver. A proportion of them pass through into the main blood circulation. The simple fatty substances are absorbed into the lymph vessels and become part of the lymph which eventually enters the main blood circulation.

The Colon and Rectum

In the canal there now remain:

1. *Undigested food*
   (a) cellulose framework of cereals, fruit and vegetables;
   (b) food inadequately chewed or digested, or non-absorbed.
2. *Water.*
3. *Bile* which gives the contents their brownish colour.

These contents are liquid in consistency and pass from the end of the small intestine into the large intestine, called the colon, at a junction which is in the lower right abdomen near to the point where the appendix is situated. The appendix is a narrow tube 5 to 7 cms in length, closed at one end, and it opens into the first section of the large intestine or caecum; it has no function in the human.

The COLON is a large puckered tube which ascends on the right side, then passes across the abdomen and descends on the left side into the pelvis. The contents pass along by peristaltic movement and *water is absorbed* through the wall of the colon into the blood circulation. This means that the contents become drier and to ensure that they pass along without causing friction, a lubricating fluid mucus is produced by cells in the walls of the colon. The results are soft solids called faeces which pass into the RECTUM.

This part of the alimentary tract is about 6 inches in length. It is situated in the pelvis and acts as a reservoir for the faeces just before it is evacuated from the body in defaecation.

Certain bacteria exist normally in the colon, e.g. *bacilli coli*. They assist in making the contents of the colon harmless to the body and also bring about the formation of vitamins B and K.

The act of DEFAECATION

When the muscle contractions of the intestinal tract are stimulated, e.g. following the eating of food, the contents of the colon pass along and enter the rectum. As this distends with faeces there is a desire to defaecate. Faeces are evacuated from the bowel by the contractions of the rectum and the dilation of the external opening, the anus. The sphincter is normally closed by contraction of its ring-like muscle. To aid in the expulsion of faeces voluntary skeletal muscles are brought into action; these are the chest diaphragm, the pelvic diaphram and the muscles of the abdominal wall. Small children learning to use a toilet article will be seen to breathe in and hold the breath momentarily indicating the forced contraction of the chest diaphragm. It may even be followed by a small 'grunt' of effort.

M

Infants empty the bowel three or four times a day, usually after feeds, but later as the child grows up it is more convenient if this action takes place regularly at suitable times. This is established during toilet training at about 18 months to 2 years of age when it comes under some voluntary control. Habits vary in different people, but it is most usual for defaecation to take place once a day after breakfast. Sometimes the habit is twice a day and occasionally every two or three days. The rhythm of individual habit is important in determining whether constipation or diarrhoea is present as a symptom of disease.

The Liver, the Gall-bladder and the Pancreas

These are organs which are joined to the alimentary tract.

The LIVER is a large, wedge-shaped organ weighing about 1 kilogramme, situated beneath the right side and centre of the diaphragm. It is red in colour, being plentifully supplied with blood from a large artery, and is divided into sections called lobes. In these are small lobules through which the blood capillaries circulate. *The portal vein* entering the liver is formed by the joining of veins from the stomach, intestines and spleen; these bring blood containing glucose, amino-acids, iron and vitamins. The liver is a very active organ. It is important in the use and storage of these food substances. It also produces bile, and destroys some poisonous substances which may be present in the body. From the liver leave two vessels, a vein and the bile duct. The former passes immediately into the major blood vessel to the heart, and the latter carries bile to the gall-bladder which lies immediately below the liver.

The GALL-BLADDER is a small sac about 7 cm in length which stores and concentrates bile. When a fatty meal is eaten, the nerve supply to the gall-bladder is stimulated and the sac contracts pushing out bile which passes through the bile duct into the duodenum. Here the bile mixes with the food and assists in the digestion of fats.

Bile is a greenish yellow fluid, sticky and alkaline. It colours and lubricates the faeces, and if absent from the intestinal tract the stools are pale and bulky due to the presence of excess fat and fatty substances.

The PANCREAS (Fig. 42) is a glandular organ which lies posterior in the upper abdomen. In the organ are two types of glandular cells. The large number of cells secrete pancreatic juice which passes to the duodenum, and the digestive substances in it take part in the digestion of proteins, carbohydrates and fats. The small number of cells in groups which can be seen under the microscope are called the Islets of Langerhans. These produce insulin, a hormone or chemical substance which, though present only in small amounts, controls the use of glucose in the body cells, i.e.

the *metabolism* of carbohydrates. Lack of this hormone in the blood causes inefficient metabolism of glucose and can produce a condition known as *diabetes mellitus*.

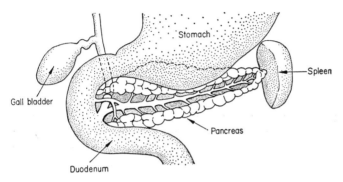

Figure 42. Pancreas.

The Alimentary Tract in Health

Cleanliness of the mouth and the sense of taste contribute to the enjoyment of food. The former prevents infection of the salivary glands and stomach. The cleanliness of food and utensils used for cooking and eating prevents infection of the gastro-intestinal tract. Teeth are necessary for mastication, and when these have been extracted dentures replace them.

The efficient functioning of the stomach and intestines requires that the diet should contain adequate fluid (approximately 2 litres a day), depending on climatic conditions and physical activity. Roughage which comes mainly from the cellulose parts of fruit, vegetables and cereal food provides bulk in the intestines.

A regular habit of defaecation ensures the complete emptying of the lower colon and rectum, thus avoiding constipation. Physical exercise generally improves appetite and digestion and aids efficient defaecation. The natural position for defaecation is squatting, and toilet seats for children and frail people should be sufficiently low for comfort. Facilities for washing the hands after defaecation are necessary in the interests of hygiene.

The Alimentary Tract During Illness

Every attention is given to the *cleanliness of food and the utensils* used in the preparation and serving of it.

CARE OF THE MOUTH

Patients who use *dentures* for eating and have their dentures with them should have them cleaned at least twice a day. In the case of patients who cannot eat solids the *mouth is cleaned* before and after fluid feeds. The dentures are removed from the mouth of an unconscious patient and he is given no fluids or food by this route or he will choke (asphyxiate).

FEEDING OF PATIENTS

The patient whose throat has been anaesthetised is not given drinks until the sensation of touch in the mucous membranes returns, the reflex action of swallowing being then possible. Helplessness in a patient such as may be associated with injuries of both hands, bandaged eyes, general physical weakness and hemiplegia will necessitate the patient being fed by the nurse. The nurse will find it necessary to allow the patient whom she is feeding to breathe easily and comfortably between swallowing sips of milk and mouthfuls of food; there is more skill in using a spouted feeder than people realise. If the patient cannot place his tongue across the spout while he breathes then it should be removed from his mouth. In many cases it is preferable to use a cup as this allows the patient to close his lips so that no milk enters the pharynx while he is breathing in.

VOMITING

The patient who vomits during illness requires some supervision. A clean bowl is quickly taken to him when he shows signs of severe nausea, e.g. 'retching' or 'heaving', and the nurse remains with him. He is most comfortable lying flat with the head turned to one side and the mouth directed downwards so that the vomit can flow away. His head is supported and the fluid is wiped away from his lips with a towel, and at the same time the patient is reassured. In a sudden attack such as may occur in an infection, he will feel faint and it is unwise for an ill patient to attempt to walk to a wash-basin or toilet when he feels sick. A vomit bowl is sometimes left at the bedside but is removed immediately after it has been used. The patient is washed and the linen changed when necessary. He often feels exhausted and needs a little time to recover.

DEFAECATION is a problem during illness. The patient in bed lacks opportunity for general exercise and possibly his prescribed diet does not contain constipation-preventing feeds and fluids. He is required to use a bed-pan, which for most people means that defaecation is incomplete, and is perhaps obliged to defaecate while he is lying flat in bed. Privacy when he is well is taken for granted but in a hospital ward is difficult. The main purpose however in the treatment of sick people is the cure or alleviation of their illness and the use of bed-pans is accepted by both patients and nurses as a natural and necessary feature of bed-treatment, the nurse making every effort for the comfort of the patient.

The ward is closed to general visitors and non-nursing personnel during any regular sanitary rounds of the day. In an emergency at other times, the nurse should be discreet in her management of the situation. Screens or curtains are drawn round the bed. The bed-pan is warm and dry when brought to the patient, the bed-clothes are loosened or turned back, and the patient lifted or assisted in raising his buttocks from the bed while the bed-pan is placed beneath him. It is centrally positioned so that it feels safe. The bed-pan supports the lower lumbar area, and the patient is more comfortable if his hips and knees are slightly flexed. The male patient requires a bottle in which to pass urine. The toilet of an ill patient is carried out by the nurse, as excreta on the skin predisposes to the formation of a bed-sore. A bowl of water is given to the patient after the removal of the bed-pan for hand washing. The screens are drawn back and the near-by windows opened for a few minutes.

As soon as the doctor considers the patient's condition is such that he can be moved out of bed, a commode at the side of the bed is made available. This should have a back rest and arms. A pillow may be placed at his back to give more support, and a bar across the front of the chair prevents him from falling forwards. A footstool is useful for a short person. The patient needs a warm jacket and slippers, and one of his blankets covers his legs and feet. His toilet afterwards is attended to by the nurse and the cleanliness of the commode is as important as that of the bed-pan and toilet. In some cases, the patient can be lifted into a movable chair which is wheeled into the toilet and over the receptacle, so that he can perform in the normal way. A patient using a commode or toilet chair should be able to contact the nurse by ringing a bell, or she should return in two minutes to attend to him. He can occasionally find the procedure exhausting or be in difficulties.

CONSTIPATION in an ill patient is prevented by the inclusion of sufficient fluid and food in the diet, and the encouragement of a regular habit of defaecation. The administration of aperients, glycerine suppositories, or enemas may be necessary.

Impacted faeces is a possible complication during the illness of an elderly patient. It is prevented whenever possible, otherwise oil retention enemas are followed by manual removal of faeces. Cleansing enemas complete the treatment.

DIARRHOEA is a symptom which causes the patient considerable distress and prevents sleep. The skin round the anus becomes sore. Application of a barrier cream such as anhydrous lanoline, zinc cream and castor oil, or a silicone cream, will prevent absorption and soft tissues or cotton wool are used for the patient's toilet in preference to toilet paper. Occasionally an incontinent pad of absorbent material beneath the buttocks is comfortable for the patient. Sheets are changed as soon as they become soiled. A person suffering from an unexpected bout of diarrhoea may faint on evacuating the bowel suddenly and needs some supervision.

Symptoms and Signs in Diseases of the Alimentary Tract

HALITOSIS is an unpleasant smell from the mouth and is due to an unhealthy mouth or some gastric upset, but also occurs in nervous tension.

The cause of LOSS OF APPETITE (anorexia) is sometimes unknown but it is common in inflammation and infections of the gastro-intestinal tract, particularly the stomach and also the liver and gall-bladder, and is a symptom associated with disease elsewhere such as congestive heart failure and infectious fevers. An emotional upset causes anorexia in some people, usually women.

There may be a simple reason in the surroundings for NAUSEA which is one type of response to an unpleasant stimulus such as a disturbing sight or a repellent smell. It may also be due to fear. It is a common symptom in disease of the digestive tract and may be combined with anorexia or vomiting. The nauseated patient dislikes fatty foods in the diet, and the nausea is aggravated by his own sudden movement or that of people near to him.

VOMITING is more likely to occur as a symptom in children, for they are not so inclined to avoid being sick as adults are. The nurse should observe the manner of vomiting. An infant may merely regurgitate milk, or the food taken during the several hours preceding the attack may be vomited to a distance of two or three feet at great speed. This is PROJECTILE VOMITING and is a symptom of disease in adults also. Abnormalities are noted in the amount of material vomited, as are its contents, for example, digested blood (HAEMATEMESIS), bile, undigested food, or something unexpected such as a round worm from the small intestine. The doctor may request to see the vomit. Occasionally, a patient will explain that discomfort in the chest or stomach is relieved by vomiting.

INDIGESTION or dyspepsia is discomfort associated with food and occurs after a meal.

HEARTBURN is usually due to a little of the acid contents of the stomach regurgitating into the oesophagus.

Difficulty in swallowing is called DYSPHAGIA. There may be some obstruction in the oesophagus, for example, muscle spasm or a tumour, but dysphagia is also a symptom of chest diseases when enlarged tissue, e.g. tumour, presses on the oesophagus.

PAIN may be vaguely present throughout the abdomen or be localised in one area, e.g. on the right side in appendicitis. Increased peristalsis causes *colic*, an intermittent 'griping' sensation, due to diet indiscretions or infection or obstruction.

CONSTIPATION is one deviation from the normal regular emptying of the bowel. It varies in degree from a very slight constipation to complete stoppage (impacted faeces).

DIARRHOEA means more frequent and more watery stools than usual. The patient may pass blood (*malaena*). In some types of diarrhoea there is little or no faeces but quantities of mucus, perhaps blood-stained, are passed. Straining to pass faeces and not being able to do so is a distressing symptom known as *tenesmus*. It is associated with either constipation or diarrhoea.

INCONTINENCE OF FAECES is a symptom associated with lack of nervous control over the sphincters.

A patient on admission may state he has passed *no wind*, i.e. no flatus. The surgeon places his stethoscope on the abdomen and listens (this is ausculation). The type of bowel sounds or their absence is helpful in making a diagnosis.

JAUNDICE is a condition in which all tissues of the body are stained yellow. It is most readily seen in the whites of the eyes. This discoloration is due to the presence of bile in the blood following liver disease or obstruction in or on the bile duct. The patient who is jaundiced usually feels ill and is nursed at rest in bed. Sight, taste or smell of fatty foods produces nausea.

Irritation of the skin in a mild degree is common, but can be sufficiently severe to cause insomnia. Swabbing the skin with sodium bicarbonate solution or adding this to water for sponging, and application of calamine lotion give relief. The doctor may prescribe a mild sedative.

Because the bile pigment is circulating in the blood and does not reach the small intestine, the colouring matter is absent from faeces. The stools are therefore bulky and pale.

In some cases of jaundice, bile is present in the urine, which appears brownish green.

Clinical Investigations

A SPECIMEN OF STOOL can be examined in the laboratory for blood and pus cells and pathogenic bacteria. The head of a tape worm is detected by sieving the stool through a fine black mesh.

GASTRIC ANALYSIS is made by the examination of a series of samples obtained from the patient's stomach. The patient has no food or drink

overnight. The samples are taken by aspiration through a naso-oesophageal tube.

For RADIOGRAPHY of the gastro-intestinal tract, the patient swallows
barium emulsion which is opaque to X-rays while he stands in front of
the X-ray screen. The radiologist observes the passage of the barium
through the oesophagus and stomach and notes abnormalities of the outline of organs and in the filling and emptying of the stomach. In preparation for this examination the patient has had an aperient 36 hours
previously and is starved overnight. He wears a loose cotton gown so
that buttons and fasteners do not cover any lesion during the screening.
As the barium emulsion passes through the small intestine, a further
X-ray examination is made. Investigation of the colon and rectum is
made by radiography following the administration of a barium enema.

Simple X-ray examination reveals opaque foreign bodies which have
been swallowed.

RECTAL EXAMINATION is a procedure frequently carried out during the
investigation of a number of conditions, not only those directly concerned with the rectum, e.g. impacted faeces and carcinoma, but also
when the prostate gland is likely to be enlarged, the appendix inflamed, or
an abscess has formed in the lowest part of the peritoneal cavity. The
patient lies in the left lateral position, the curtains having been drawn
round the bed, and the anal area is exposed.

The doctor inserts a gloved finger lubricated with paraffin molle
through the anal canal and into the rectum. The abdomen may be palpated at the same time, and any pain or discomfort experienced by the
patient is noted in addition to any abnormality felt by the surgeon. The
patient is more comfortable if he has passed urine prior to the examination.

OESOPHAGOSCOPY AND GASTROSCOPY are examinations by means of
metal tubes which can be inserted through the mouth into the oesophagus
or stomach. A small electric bulb at the end of the tube provides illumination. Some foreign bodies can be removed through an oesophagoscope.
Anaesthesia of the mouth and throat is included in the preparation of the
patient and the procedure is carried out in the operating theatre.

In SIGMOIDOSCOPY the surgeon examines the sigmoid colon. He usually
prefers the patient to be in the chest-knee position, i.e. kneeling with
the hips and knees flexed so that the body is inclined downwards and the
face rests on a pillow placed on the examination couch in front of the
knees. The instrument used is a sigmoidoscope.

Examination of the rectum using a proctoscope is PROCTOSCOPY and
the patient lies in the left lateral position with both legs fully flexed or
drawn up towards his chin.

In these examinations a small piece of tissue may be removed (biopsy) and a section of this is later examined beneath the microscope.

Medical and Surgical Conditions of the Alimentary Tract

The Mouth

Micro-organisms grow normally in the mouth but infection is not likely unless the mucous membrane becomes dry or inflamed. Breathing through the mouth, not eating food and dehydration are reasons for the mouth becoming dry in debilitating illnesses. Infection can spread to a parotid gland which shows as a red, painful swelling in front of the ear. Regular, careful oral toilet and cleanliness of utensils prevent this complication.

Penicillin and several other antibiotics destroy bacteria in the mouth but THRUSH due to a yeast and insensitive to penicillin appears to be more common. The rash looks like milk clot on the mucous membrane but cannot be removed easily. It can spread quickly through the gastro-intestinal tract.

HERPES SIMPLEX is the result of a virus infection and appears on the lips and surrounding skin after a cold or in pneumonia. The shallow superficial blisters become painful ulcers. These lesions should be kept dry, and touched as little as possible. It can also occur in the mouth.

The Oesophagus

Large pieces of food can cause OBSTRUCTION OF THE OESOPHAGUS and are removed during oesophagoscopy.

Other causes of obstruction include CARCINOMA of the oesophagus which is treated by a tube passed through the constriction and deep X-ray therapy or surgical removal (oesophagectomy).

CARDIO-SPASM is thickening and spasm at the lower end of the oesophagus, causing difficulty in swallowing (dysphagia). Later the oesophagus dilates and the patient vomits the stale food which collects in it. In surgical treatment the muscle fibres are divided to relieve the thickening.

In HIATUS HERNIA a small amount of the stomach near the lower end of the oesophagus protrudes through the oesophageal opening in the diaphragm. Small amounts of acid stomach contents regurgitate into the oesophagus which becomes inflated causing 'heartburn'. The patient prevents the regurgitation by sitting upright while he sleeps, and he avoids bending, stooping and lifting. Surgery may be necessary. The condition is seen occasionally in infants. They are nursed in a special chair which supports them in an upright position.

M*

Swallowing of corrosive acids and alkalies results in severe OESOPHA-
GITIS followed later by STRICTURE OF THE OESOPHAGUS. This frequently
interferes with nutrition and the patient may need extra nourishment
through a gastrostomy tube. Refashioning of an oesophagus beneath the
skin is possible on some occasions.

The Stomach
Symptoms of narrowing at the emptying end of the stomach (pyloric
stenosis) appear in infants three to six weeks old who have thickening of
the pylorus muscle. The stomach dilates and the baby vomits large
amounts of stale material in a projectile manner. He quickly becomes
dehydrated. The surgeon, in an abdominal operation, divides the pylorus
muscle and the opening from the stomach becomes effective.

FOREIGN BODIES swallowed, usually by children, pass through the alimentary tract if they are smooth and round. Others may damage the
oesophagus and stomach. Open safety pins are dangerous (one reason why
a nurse never leaves a safety pin opened). The patient who has swallowed
a foreign body is X-rayed. A stodgy diet of thick porridge and bread may
be advised and the patient remains in bed. Stools are examined. If the
foreign body is not recovered, another X-ray film is taken and, should
the object not have moved, abdominal surgery for removal is performed.

INJURIES of the stomach are usually penetrating wounds caused by
bullets or knives, or crash injuries. Repair is performed by the surgeon
without delay to prevent extensive peritonitis. The patient may have sustained other injuries at the same time.

GASTRITIS is inflammation of the stomach. This is a cause of acute
vomiting. It is the result of infection, e.g. food poisoning, or an unsuitable
diet with excess of unripe fruit, spiced foods or alcohol. Smoking can
produce this condition and gastritis may follow a long course of salicylates
(including aspirin).

PEPTIC ULCERS are ulcers of the stomach and duodenum. These are a
common condition and appear in people who are inclined to be anxious,
to worry or overwork. Irregular meals are another factor. Many of the
patients are 25 to 35 years of age. In the acute attack the patient complains of sudden dyspepsia. Pain is associated with food and is relieved
by vomiting or taking alkali medicines. Because roughage and spiced
foods increase the pain he leaves these out of the diet and takes plenty
of milk and milk puddings. In many cases the ulcer heals following treatment by a milk diet and alkalies (magnesium trisilicate). *Complications*
in an acute attack include bleeding from the ulcer; the patient either
vomits blood (haematemesis) or passes blood in the stools (malaena).
Perforation of the stomach is another complication. In some cases the

attacks of pain return and eventually the patient has a chronic ulcer which is deeper and more penetrating than the first ulcer. The pain in chronic gastric ulcer is continuous and food, especially hard food and pickles, makes it worse. Vomiting leads to loss in weight. The diagnosis is made with the aid of gastric analysis and radiography.

The treatment usually includes six weeks' mental and physical rest and a non-irritating, easily digested diet. Alcohol and smoking are avoided. Alkalies are prescribed as medicines. Subsequent attacks are treated in the same manner. In cases which do not respond to treatment or in which the treatment interferes with work, the surgeon may consider operative treament in which the ulcer is removed but the function of the stomach is changed as little as possible, e.g. the remaining part of the stomach is partially closed and then joined to the duodenum.

CHRONIC DUODENAL ULCER is related to a high acid content of the stomach and pain is relieved by food, water and alkalies which mop up or dilute the acid. The patient has frequent milk drinks and these relieve pain during the night.

Medical treatment is similar to that for gastric ulcer. In surgery, part of the stomach is removed to reduce the acidity together with the duodenal ulcer, and the remaining part of the stomach is joined to the small intestine. This is partial gastrectomy. Preparation for these operations is mainly to prevent complications. The stomach is washed out if there are unpleasant contents as in pyloric stenosis. The patient has breathing exercises and if there is a chest infection it is treated. An intra-gastric tube is passed into the stomach and aspirated at frequent intervals after operation. This prevents the stomach filling up with fluid and also indicates possible haemorrhage. As the amount of aspirated fluid becomes less, the intake by mouth increases. In the meantime an intravenous infusion supplies fluid to maintain a correct balance, for example 1 litre of 5 per cent Dextrose in the first 24 hours. Mouth toilet is important and the patient is encouraged to cough.

When the patient recovers from his operation, the ulcer having been removed, he avoids large meals but increases their number by eating another meal or snack, and in two to three months he is having a mixed diet of ordinary food.

HAEMATEMESIS resulting from a peptic ulcer occurs frequently without warning and the patient is admitted to hospital for blood transfusions. He is nursed at absolute rest and when the emergency is over treatment for the ulcer commences. Occasionally surgery is performed after admission to remove the ulcer.

MALAENA is treated in a similar manner.

PERFORATED GASTRIC OR DUODENAL ULCER is a surgical emergency. The patient is extremely ill with abdominal pain and rigidity of the abdomen. Peritonitis develops rapidly if the perforation is not sutured quickly. The patient is prepared for operation with all speed.

CANCER of the stomach occurs most often in men betwen 50 and 60 years of age. The patient has loss of appetite followed by loss of weight, and anaemia. Diagnosis is by radiography and gastric analysis shows a low gastric acidity. Treatment depends on early diagnosis, the malignant growth being removed in partial or total gastrectomy. When the condition is found to be inoperable the patient needs sympathetic and skilled bedside care during his illness.

GASTROSTOMY is an artificial opening in the stomach. This operation is performed when obstruction or stricture of the oesophagus does not permit food to enter the stomach. It may be a temporary or permanent operation and the opening is maintained by a tube sutured into it. A varied, well-balanced diet is reduced to a liquid consistency and administered at the usual meal times through this tube which is then closed by a spigot or clip.

PERNICIOUS ANAEMIA follows the failure of the gastric glands to produce the anti-anaemic factor due to inability to absorbe vitamin B_{12}. This condition is treated by the administration of vitamin B_{12} in intramuscular injections.

The Small Intestine

ENTERITIS, i.e. inflammation of the small intestine, is caused in this country by eating unsuitable food or by infection from food-poisoning or typhoid bacilli. It is accompanied usually by gastritis which results in vomiting. Food poisoning is characterised by colic which begins in the centre of the abdomen, each wave of pain being followed by a bowel action. The loss of fluid in the frequent watery stools is dangerous, particularly in children, who are affected quickly by dehydration. Food poisoning is an infectious condition and the patient is isolated. Careful instructions are given to the relatives nursing the patient at home. A child has a receptacle for his own use and the stool is emptied in the toilet and flushed away immediately, taking care not to contaminate the outside of the toilet. The receptacle is disinfected using a mop with a white fluid solution 1 in 10. It is rinsed in hot water using a second mop. Towels, flannels, and a roll of toilet paper or tissues are reserved for the patient. The bed linen and clothing are collected in a bag and boiled, washed and ironed separately from the other linen in the house. Hands are washed immediately after using sanitary equipment and before any person leaves the sick room. Everyone in the house uses his own knives, forks or spoons. Visitors are discouraged.

The infection is treated by sulphonamides or antibiotics for about a week. Diet consists of clear fluids, with glucose, then as the gastritis improves thickened fluids such as cornflour, Benger's food and thin custard are often tolerated more easily than water and milk. To these are added at intervals a little cereal, thin bread with a little butter, honey, lightly boiled or coddled eggs, steamed fish and egg sauce, boiled or casseroled chicken drained of the cooking fluid, creamed potatoes and purée of vegetables and fruit. Small children and infants who become dehydrated are admitted to hospital for intravenous replacement of fluid. Patients with *typhoid fever* are taken to an Infectious Diseases Hospital as the disease can be serious and prevention of spread of infection is necessary.

INTESTINAL PARASITES are not common in this country. The *tape worm* is the largest, being many feet in length and consisting of a very tiny head joined to greyish white sections. It causes colic and interferes with nutrition, the patient becoming thin. Parts of the worm can be seen in the stools. Treatment is by a drug, filix mas, and is not finished until the head has been moved from the wall of the intestine and identified in the faeces.

A *round worm* is similar to an earth worm and exists in the small intestine, giving rise to few symptoms. It may be passed with a stool or be vomited. Santonin is a drug used in treatment.

Thread worms are produced in very large numbers in the small intestine but they move to the rectum, and the eggs escape from here to the skin around the anus. The area itches particularly at night and a child soon reinfects himself by his hands which carry the ova to food and to his mouth. It is possible for other members of the family to become affected. This condition is most common in children of toddler age and occurs in some old people. Hygiene regarding toilet of the anal area, hands, nails and cleanliness of clothing and sanitary utensils is necessary. Treatment is by drugs—piperazine in tablet form, prescribed by the doctor. Unless each member of the family with the infestation has been successfully treated, reinfection will occur in the family.

COELIC DISEASE is a condition which occurs in early childhood. The infant is sensitive to gluten, the protein in wheat flour, and when he begins to eat cereals, bread and biscuits the symptoms appear. He is unable to absorb fat from the small intestine and passes frequent large fatty stools. This form of malnutrition due to his not being able to absorb fat causes him to become weak and apathetic, with wasting of the muscles and anaemia. Treatment is to leave wheat flour out of his diet. Bread, biscuits and cakes are made from gluten-free flour which the mother can buy from firms which supply flour. This may be done by post if the family lives away from a large town. The mother is given instructions regarding recipes before the child leaves hospital. As he grows older the disease becomes less obvious.

ACUTE APPENDICITIS is a serious condition having a mortality rate of 3 to 4 in a hundred cases. There is usually a sudden onset with central abdominal pain and vomiting. The pain settles in the right lower abdomen and there is tenderness in this area. In children the temperature and pulse rate are raised. The surgeon takes a medical history and examines the patient (including a rectal examination), and he may wish to observe the patient to exclude other causes for the symptoms. As soon as a diagnosis of acute appendicitis is made, he performs the operation appendicectomy.

Complications of the disease include appendix abscess and peritonitis. If the former be diagnosed operation may be delayed until the abscess has been localised. The patient is nursed in bed, having only fluids by mouth, no aperients, and the temperature and pulse rate are recorded.

Peritonitis (inflammation of the peritoneum) is caused by an inflamed appendix which becomes gangrenous, perforation of the stomach or intestine, or by ruptured organs, e.g. spleen, bile duct. The patient is very ill with fever and becomes dehydrated. Paralytic ileus occurs when the intestines cannot contract due to oedema of the peritoneum which covers them. Antibiotic therapy is prescribed. An intra-gastric tube is passed and gastric aspiration is performed to keep the stomach empty. Fluids are given by the intravenous route. Oral toilet is necessary and the patient needs general nursing care. He is nursed in an upright position in bed so that any pus in the abdomen may localise in the pelvis from where it may be drained more easily than elsewhere in the abdomen. Gonococcal peritonitis may occur in women with untreated gonorrhoea following spread of infection from the uterus through the uterine tubes. Tubercular peritonitis is uncommon now but in some chldren peritonitis is associated with pneumonia or influenza.

HERNIA is the bulging of part of an organ through the wall of the cavity in which it is ordinarily contained.

Examples in which intestine bulges through the abdominal wall:

Umbilical hernia in infants, treated by a pad and Elastoplast. When this persists or occurs at a later age, surgery is performed to reduce the size of the umbilical scar.

Inguinal hernia (in the groin) is more common in men as the inguinal canal is open to allow the passage of the spermatic cord.

Femoral hernia (at the top of the thigh near to the groin) is more common in women because the femoral ring is large owing to a wide pelvis.

The bulge appears as a swelling which becomes bigger on coughing.

Usually the swelling disappears when the patient stops coughing or lies down flat. Eventually it may not disappear and occasionally the hernia strangulates. A truss is one form of treatment. It should be put on while the patient is lying down and there is no swelling. The pad is placed exactly over the opening where the bulge occurs. It can usually be worn indefinitely. Operative surgery reinforces the opening through which the intestine bulges, strengthening the muscle and tendon at that point; this operation is called *herniorraphy*.

Strangulated hernia. The part of the intestine bulging through the abdominal wall becomes oedematous, the blood supply to it stops and it becomes gangrenous. This gives rise to symptoms and signs of INTESTINAL OBSTRUCTION. The patient complains of colicky abdominal pain and there is some pyrexia and he feels ill. Fluid collects in the abdomen, which becomes distended. This fluid has been withdrawn from the general circulation and the patient can develop signs of shock. No flatus or faeces are passed, and no bowel sounds are heard through a stethoscope on the abdomen. The patient's abdomen is X-rayed.

Treatment of this acute condition is immediate surgery in which the cause of obstruction is removed (resection of gut), and the small intestine is repaired.

Foreign objects in the small intestine, inflammation and adhesions can also cause intestinal obstruction. In children it may be due to inflammation surrounding an infected appendix, loops of small intestine becoming twisted, or by one section doubling up inside the following section of gut.

The Large Intestine and Rectum

ULCERATIVE COLITIS (inflammation of the colon with ulcers forming in the mucous membrane) occurs in young people and is a debilitating disease. The cause is unknown. Diarrhoea is the main symptom and the patient passes mucus and blood in the stools. Because of this there is loss of weight and anaemia with general weakness. Frequency of defaecation causes physical and mental distress and the fastidious and sensitive patient becomes depressed.

The diagnosis is made following radiography (barium enema) and sigmoidoscopy, which show an ulcerated colon.

In less severe cases the patient has a low-residue diet containing very little roughage or residue. Milk and eggs may form the basis of the diet but it is essential that the diet is well balanced and varied, including protein to replace that lost as mucus in the stools and vitamin C to promote healing. Occasionally a patient has an allergy to milk associated with colitis and this patient is given a milk-free diet.

Sulphonamide or antibiotic therapy deals with infection associated with the ulcer formation.

Anaemia is treated by blood transfusion or iron injections when necessary and the patient's comfort in bed is maintained. The nurse reassures the patient regarding frequent use of bed-pans and endeavours to increase his confidence and optimism by a constant interest in his progress.

In more severe cases, the affected colon is removed by *hemicolectomy*, but the operation *ileostomy*, an opening on to the skin from the small intestine, is less advanced and can be performed in a large number of patients. Through this opening the liquid contents of the intestine are discharged. The disease is not cured but the symptoms are relieved and the condition of the colon improves. However, if the ileostomy is closed later it has been found the ulceration recurs and it is necessary for the patient to understand before the operation that this is likely to be a permanent method of emptying the bowel. It encourages him to know that many others with the same complaint now lead normal lives apart from the wearing of an appliance (a rubber bag) over the ileostomy opening in the abdomen.

CANCER OF THE LARGE BOWEL AND RECTUM occurs usually over 40 years of age. Symptoms include alternating constipation and diarrhoea with loss of some blood in stools. As the malignant growth develops there will be signs of increasing obstruction. The affected part of the large bowel may be removed in operative surgery. When the rectum is involved it is removed together with the sigmoid colon in *abdominal-perineal resection of rectum* by two surgeons, one approaching the site through the abdomen and the other through the perineum. A colostomy is necessary in this operation. A part of the large bowel is brought to the surface of the abdomen and the patient empties the bowel through an opening on to the skin. Preparation for operation is intensive as the patient is not young and his general health should be as satisfactory as possible. It is important that he and his relatives should understand before the operation what having a colostomy means and its management is explained before he leaves hospital. In many cases this form of treatment comes as a shock to older people and reassurance is necessary with a simple and practical explanation first, followed by details later and an opportunity to ask questions.

In cases where carcinoma of the rectum is inoperable the surgeon performs an operation to by-pass the growth or a colostomy, and this relieves symptoms of obstruction. Whenever possible the growth is removed so that the pain and diarrhoea it would cause are avoided.

Colostomy management. The contents of the colon are fairly solid and the colostomy acts twice a day, the action being associated with the taking of food. Diet is adjusted to prevent loose or dry stools or actions that are too frequent or irregular. The skin is protected by washing gently with soap and water and drying well. Barrier creams or an aluminium paint such as Baltimore paste are useful. The dressings or rubber bag placed over the opening are supported by a belt, and changing of these takes place as soon after the bowel action as possible. The habit of emptying the colon can be arranged to suit the patient so that he is at home or can visit a works surgery to change the dressing when the colostomy has acted.

Several hospitals have produced pamphlets which contain instructions and advice and are given to patients as they are discharged home. Additional aid can be offered by the district nurse whose services will be requested when there is no bathroom in the house and he lives with a number of people.

HAEMORRHOIDS are dilated veins in the anal canal, associated with straining at stool and standing a great deal. There is swelling of the mucous membrane followed by *internal piles* which are bluish and bleed. There is no pain unless they become inflamed. When untreated the haemorrhoids swell and are visible. Treatment is by injection into the mucous membrane which then shrinks and the swelling disappears, or by injection (e.g. 5 per cent phenol in almond oil) into the bulging piles (haemorrhoids).

There is considerable post-operative pain and discomfort following a *haemorrhoidectomy* (excision of piles). Sometimes a small tube is left in the anal canal for a few days to allow the patient to pass flatus and this would reveal bleeding that might occur. The wound is redressed after daily hot baths. Retention of urine is common.

An *external haemorrhoid* contains blood which has collected during straining at stool. This is incised to release the clot of blood.

Medical and Surgical Conditions of the Liver

Acute inflammation of the liver (ACUTE HEPATITIS) is caused by a virus, the symptoms including depression, anorexia and jaundice. The patient is nursed in bed and given a low-protein diet (about half the normal amount each day) with very little fat and plenty of carbohydrate. The patient feels rather ill and some convalescence is necessary afterwards.

CIRRHOSIS OF THE LIVER means the liver tissue has changed to fibrous tissue and is permanently damaged. It may follow acute hepatitis but is also associated with lack of protein in the diet. The patient loses weight but develops ascites (increased amount of peritoneal fluid in the abdomen). This is extremely uncomfortable and the doctor relieves the patient

by draining the fluid away through a metal tube introduced through the
skin of the abdomen (tapping of the abdomen).

Medical and Surgical Conditions of the Gall-Bladder

In an attack of ACUTE CHOLECYSTITIS, the cause of which is not always
known, the patient is ill with pyrexia and complains of pain under the
right lower ribs. This condition is more common in women. The patient
is nursed in bed and her diet consists of clear fluids with plenty of glucose
until the attack is over. The gall-bladder is removed in many cases at a
later date (cholecystectomy).

CHRONIC CHOLECYSTITIS due to gall-stones causes pain in the right side
of the upper abdomen with pyrexia and loss of appetite. The patient dislikes yellow and fatty foods which make her feel sick. Presence of gall-
stones is diagnosed by cholecystogram. After the inflammation has sub-
sided cholecystectomy is performed. After this operation the surgeon
often leaves two tubes in the wound. A short tube drains the cavity which
the gall-bladder occupies and is removed in 24 to 38 hours. The longer
tube drains bile from the common bile duct into a bottle; this is a
T-shaped tube and is removed in five to ten days, depending on drainage.
After cholecystectomy, the bile flows directly into the duodenum. The
patient eats a normal diet but may find that a very fatty meal, e.g. fried
fish and chips, causes some dyspepsia.

When a small gall-stone passes down the common bile duct to the
duodenum the patient suffers from intense pain. This passes in waves
from the area of the gall-bladder to the centre of the abdomen above the
umbilicus, and may radiate to the left shoulder. It is called *biliary colic*
and the doctor may prescribe an analgesic such as pethidine.

Diseases of the Pancreas

These are not common. The pancreas may become inflamed (ACUTE PAN-
CREATITIS).

CARCINOMA OF THE HEAD OF PANCREAS causes pressure on the common
bile duct and the patient becomes deeply jaundiced. Operative surgery
may follow in some cases of these conditions.

The *spleen* may be ruptured by direct violence in injury, and internal
haemorrhage is severe. The surgeon replaces lost blood and removes the
spleen (splenectomy). This operation is also performed in an unusual
form of anaemia.

Nursing Procedures

GASTRIC ASPIRATION is the withdrawal of fluid from the stomach through a naso-oesophageal tube.

The reasons for this procedure are:

1. To prevent a collection of blood and gastric secretions after an operation on the stomach.

2. To prevent vomiting by keeping the stomach empty.

3. As part of the treatment in persistent vomiting.

4. To empty the stomach before emergency operation when the patient has eaten recently.

5. To keep the stomach empty when there is intestinal obstruction. The contents of the stomach cannot pass through the intestine and would cause the patient pain, discomfort and distress.

A Ryle's tube is often the type of tube used and the end of this is passed through the nose into the stomach as described in naso-oesophageal feeding. The other end is secured to the cheek by *adhesive tape* when fluid is to be withdrawn at intervals. It is left unsealed so that gas or excess liquid in the stomach can escape, thus preventing abdominal discomfort in the patient.

A *20-millilitre syringe*, preferably kept for aspiration only, is used to withdraw the fluid, which is ejected into a *measure*. A polythene syringe and measure are useful when the fluid may be bloodstained after operation, as this avoids distressing the patient who would be able to see the fluid in a glass measure.

The amount of fluid is recorded on the *Fluid Balance Chart* and a *report* made to the sister of the amount and any abnormality such as blood (dark or bright red) or bile (green and slimy). As the patient is taking nothing or only small amounts of water by mouth, *oral toilet* is necessary. This is carried out immediately following the aspiration either by mouthwash or using swabs and forceps.

Gastric aspiration may be requested at regular intervals such as every two hours. Sometimes, when the gastric fluid has been removed, the patient is allowed 30–60 ml of boiled water to drink.

GASTRIC SUCTION is continuous removal of the contents of the stomach. The method most commonly in use is that employing a small suction pump which is on the patient's locker, or a wall suction supply. The pressure is low, e.g. $1\frac{1}{2}$ lb to 3 lb per square inch. The patient drinks small amounts of water. Suction is not applied when the stomach is completely empty, as it may cause some inflammation of the stomach wall. The equipment is supervised by a State Registered Nurse.

STOMACH WASHOUT

The purposes of this procedure are:

1. *To cleanse the stomach* (pyloric stenosis). The opening out of the patient's stomach is narrowed due to chronic ulcers and food is retained in the stomach where it becomes stale and sour. The patient vomits but the stomach is unhealthy and the surgeon may request stomach washout before he operates. When there is adequate time for preparation for operation the procedure is rarely necessary.

2. *To remove poisons from the stomach.* The patient may be unconscious. The procedure is carried out by a doctor, sister or experienced staff nurse and some assistance is required.

Equipment. This is a *clean* procedure. Stomach tube of suitable size, tubing, glass connection and large funnel. A tubing clip may be requested. Large jug containing 3 litres of fluid at 38°C. The fluid may be tap water, salt and water 1 teaspoon to 500 ml, or sodium bicarbonate and water 1 teaspoon to 500 ml. A small jug for pouring the fluid into the funnel. Waterproof cape and absorbent towel to protect the patient's skin and clothing. A pail into which the returned fluid is poured.

If specimens of stomach contents are required as in cases of poisoning, specimen containers, labels and laboratory forms and the patient's case notes will be required. If the patient is unconscious and his name is known an identification label has been fixed to his wrist.

PROCEDURE to cleanse the stomach if the patient is conscious.

An explanation is given to the patient so that his co-operation is assured. The curtains are drawn round the bed and he sits upright if possible, well supported by pillows. The protective capes are arranged to cover his neck and chest and if dentures are worn it may be wise to remove them to a denture carton as he may feel a little nauseated as the tube is being passed.

The point of the stomach tube is passed through the mouth, at the side of the tongue to prevent retching, into the oesophagus. The patient swallows and as he does so, the end of the tube can be passed a little farther until it reaches the stomach (45 to 50 centimetres). The tubing, connection and funnel are attached. The funnel is held at the level of the patient's stomach and 250 ml of fluid is poured in. Then the sister or staff nurse raises the funnel to her shoulder level and the fluid flows into the stomach. When it has almost run through the funnel is lowered to mattress level and the fluid returns into it. While at this level the funnel is inverted so that the contents flow into the pail. Then it is refilled, raised to shoulder level and the procedure repeated. This continues until the returned fluid is clear.

The tube is withdrawn. If the patient swallows while this is being done there is less discomfort.

A mouthwash is given to the patient.

Report:
>Amount of fluid used.
>Any abnormalities observed such as food debris, bloodstained liquid.
>The general condition of the patient.

WHEN REMOVING POISONS FROM THE STOMACH:

(a) The patient may be a child who has swallowed an antiseptic or disinfectant. If there is burning of the lips, the stomach is *not* washed out.

If there is no burning of the lips, the stomach is washed out with a soothing alkaline fluid such as milk or sodium bicarbonate 1 teaspoon to 500 ml of water.

(b) If a child has swallowed several tablets, e.g. iron medicines, the stomach is washed out, using a wide-bore tube through which the tablets can pass.

(c) If the stomach contains fluid poison, this is removed before the stomach is washed out and it is reserved for examination.

(d) In barbiturate or aspirin poisoning the patient is usually unconscious and treatment is urgent.

THE PROCEDURE WHEN THE PATIENT IS UNCONSCIOUS is usually carried out by the doctor with the assistance of a nurse.

Equipment is as before with the addition of a tongue depressor and mouth gag. 10 litres of fluid should be available. Specimens of stomach contents are important as the identity of the poison may not be known.

Preparation of the patient. The dentures have usually been removed already. He is laid flat with his head lower than his stomach, i.e. with his head over the side of the casualty trolley or bed. The nurse supports his head. His mouth is held open with the mouth gag, and the tongue depressor is used when the tube is passed through the mouth into the oesophagus. The nurse observes the patient's colour and pulse, indicating any blueness or a rapid feeble pulse rate.

Sometimes the stomach is emptied of large amounts of alcohol (the patient may vomit copiously with the same effect) by passing the stomach tube and attaching the funnel. This is inverted below the level of the stomach, the fluid flows out of the stomach, which is then washed out. This patient may be aggressive and unable to co-operate.

ADMINISTRATION OF FLUID INTO THE RECTUM

ENEMAS are usually purgative in action, i.e. the rectal administration results in a bowel action.

RECTAL INFUSIONS are given more slowly. Electrolytes, glucose or drugs contained in the fluid are absorbed.

Enemas are either:
> (a) *Given quickly and returned at once.* Examples are:
> Salt: 2 teaspoons to 1200 millilitres water.
> Green soft soap; piece as big as a walnut, and 1200 millilitres water.
> (b) *Given slowly* to soften faeces (*retained enema*). The patient has his bowels opened 20 to 30 minutes later. Examples are:
> Arachis oil: 170 millilitres, which soften the faeces and lubricate the rectum.
> Glycerine: 30 millilitres with the same amount of warm water. This attracts mucus from the bowel wall and softens the faeces.

A *strong phosphate solution* 135 ml attracts water into the rectum, softens the stool and increases its bulk, causing evacuation from the lower bowel. This is prepared in a disposable packet for immediate administration.

Rectal infusions include:
> Salt: 1 teaspoon in 600 millilitres water, 180 millilitres fluid administered slowly, or given by continuous method 100 millilitres an hour. This is a suitable electrolyte solution to introduce into the rectum.
> Salt as above with addition of glucose 20 grammes. Glucose provides some calories.
> Drugs, e.g. prednisone (ordered in ulcerative colitis), paraldehyde (to sedate restless patients), pentothal sodium and avertin (before general inhaled anaesthetics to sedate the nervous patient).

The efficiency of ENEMAS in which the fluid is returned immediately depends on sufficient fluid being introduced into the rectum. 750 to 1000 ml of fluid are necessary to ensure distension of the rectum so that the nerve endings are stimulated and there is a reflex action of increased muscle contraction in the bowel and in the abdomen to empty the bowel.

Equipment. 1200 millilitres of salt and water or soap and water 38°C. A funnel, tubing, glass connection and large rectal catheter. A bed-pan and cover are brought to the bedside.

The procedure is explained to the patient and the curtains drawn round the bed for privacy. The patient will not be so uncomfortable if he empties his bladder before the procedure begins. Heavy bed-clothes are turned back and the patient lies in the left lateral position. This allows the injected fluid to flow downwards into the rectum and lower part of the bowel. A towel beneath the buttocks protects the bed.

The catheter is lubricated and the assembled apparatus filled with fluid so that no air is introduced into the rectum to cause unnecessary distension and discomfort. A tubing clip may be needed to clamp the tubing and prevent the fluid leaving the apparatus while 7 centimetres of catheter are passed into the anal canal. The patient is relaxed. The fluid flows into the rectum from the funnel which is held at the nurse's shoulder height. As soon as the level falls to 3 cms in the funnel, this is lowered to mattress level and filled, then raised again to shoulder level. This is repeated until the total fluid has been used, or the patient cannot tolerate more.

The catheter is withdrawn through a wool swab held over the anus and the patient turns on to his back so that the bed-pan can be placed beneath the buttocks. It may be possible for him to use the commode at the side of the bed. In either case he is properly supported by pillows and the nurse does not disappear from the vicinity. The patient may feel faint as he returns the enema rapidly and the nurse's assistance is needed to lay him flat or help him into bed.

If fluid from an enema is not returned, the nurse informs the ward sister. She may request that a rectal tube be passed. If no fluid is produced by this method, the surgeon is informed.

Occasionally the soap solution causes a rash. For this reason the area round the anus is cleaned carefully with wool or tissue after the enema has been returned.

The patient is made comfortable after the bed-pan has been removed and he washes his hands.

Report to sister includes the patient's general condition, the faecal result of the enema and any abnormalities of stool. The equipment is washed well and the catheter disinfected by immediate immersion in Chlorhexidine 0·5% later boiling for 5 minutes or preferably autoclaving. Disposable rectal catheters are available.

Enemas to be retained are given slowly and in small amounts so that the reflex action of defaecation does not occur until the hard faeces in consideration have been softened.

Equipment includes a funnel, short tubing and medium-size rectal catheter. A syringe reserved for this purpose and a rectal catheter may be used to administer the small amount of glycerine and water. The method is the same as before except that the patient uses the bed-pan 20 to 30 minutes later; otherwise a simple salt and water or soap and water enema is prescribed.

Disposable retention enemas are now available, e.g. arachis oil,

magnesium sulphate and phosphate solutions. To the plastic bag containing the fluid (130 ml) is attached a short rectal tube. This is inserted into
the rectum and the pliable plastic bag is compressed. The equipment is
discarded after use into a strong paper bag for disposal.

RECTAL INFUSIONS are given slowly in small amounts so that the fluid
can be absorbed.

Equipment is as for retained enema with a small-size rectal catheter.
A syringe and small tube are suitable equipment in this procedure prescribed for an infant or child.

Drugs Given per Rectum

A drug is given on the prescription written by the doctor, and a witness
assists in the checking of sedatives with the patient's prescription sheet.

Preparation of the patient includes the emptying of the bowel either in
a normal bowel action or by aperient, enema or rectal washout. If there
is any distension due to flatus, a flatus tube is passed. The patient empties
his bladder so that he is comfortable during the procedure.

The procedure is as for retained enema but the fluid is absorbed and
no bed-pan is necessary. Observations are made of the effects of the drug
on the patient.

Water, salt and glucose are administered in this way when the patient
is dehydrated but is unable to have fluids by mouth, naso-pharyngeal
tube, subcutaneous or intravenous infusion. The appropriate entry is
made on the fluid balance chart.

Continuous rectal infusion is a more suitable method of giving fluid
through the rectum to the dehydrated patient than rectal infusions at
intervals of say, 4 hours.

Continuous Rectal Infusion

In this procedure normal saline solution (0·9% sodium chloride in water)
flows slowly into the rectum, where it is absorbed. When the patient is
unable to take fluids by mouth, this is one method by which dehydration
may be prevented. Dehydration may also be treated in this way if intravenous therapy is not possible.

Saline solution (0·9%) is necessary because this is the strength of
sodium chloride in the body fluids and tissues, and the administration of
water with this amount of sodium chloride prevents alteration from
the normal electrolyte balance. The dispensary may prepare the solution
ready for administration.

Equipment. 30 millilitres of normal saline warmed by standing the
measure in a bowl of warm water. The temperature should be about
37°C. The *solution* will be held in a *flask or bottle* from which it will

flow through *tubing, a drip connection, tubing, glass connection* to a fine *rectal catheter* No. 14. The catheter will be *lubricated* so that it can be passed easily into the rectum. A *tubing clip* will control the flow. A *towel* protects the bed, a piece of *adhesive tape* may be necessary to secure the catheter to the skin near the anus, and a *stand with hook* is required to hold the flask or bottle.

Preparation of the patient. Absorption of water in the rectum will not be satisfactory if the rectum contains faeces. If this situation is likely, Sister may request that the patient has an enema of salt and water 1 teaspoonful to 1 pint (soap enema solution will not improve the absorption in the rectum), or a rectal washout.

After this preliminary preparation, should it have been necessary, the rectal infusion procedure is explained to the patient (he may know the rectum as the 'back passage') and curtains are drawn round the bed for privacy. He is given an opportunity to empty the bladder to prevent avoidable discomfort.

He is assisted into the left lateral position; this may be difficult if he is very ill but he needs to be relaxed with the lower limbs drawn up. The bed is protected by the towel and the patient is not exposed unnecessarily.

Procedure. The flask of solution hangs on the stand and the fluid is allowed to flow through to the catheter. Then the tubing clip is closed. The end of the catheter is lightly lubricated and introduced (7 to 12 cm) into the rectum (the anal canal is 4 to 5 cm in length). The patient is made comfortable in his usual position in bed, with the catheter secured to the skin by adhesive tape so that he is not lying on it, neither is it beneath any bed apparatus. A bed cradle may be useful. The tubing clip is released until the flow through the drip connection is 20 to 30 drops a minute according to the doctor's prescription. About 120 millilitres should pass through in 2 hours, and this amount can be added to the flask at these intervals. The apparatus should not be allowed to fill with air, so if the patient has been given the desired amount, e.g. 20 millilitres; the tubing clip is turned off just before the flask is empty and kept closed until the next amount is due. If the solution flows in too quickly there will be leakage from the rectum and the catheter will come out. The amount of normal saline is entered on the fluid balance chart.

This procedure can be continued for some days. Usually the patient's treatment changes after 24 to 48 hours. His bed is made with extra care so that the tubing is not disturbed. If the tubing is inclined to move about a loop of it can be fastened to the bottom sheet with a large safety-pin.

After the procedure the total amount of fluid is recorded. The equipment is washed thoroughly and disinfected by boiling or autoclaving.

The catheter is discarded if possible, otherwise autoclaved and reserved for rectal use only.

RECTAL SUPPOSITORIES are medications prepared for rectal administration. They are cone-shaped, 3 to 4 cm in length.

Glycerine suppositories have a gelatine base which dissolves in the rectum. Glycerine attracts mucus from the rectal wall; this softens the faeces and causes sufficient stimulation for the rectal wall to contract and expel faeces in a bowel action about 20 minutes later.

Dulcolax suppositories are ordered as treatment in constipation, producing an irritant effect on the bowel which results in faecal evacuation.

Anusol suppositories are prescribed for the relief of pain and discomfort in haemorrhoids (piles).

Methods of administration. Following an explanation of the procedure and the curtains having been drawn round the bed, the patient lies relaxed on his left side with the lower limbs flexed at hips and knees. The nurse wears a disposable glove or finger-stall. A glycerine suppository is dipped into warm water to soften the gelatine in the suppository so that it is more easily inserted. The suppository is held in a swab and the pointed end is introduced into the anus. The anal canal is 3 to 4 cm long, and to be effective the suppository is introduced 7 to 9 cm into the rectum. Any slight discharge is wiped from the anus with a gauze swab. The glove or finger-stall is discarded.

A report to the sister states that the suppository has been administered as requested, and the result, i.e. a satisfactory bowel action, or in the case of Anusol suppositories, relief of pain.

Rectal Washout

The PURPOSE of this procedure is to cleanse the rectum and it is performed in preparation for operations on the rectum, barium enema (which is given before an X-ray of the colon and rectum), and sigmoidoscopy (in which an instrument is passed into the rectum and lower colon; the sigmoidoscope contains a tiny electric light at the end of a tube so that the lining tissue of the sigmoid colon can be seen).

Equipment. It is a clean procedure. *Rectal catheter* to which is attached a *glass connection, rubber tubing*, tubing clip and a *funnel*. The end of the rectal tube will be *lubricated*. A towel protects the bed.

The *lotion* used is normal saline, 1 teaspoon of salt to 1 pint of water. 2 to 3 litres are prepared at a temperature of 38°C, and a small jug will be needed for pouring. The fluid will be returned into a *pail*.

The *procedure* is explained to the patient and curtains are drawn round the bed for privacy. He lies in the left lateral position and is not exposed unnecessarily. 500 ml of fluid is poured into the funnel, the air removed by allowing the fluid to flow through the apparatus, then closing the tubing clip. The end of the rectal catheter is lubricated and passed 12 to 16 cm into the rectum. The funnel is held at shoulder level, the tubing clip released and the fluid flows into the rectum. When the funnel is almost empty it is lowered to mattress level, the fluid returns to the funnel which is then inverted to allow the fluid to flow into the pail. This procedure is repeated until the returned fluid is clear.

The rectal catheter is removed gently through a wool swab or tissue held over the anus to clean it. Any moisture around the anus is mopped with tissue or towel. The equipment is washed thoroughly, and is disinfected before storing and is reserved for rectal use.

Report. Amount of fluid used and amount returned, any abnormalities such as fresh blood (red) or digested blood (black), excess mucus. General condition of the patient.

Colon Washout

This is a similar procedure but is ordered as a special preparation for operations on the colon, the lotion being prescribed by the surgeon. The patient's position is changed during the procedure, e.g. left lateral to right lateral to dorsal (on his back). The foot of the bed may be raised. 500 ml of fluid is poured in from a level of 50 cm above the mattress at each change of position. The total amount of fluid is returned through tubing and funnel, or the rectal catheter is removed and the contents of the colon and rectum are returned into a bed-pan.

Changing the patient's position enables the fluid to pass from the rectum into the sigmoid colon, then descending, then transverse, then ascending colon before it is emptied.

CHAPTER 35 | METABOLISM

The body tissues are supplied with *foodstuffs* and *oxygen* from the blood as they require them. These substances in solution pass through the walls of the blood capillaries into the tissue fluid which surrounds the tissue cells. From these they are drawn through the cell walls into the cell substance itself. A series of chemical changes takes place. The oxygen and food are converted into *energy* so that the cell can live and function. *Heat* also is produced and this contributes to the maintenance of body temperature. The waste products which remain are *carbon monoxide* and *water*, with the addition of *urea* from the protein metabolism. These return in solution to the blood and are excreted by the lungs, kidneys and skin.

$$OXYGEN + FOOD \longrightarrow WATER + CARBON\ DIOXIDE + UREA$$

Energy and heat are produced.

This series of chemical changes within the tissue cells is known as METABOLISM.

The rate at which the chemical changes take place is referred to as the *metabolic rate*. This can be assessed in a person *at rest* and the resulting figure is used as the person's *basal metabolic rate*.

The patient is prepared by having no food or exercise previous to the test, and during the test oxygen consumption is measured.

The rate of metabolism is controlled by the secretion of the thyroid gland, THYROXINE.

The basal metabolic rate is increased in exercise, and in fevers, infection and over-secretion of the thyroid gland. It is lowered in sleep and in old age, and decreases in under-secretion of the thyroid gland. In treatment, hypothermia may be used to lower the metabolic rate (see treatment of head injuries).

DIABETES MELLITUS is a disease affecting the metabolism of carbohydrates. The cells in the body are unable to *use* digested and absorbed carbohydrate and the blood sugar rises. There is a lack of insulin in the blood. This disease appears at all ages but becomes common in both men and women after the age of 45 years. Symptoms and signs appear gradually but may be brought about by an acute infection such as gastroenteritis. The patient complains of thirst as he passes large amounts of urine in order to rid the body of the excess sugar in the blood. He is not able to use all the food he eats and consequently he *loses weight and feels very weary*. In women particularly, the urine containing sugar comes in contact with the skin of the vulva causing irritation (pruritus).

Diagnosis. The urine is tested for glucose (using Clinistix). A positive result will be obtained then a quantitative test is carried out using Clinitest to show the amount of glucose. Accuracy is important and an early morning specimen is more informative. Acetone may be present as shown by the Acetest reagent. A blood sample is collected and this is tested by the laboratory technician for excess glucose in the blood.

The disease cannot be cured and although the discovery of insulin has meant reasonable health and activity for the person affected, the treatment is necessarily continuous and life-long. For this reason it is essential that the hospital clinic staff create a feeling of confidence in the patient.

Treatment. An overweight patient with mild diabetes often responds to a diet with less carbohydrate. An important advance in treatment has been in the use of drugs which stimulate the production of insulin, the hormone produced in the pancreas. Patients are prescribed drugs such as Tolbutamide or Chlorpropamide which are taken by mouth and are often suitable for slightly more severe cases.

In severe diabetes, however, insulin is given by injections every day (Fig. 43). The patient in this instance may be young and it is necessary

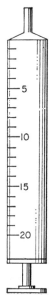

Figure 43. Insulin syringe.

for him to have an adequate diet for growth, some exercise and average physical work. The carbohydrate foods, bread, potato, cereals, are given in definite amounts each day and some of these are included in each meal during the 24 hours. Diets include more protein than in the average person's diet as the young diabetic person tends to be thin and underweight. Fat is not cut down but given in average amounts and vitamins are necessary. Food must always be given on time and the patient should not go on too long without a meal. The dosage of insulin depends on the needs of the patient and is prescribed by the physician. This substance is destroyed in the stomach and therefore given by subcutaneous injection. There are several preparations:

Soluble insulin acts quickly and its effect last about 6 hours. It is injected half an hour before a meal, usually breakfast and supper.

Protamine zinc insulin. The effect begins in 6 hours after administration and lasts 24 hours. It is ordered to be given before breakfast with a quick-acting soluble insulin. Repeated injections of this insulin in one site may cause hard swelling under the skin.

Insulin zinc suspension is a combination of a rapid-acting and a slow-acting insulin, and one injection a day is required.

Insulin is measured in units and the method of measurement is universal so that no problems arise from this point of view when the diabetic person travels abroad.

The *strengths* of the preparations vary:

20 units per millilitre
40 units per millilitre
80 units per millilitre

and each type of insulin has a distinctive label. To avoid any confusion when a number of injections are being given, as in the hospital ward, the nurse preparing the injection requests another nurse to check the drug and its dose with the prescription sheet and confirms the identity of the person to whom it is to be given. It is important also that the injection is given exactly at the ordered time and that it is followed by the prescribed meal in half an hour.

Observations during treatment. Especially in severe diabetes, the patient's urine is tested *before* meals and it should be glucose-free. It is also tested before he goes to bed. Then it should contain $\frac{1}{2}$ to 1% glucose so that hypoglycaemia (too little sugar in the blood) does not occur during the night.

He is weighed every week and his energy and general well-being are noted. Possible complications are borne in mind by the nurse (see later) and appropriate observations made.

The PATIENT'S morale is of great importance throughout treatment, supervision and guidance, as he needs to learn to live with his condition. He is encouraged to lead as normal a life as possible. The dietitian explains his diet, and the clinic sister or nurse teaches him to give his own injections in the thighs, arms, or lower abdomen. He learns how to test his urine and recognise approaching hypoglycaemia attacks. Toes and feet need to be cared for so that the skin is not damaged, for injury, even very slight abrasions, may result in gangrene. A chiropodist's advice is helpful.

His work is altered if necessary to fit in with his standard of fitness, and also to allow management of diet and insulin injections. He learns to take glucose drinks of the same value as his meal when he cannot eat, and when he has an infection or is vomiting he sees his own doctor. In case of accident he carries a card which states that he is a diabetic and his insulin dosage and times of administration. There is an active Diabetic Association of which he can become a member. In most cases dietary or insulin treatment is quite satisfactory and the patient can lead a normal life. However, there are a number of serious complications which can occur in this disease after a number of years. The eyes may be affected (retinopathy and cataract), the kidneys (nephropathy) or the nerves (neuritis), and in addition coronary heart disease commonly complicates diabetes mellitus. Small abrasions on toe or foot can predispose to gangrene.

KETOSIS COMA. In diabetes the carbohydrates are not used up, and because of this fats are not metabolised completely. This leads to the presence in the blood of partly metabolised fats called ketone bodies, one of which is acetone. This condition is called *ketosis*, and, if untreated, leads to coma, which is a medical emergency. The patient becomes gradually ill and *dehydration* is obvious with dry skin, furred tongue, and a rapid, feeble pulse. The patient has air hunger.

After diagnosis the doctor's treatment includes administration of large doses of soluble insulin, then water and saline by intravenous infusion. Samples of blood are taken for estimation of blood sugar level.

The urinary bladder is sometimes catheterised when urine specimens are requirel for testing. The nurse should empty the patient's bladder completely when obtaining a specimen otherwise later specimen tests will be inaccurate.

Instructions for treatment are carried out promptly and accurately, and observations made regarding depth of unconsciousness and signs of possible hypoglycaemia.

HYPOGLYCAEMIC COMA. This occurs when the patient is being treated with insulin for diabetes mellitus. It is helpful if he recognises the symptoms of hypoglycaemia, which include faintness, weakness, trembling, peculiar behaviour, etc. Four lumps of sugar taken into the mouth will dissolve and when swallowed are absorbed into the blood, to raise the very low level of blood sugar. Coma is prevented in this way. The attack occurs quickly and if unrecognised the patient begins to sweat, becomes pale and may be delirious. He becomes stuperose and then passes into coma.

Treatment given by the doctor is glucose administered by intravenous injection, followed by a return to the combination of glucose or carbohydrate food and insulin with some investigation as to why the attack occurred, so that advice may be given to avoid this situation from occurring again.

Emergency diet. When the nurse is responsible for the diet of a diabetic patient it is necessary for her to understand the amounts of carbohydrates he has in each meal. If the patient does not eat his meal the dietitian is informed and she will replace the food by a drink of the same carbohydrate value as the meal. If a dietitian is not available, the nurse consults the list of equivalent foods and prepares an appropriate fluid feed. If he does not drink this or vomits, the sister (this may occur during the night) is informed. It is obvious that a diabetic's diet should be one he enjoys and one which is satisfying but not too much for his appetite.

Some Emergency Equivalents

15 *grammes* of carbohydrates is equivalent to:
3 rounded teaspoons of glucose or sugar, *or*
300 cc of milk, *or*
1 heaped teaspoon of Horlicks and 1 teacup of milk, *or*
1 level teaspoon of Benger's and 1 teacup of milk, *or*
half tumblerful of fresh orange juice, *or*
gruel from $\frac{3}{4}$ ounce oat flour.

CHAPTER 36 | EXCRETION

The main waste products of metabolism are water, carbon dioxide and urea. The organs by which they are excreted from the body are as follows:

Water H_2O—by the kidneys, lungs, skin.
Carbon dioxide CO_2—by the lungs.
Urea—by the kidney, and a very small amount through the skin.

The Urinary System

EXCRETION of water and urea is the main function of the urinary system (Fig. 44). There are other unwanted or harmful substances which the body rids itself of in the same way. The organs in the urinary system are the two kidneys, which secrete urine, from each of which passes a tube or ureter carrying urine to the bladder, which is a reservoir for urine. At intervals the urine is evacuated from the bladder through another tube, the urethra. The act of emptying the bladder is known as MICTURITION.

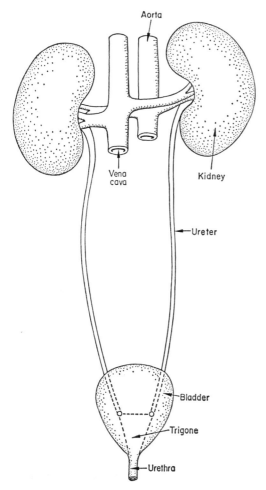

Figure 44. The urinary tract.

The KIDNEYS (Fig. 45) are situated one on either side of the vertebral column in the abdominal cavity but behind the peritoneum. They lie on the thick muscles of the back, the right kidney is lower than the left, and they are protected by the muscles on which they lie and to a small extent by the ribs. Each kidney is shaped like a bean and is about 10–12 cm in length, 5 cm wide and 2·5 cm thick. It is dark red in colour, being well supplied with blood, and is covered by a thin fibrous capsule. The organ is embedded in fat and fibrous tissue which supports it. At the medial curve of the kidney enters the renal artery, which is a branch of the abdominal aorta, and close to this, the renal vein passing to the inferior vena cava. Posteriorly, there is the ureter, which transports the urine to the bladder.

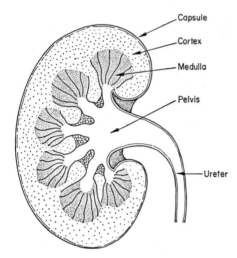

Figure 45. The kidney.

When the kidney is cut in longitudinal section, its various parts can be identified:

(a) *a fibrous capsule* which covers and protects the kidney tissue on the outside;

(b) *the cortex* which is dark brown;

(c) *the medulla*, the inner portion, is pale and streaked in appearance; the streaks are tubules, some of which open into trumpet-shaped tubes entering the *pelvis of the kidney*, which is the upper dilated part of the ureter.

Microscopically the kidney substance is a mass of tubules. The beginning of each tubule is enlarged like a cup and in each cup there is a tuft of blood capillaries. This part of the tubule is in the cortex of the kidney. A loop of tubule and the collecting tubule are in the medulla. Parts of each tubule are surrounded by blood capillaries.

The blood in the tuft of capillaries is under pressure and filtration takes place. Water, sugar and salts in solution are forced from the plasma through the walls of the capillary into the tubule. In the remainder of the tubule, some salts and the sugar and some water are absorbed into the blood stream (the volume of fluid in the tubule becomes concentrated), and lastly excess urea is removed from the blood and enters the tubule fluid which is now *urine*.

The composition of urine:
Water, 96%; Urea, 2%; Some salts.
The reaction is slightly acid.

Average amount excreted in 24 hours:
Water, 1,500 millilitres; Urea, 30 grammes.

The Functions of the Kidneys

These organs regulate the composition of the blood plasma. Excess water is removed and the amounts of sodium chloride, bicarbonates and potassium are controlled. Any slight alteration in the level of electrolytes in the blood from the normal can cause the individual to become very ill. These functions concerning excretion of water and sodium chloride are under the control of the pituitary and adrenal hormones.

Waste products of metabolism, e.g. urea, are removed from the blood, also abnormal substances such as drugs, e.g. barbiturates, and excess glucose in patients with diabetes mellitus.

The *ureters* are 25 cm. in length and pass from the kidneys to the bladder. They are composed of unstriped muscle tissue, covered by protective fibrous tissue and lined by epithelium. Urine passes to the bladder by peristaltic action.

The BLADDER (Fig. 46) is in the pelvis but when distended it rises into the abdomen. In front of it are the pubic bones of the pelvic girdle. Behind the bladder in the female is the uterus, and in the male the rectum, and above it is peritoneum. It is formed from unstriped muscle, with an inner epithelium which lies in folds to allow for distension.

The ureters enter the base of the bladder at an angle and the area between the entry of those tubes and the exit of the urethra, the trigone, is smooth and sensitive to irritation. In the male, the neck of the bladder is surrounded by the prostate gland.

The URETHRA in the male is 15 to 20 cms long and passes from the neck of the bladder through the penis. At the tip of the penis is a fold of skin called the foreskin.

In the female, the urethra is 4 cms long and opens into the vestibule in front of the vagina.

The urethra has internal and external sphincters, the latter under voluntary control.

Micturition

This is the passing of urine from the bladder. It is primarily a reflex action which, after infancy, can be controlled consciously by impulses from the higher centre of the brain.

As urine accumulates, the pressure in the bladder increases and sensory nerve endings are stimulated. Impulses pass from the bladder to the spinal cord, then to the brain and there is a desire to micturate.

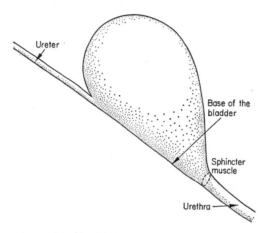

Figure 46. The bladder.

The diaphragm and abdominal muscles contract, increasing pressure in the abdomen, the bladder unstriped muscle contracts, the sphincter muscle relaxes and urine is evacuated.

Common Symptoms and Signs in the Urinary Tract

PAIN may be colicky as experienced when a small renal stone passes from the pelvis of the kidney down the ureter. The patient may complain of scalding pain when he passes urine; this occurs in cystitis.

FREQUENCY OF MICTURATION is a common symptom. Small amounts of urine are passed. It may be associated with *dysuria*, which is pain in passing urine.

INCONTINENCE OF URINE is the continual passing of urine when the bladder is unable to retain the urine. The sphincter muscles of the urethra are not contracting efficiently.

RETENTION OF URINE. The bladder is distended, but the patient cannot micturate, and is uncomfortable or distressed. There is a possibility that older patients with retention of urine dribble a little urine continuously; this is RETENTION WITH OVERFLOW due to lack of sphincter control.

HAEMATURIA, i.e. blood in the urine, occurs either at the beginning, during, or at the end of the urine stream.

In damage to the bladder following fracture of the pelvis, a little blood is passed but no urine.

Observations

PALPATION OF THE ABDOMEN of an unconscious patient or one who is restless while mentally confused, may reveal a bladder distended with urine. This reservoir of urine can enlarge from the level of the symphysis pubis, when empty, to the level of the umbilicus and would then contain about 1 litre of urine. A distended bladder causes a great deal of discomfort and the patient with retention becomes very distressed.

URINE OUTPUT is recorded in 24-hour periods. Not only must all amounts be charted, but it is also useful to observe whether there are any abnormalities of micturition such as frequency or incontinence. When the bladder is distended any incontinence is due to retention with overflow.

Following pelvic operations, the patient may be unable to empty the bladder completely. This means residual urine and may predispose to infection.

Passing no urine, i.e. *anuria*, is rare. This and *oliguria*, which means passing a little urine, usually less than 500 millilitres a day, are observations to be reported without delay. These two terms indicate that the kidneys are secreting little or no urine if the bladder is empty. The patient begins to show signs of uraemia and electrolyte imbalance.

URINE. The colour and specific gravity are noted and also whether a sediment is present. Albumin and glucose tests are made and the urine microscoped.

In the Outpatients' Clinic, or after the patient's admission to the ward, the doctor may wish to make a RECTAL EXAMINATION, which assists in diagnosing an enlarged prostate gland.

Clinical Investigation

In suspected infection of the urinary tract, an UNCONTAMINATED SPECIMEN OF URINE is required in the bacteriology laboratory. Organisms in the urine will be grown in the culture media and the resulting colonies examined by the naked eye and beneath the microscope. The sensitivity of the bacteria to different antibiotics is also assessed.

Catheterisation of the bladder predisposes urinary infection, so the urine is usually collected as a MID-STREAM SPECIMEN (for method of procedure see later). Certain varieties of organisms survive only a short time after leaving the body and it is important, when a special request has been made, to ensure the immediate delivery of the specimen to the laboratory.

Examination for blood cells in urine is made in the laboratory. A 24-hour specimen is preferred when a test is being made for tubercle bacilli. The outline of the kidney and bladder can usually be seen in an X-RAY FILM of the abdomen and pelvis, together with parts of the skeleton. Nearly all renal calculi (stones) show on straight X-ray. In an intravenous pyelogram, a dye which is opaque to X-rays is injected into a vein. The drug circulates in the blood and then is excreted by the kidneys. As this is taking place X-ray films are taken and reveal details of the kidneys and their function.

CYSTOSCOPY is the examination of the interior of the bladder through a special instrument called a cystoscope. This is a straight metal tube, containing a telescope and a small electric bulb at the tip. The urethra is anaesthetised and the cystoscope is introduced into the bladder. 240 millilitres of sterile water are introduced to distend the bladder so that the surgeon can see the whole of the interior by the small light. He will then be able to see any abnormalities such as growths or stones.

During cystoscopy, very fine catheters may be introduced into one or both of the ureters and individual specimens of the urine obtained, either for bacteriology or electrolytic studies. For a retrograde pyelogram, the surgeon may introduce a radio-opaque dye through one of the ureteric catheters into the pelvis of the kidney. The patient is then X-rayed and the architecture of the kidney is shown. Renal calculi may prevent the pelvis from being filled by the dye. Sometimes, the non-radio-opaque stones are surrounded by the dye, showing their outline clearly as negative shadows.

When *patients are being prepared for X-ray examination* of the urinary tract, it is advisable for them to have their bowels open normally in the morning with no aperient or enemata, and then whenever possible to get up and walk in the ward. These two precautions prevent a collection of gases in the colon which would appear dense on the X-ray films and cover the outline of the urinary tract which lies posterior to the abdomen.

Medical and Surgical Conditions in the Urinary Tract
The kidneys are protected by fat and to some extent by muscles of the back and lower ribs, but in accidents when the lumbar region is exposed to INJURY the protection is inadequate. Haemorrhage is usually severe and may not be visible so recognition of signs indicating haemorrhage is important. A patient who has been involved in a major accident probably has a number of different injuries. The patient is moved as little as possible at the time of accident, the cause of injury removed if possible and

wounds covered with clean handkerchiefs or towels. When the doctor assesses the patient's condition blood transfusion may be necessary to restore the blood volume. On arrival in hospital, specimens of urine are collected to ascertain the severity of the haematuria. Treatment is conservative unless the bleeding is severe. An intravenous pyelogram may show the damage and confirm that the other kidney is present and normal. If operation is necessary, repair or removal may be carried out. Occasionally, there is temporary cessation of function—anuria—and the 'artificial kidney' machine may be required to dialyse the patient's blood until his own renal function recovers. On a few occasions the patient has only one kidney from birth or a nephrectomy has already been performed. Where irretrievable damage has occurred to a solitary kidney, a renal transplant may be considered.

A streptococcal infection of the throat or scarlet fever may be followed by ACUTE NEPHRITIS. The patient is feverish and passes a little blood in the urine which looks smoky. Puffiness of the face and hands (oedema) is accompanied by decrease in the amount of urine excreted. There may be headache, vomiting and drowsiness. Most patients recover completely, but a few patients continue to a sub-acute or chronic phase. In the treatment of acute nephritis the cause of the inflammatory process may be dealt with by using cortisone, and injections of penicillin are prescribed for the streptococcal infection. The patient is made comfortable in bed. usually with 3 or 4 pillows. A patient with oedema sometimes feels cold and benefits from warm bed-clothes and a flannelette sheet next to him, but hot-water bottles are avoided as the skin is easily damaged. Due to the inflammatory process, the function of the kidneys is lessened and in adapting the diet to this, the fluid content is restricted and contains no protein but some sugar for two to three days. For example, the diet may consists of 1100 millilitres of water a day for two days if the urine volume is less than 600 ml per day, the fluid being flavoured with orange juice or blackcurrant juice or rose hip syrup (vitamin C aids the healing process) and sugar or glucose added. Chewing a little raw apple or tinned pineapple assists in keeping the mouth in satisfactory condition and boiled sweets can be given to the younger patient. After two or three days the diet is increased to include a *little* protein, milk, milk puddings, a biscuit, thin slice of bread and butter, cereal, and finally small helpings of easily digested egg, fish and meat dishes. Mouthwashes and mouth treatment are necessary while the diet is restricted.

Recovery takes place in a large number of patients, but sometimes the disease continues as SUB-ACUTE NEPHRITIS. The patient passes large amounts of *albumin in the urine* as a result of kidney glomerular damage. Because of the protein loss from the blood, the water in blood plasma leaks out into the tissue spaces giving rise to *oedema* not only beneath the skin, but in the lungs, which become congested, and in the abdomen, where ascites develops. The patient is short of breath and is more comfortable sitting upright well supported by pillows. The oedematous areas need protection, the sacral area and the lower limbs by a type of air-bed, and the swollen arms supported from pillows placed beneath them.

The patient is pale and iron medicines may be prescribed for anaemia. As there is loss of protein in the urine, he is given a high-protein diet containing extra meat, fish, eggs and cheese, but it is difficult to arrange meals when the patient's appetite is below normal, and he is offered small helpings. Salt is retained in the body tissues associated with oedema, and this must be reduced in the diet. The condition frequently becomes chronic and skilled nursing care is required in the long illness.

PYELONEPHRITIS, i.e. inflammation both of the pelvis and the kidney tissue, is due to acute infection and the onset is characterised by rigors in which the temperature rises to 40°C. There is pus in the urine. The patient needs 2 or 3 litres of fluid to drink in each day, mostly water flavoured with tea or fruit juices. Barley water with lemon juice added is pleasant. Appropriate antibiotic or sulphonamide therapy is prescribed to deal with the infection.

RENAL CALCULI are stones in the kidney and give rise to haematuria or pain. The types of stone vary from a single large irregular-shaped calculus—staghorn—to a variable number of very small stones. If one of the latter escapes into the ureter, its passage to the bladder causes intense colicky pain along the line of the ureter. The doctor prescribes an analgesic to relieve this pain. As the stone enters the bladder the pain disappears. Most small stones are passed through the urethra. Large renal calculi are removed by incising through the pelvis (pyelolithotomy) or through the kidney itself (nephrolithotomy). Where the kidney is damaged, the whole or part of the organ may be removed.

CANCER is a disease which may occur in the kidneys as in other organs and is treated by surgery, e.g. nephrectomy.

Conditions of the Bladder

The bladder may be damaged by bone fragments in a fracture of the pelvis, so after such an accident, the patient's urinary output is observed carefully. RUPTURE OF THE BLADDER causes escape of urine into the pelvic tissue with consequent inflammatory changes. A little blood but no urine is passed from the urethra. Surgical repair is performed, with drainage of the bladder.

Frequency of micturition with dysuria and haematuria are symptoms and signs of inflammation of the bladder—CYSTITIS. Chronic cystitis may be associated with diseases in the urinary tract such as an enlarged prostate gland, stones in the bladder, infections from kidney or urethra or paralysis of the bladder in spinal diseases or injury. Infection via the urethra is more common in women as this channel connecting the bladder with the exterior is only 4 cms in length.

Aseptic technique in urinary bladder catheterisation is necessary to avoid infection by this method.

An uncontaminated specimen of urine will be examined in the bacteriological laboratory which will indicate the best antibiotic to be given. Sulphadimidine is a drug frequently prescribed to treat infection causing this condition. Alkaline medicines are given and the patient requires 2500 millilitres of fluid each day. The condition is sometimes recurrent. In severe attacks the patient may need analgesics.

STONES IN THE BLADDER cause frequency of micturition with pain and haematuria. Later cystitis develops. Small stones are usually passed through the urethra and large stones are removed either through an incision in the bladder or by crushing the stone in a special instrument, then washing out the fragments from the bladder.

PAPILLOMA and CARCINOMA are tumours of the bladder. The patient usually has painless haematuria, dysuria, and then the symptoms of cystitis may appear in the later stages. The growth can be seen through the cystoscope and a specimen from it is removed for identification of type (biopsy). Papilloma is removed by diathermy, usually through an operating cystoscope, but if it is very large it may be necessary for the bladder to be opened suprapubically. Carcinoma is treated by partial cystectomy or radiotherapy. When total cystectomy is necessary, the ureters are transplanted into the pelvic colon and micturition is controlled by the anal sphincter, or a bladder is fashioned from a part of the ileum (small intestine).

ENLARGEMENT OF THE PROSTATE GLAND is a possible occurrence about the age of 60 years. The man complains of difficulty and frequency of micturition during the night as well as in the day. There is a poor stream of urine. If untreated, retention of urine may develop. This becomes acute after a suddenly increased intake of fluid, and catheterisation is necessary, otherwise the retention occurs with overflow and a little urine escapes continually. Pain is due to retention of urine or secondary cystitis.

Diagnosis is made following clinical examination, rectal examination, and cystoscopy. Tests like intravenous pyelography and blood urea indicate efficiency of the kidneys and a mid-stream specimen of urine is examined in the bacteriological laboratory.

N*

Treatment is by surgery when the patient is fit for operation. His chest is examined and haemoglobin estimated. There are various methods of performing prostatectomy, the most common being by an incision in the abdomen, when the gland is approached from behind the pubis—retropubic, or across the bladder—suprapubic. Another method involves passing an instrument through the urethra by which the gland is removed in small sections: per-urethral resection. An alternative when the patient is seriously ill, is an operation in two stages: (i) suprapubic opening is made into the bladder which is drained by a tube, and (ii) the prostate gland is removed and the previous wound sutured—an uncommon practice these days.

In ACUTE RETENTION OF URINE, the surgeon may decide to remove the enlarged gland in an emergency operation, but only if a catheter cannot be passed. Following operation, the nurse observes the patient's general condition and records his pulse in the first 12 hours in case of complications, which include haemorrhage and shock.

Fluid intake should be 3,500 millilitres (3½ litres) a day as this assists the function of the kidneys and aids adequate bladder drainage. Drainage takes place through an indwelling urethral catheter fixed in position by waterproof plaster attached to the penis to prevent leakage of urine. The urine drains into a closed plastic bag at the side of the bed. In the first 48 hours the urine is blood-stained. The catheter is removed in 2 to 3 days when there may be slight difficulty in passing urine, but if the patient can continue the catheter is not replaced. The bladder is irrigated when an obstruction, e.g. a blood clot, in the catheter is suspected. Possible infection in the urinary tract is dealt with by antibiotic cover or sulphathiazole administration.

While he is in bed the patient's position is changed every 2 hours and he drinks fluid every half hour. His pressure areas may need special attention. He becomes ambulant as early as possible, sitting out of bed on the first post-operative day, using the commode, then walking in the ward. It is reported if the patient has difficulty in micturition when he goes home, as it may be necessary for bougies to be passed. (A bougie is like a catheter but solid, not hollow, and is made from rigid material such as some plastics.)

Conditions of the Urethra

INJURIES TO THE URETHRA in the male are the result of a fractured pelvis; or a child, for example, may fall astride a fence. The patient bleeds from the urethra and develops retention of urine. URETHRITIS is due to infection by a virus or organism such as bacillus coli, staphylococcus and gonococcus. These infections can occur in either sex. An indwelling rubber catheter may cause urethritis in the male patient—a plastic catheter does not.

STRICTURE OF THE URETHRA is a possible complication from injuries and inflammation of the urethra but it is rare in women. There is increasing difficulty in passing urine and later retention may develop. Treatment is usually by dilation or by a plastic operation on the urethra. Bougies are passed at intervals after the operation to maintain the opening.

PHIMOSIS is a condition in which the foreskin (prepuce) of the penis cannot be drawn back from the opening of the urethra. It may be present at birth and the male infant sometimes cannot pass urine easily. The operation is *circumcision* in which the excess of foreskin is excised, and the skin and mucous membrane edges are sutured with catgut. The operation is occasionally performed in young adults under local anaesthetics.

NEPHRECTOMY, removal of the kidney, is performed for renal calculi, deformity or tumour of the organ, and occasionally in injury to the kidney. During the preparation for operation, blood samples are examined for blood urea and haemoglobin estimation. The blood groups are identified. Tests are carried out to ensure efficient function in the other kidney. The urine is measured daily and tested for albumin; the presence of blood is reported to the ward sister. The doctor usually prescribes urinary antiseptics—medicines which prevent the growth of pathogenic bacteria in the urinary tract, e.g. sulphonamides.

The surgeon indicates the area of skin to be prepared for the incision, otherwise the patient is bathed using a bacteriocidal soap. The site of operation is prepared again in the operating theatre.

After operation the patient lies inclined towards the affected side, but in a few hours is supported by back-rest and pillows, though still leaning towards the side of operation, to allow drainage from the tube, which must be protected from pressure or kinking.

The wound dressing is observed for signs of haemorrhage and repacked with extra wool when necessary. The tube drains serum from the cavity formed by the removal of the kidney, and allows the escape of blood should haemorrhage occur. This tube is removed in two or three days and the wound re-dressed.

Adequate fluids are administered into a vein or beneath the skin. The urine output is measured each day and the presence of albumin or blood noted.

Complications of this operation are shock due to haemorrhage (which will be observed in the urine or from the tube), aggravated by pain, anuria, or retention of urine.

RENAL FAILURE may follow situations in which great stress is placed upon the kidney function. A predisposing factor is previous damage by infection, abnormality, or injury.

Causes of renal failure include:

1. *Toxaemia* associated with infections, e.g. by haemolytic strepto-coccus, or extensive tissue damage such as that resulting from burns. In these cases, infection is dealt with by antibiotic therapy which assists in maintaining renal function. Some poisons irritate renal tubules, and in excess cause damage. During treatment by drugs containing metals like gold, the urine is tested for albumin.

2. *Certain sulphonamides* crystallise in the renal tubules when the fluid intake is insufficient. For this reason, the nurse makes sure the patient drinks 2,500 millilitres of fluid each day and reports a lowered output of urine, a dry skin and mouth and drowsiness.

3. *Overdose of some drugs*, such as barbiturates and salicylates (aspirin), causes a rapid increase in kidney function in an effort to excrete excess poison, and renal failure is possible in these cases. After stomach washout, this patient is given large amounts of fluid—3,000 millilitres or more a day.

4. *In shock* the general vitality of the body is lowered, including the blood circulation. This results in an insufficient flow through the capillaries of the kidneys, and the extraction of waste products and water does not take place. This situation is prevented by maintaining the blood volume. This is done by replacing blood, plasma or water with appropriate fluids. Shock may also cause renal failure due to acute tubular necrosis—this causes anuria, which can be corrected by the artificial kidney.

5. *An inadequate intake of fluid* when the patient is unable or un-willing to drink, or an abnormal loss by vomiting, diarrhoea, or by sweating in fever, lead to renal failure unless treated. So too, does loss of fluid in burns.

6. *Any obstruction* which prevents the passage of urine from the pelvis of the kidney, such as stones in the ureter or enlarged prostate gland, will interfere with renal function.

The effect of renal failure is a decrease in the amount and quality of urine passed, and the signs of URAEMIA appear. This means that the blood urea is rising above normal but in actual fact this does not produce the toxic signs. These are thought to be due to the electrolyte imbalance in the blood, and other factors yet unknown. The patient complains of thirst and headache, his skin and mouth (particularly the tongue) are dry. Nausea and vomiting are common and the patient may have hiccough. He becomes drowsy, occasionally is mentally confused, and the nurse may see twitching of the face muscles or possibly convulsions. Coma occurs in the late stages. During the illness, the blood urea rises and the patient may pass less than 500 ml urine in 24 hours (oliguria).

In possible renal failure the condition causing the loss of kidney function is treated, while the patient is given the nursing care of any very ill patient with special attention to the mouth, and prevention of bed-sores, pneumonia and venous thrombosis. The patient feels extremely ill and when treatment takes some time, becomes depressed. Children and young adults, in particular, need a cheerful nurse whom they see frequently. The doctor prescribes a diet which is necessarily restricted and perhaps not attractive to the patient, he has no appetite, is thirsty and his mouth is often unpleasant. It is the nurse's help, encouragement and supervision which makes this part of the treatment successful.

The patient is nursed at rest in bed, to reduce tissue activity. Fluid intake is reduced to 500 to 600 ml in 24 hours. As the diuresis improves, the fluid intake is raised to keep pace, and for this reason the importance of accurate fluid balance charts cannot be over-stressed. The diet includes a minimum of protein to prevent breakdown of the patient's own body protein as well as some fat and carbohydrate. The electrolyte balance is assessed daily so that any alteration can be corrected.

It may be considered advisable that the 'artificial kidney' apparatus should be used, to remove unwanted substances from the blood and relieve the kidneys temporarily of this function. This treatment takes about 5 hours. The procedure is referred to as DIALYSIS and may be repeated as necessitated by the patient's condition until his own kidneys are able to resume their normal function. In the meantime, he requires general nursing care, his diet is carefully controlled, infection prevented by a high standard of cleanliness and aseptic technique, and accurate fluid balance charts are maintained.

Nursing Procedures

Catheterisation of the Urinary Bladder
Catheterisation of the urinary bladder is the passing of a catheter through the urethra to empty the bladder or to obtain an uncontaminated specimen of urine for laboratory examination. This procedure is carried out using an aseptic technique to prevent infection. Cystitis following infection causes discomfort, sometimes pain, and does not always respond quickly to treatment. The infection may also spread to the kidneys. The nurse should be familiar with other methods to encourage a patient to pass urine so that catheterisation may be avoided, and mid-stream specimens are obtained where possible. There are, however, occasions (e.g.

when the bladder must be empty during pelvic operations, or an enlarged prostate gland partially obstructs the urethra) when catheterisation is necessary.

This procedure in the male patient is performed by the doctor or male nurse. It requires considerable skill as the urethra is 20 cms long and is curved before it enters the bladder. A sterile lubricant containing a local anaesthetic is used to facilitate passing of the catheter.

The female urethra is 4 cms in length and the orifice opens into the vestibule between the labia. It is situated in front of the vaginal opening and is not always easy to see, so adequate lighting is necessary.

PREPARATION OF EQUIPMENT. *Catheters* are made of rubber or plastic. They are sterilised by:

(a) autoclave after being sealed in a packet;

(b) industrial methods. The catheter is purchased already sterilised in a sealed packet, and is the disposable type.

(c) formaldehyde gas, applied for 30 minutes in an electrically heated formalin cabinet, after which the catheter is rinsed and placed in a sterile container. This method is useful for catheters which become distorted when exposed to heat.

(d) boiling for 2 to 5 minutes immersed in water.

Methods (c) and (d) are rarely used at the present time.

Sterile towels are needed to surround the area round the urethral orifice.

Sterile swabs are required for cleaning the area.

An antiseptic is occasionally requested, but warm boiled water is often sufficient when the patient has recently been to the bath or bed-bathed and the area has been washed well with soap and water.

Sterile forceps, either dissecting or dressing-forceps, are needed to hold the catheter.

A large receiver or a sterile jar is required for collection of urine.

THE MAIN POINTS TO BE OBSERVED IN THE PROCEDURE. The patient may think this will be a painful procedure and can be reassured that this will not be so. Privacy by the use of curtains or screens reduces embarrassment. A small child, especially if her injury or disease is associated with this area, may be extremely frightened. If the nurse suspects this situation she does not proceed but informs the ward sister, who will discuss the matter with the doctor.

The position of the patient. She lies relaxed on the bed or couch with two or three pillows under her head and her legs drawn up and separated, her feet are flat on the bed or turned inwards and she is covered by bed-clothes except the area round the urethral orifice. Adequate lighting is available.

Methods of swabbing the vulva. The nurse washes and dries her hands.

The fingers of the left hand separate the labia, and with the right hand she swabs the labia majora, labia minora and vestibule (Fig. 47) in an anterior to posterior direction using each swab for only one stroke.

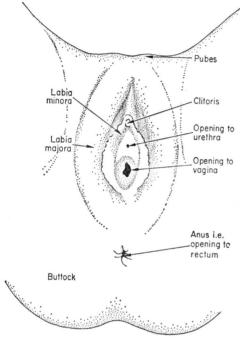

Figure 47. The vulva.

Handling the catheter. The catheter is held by forceps or in a sterile gloved hand about one inch from the eye and this end is introduced directly into the urethral orifice without touching any skin or mucous membrane around it. The urethra contracts round the catheter, the forceps are moved along the catheter so that the catheter may be inserted farther, about 8 cm in all. When the catheter is in a sterile packet, the end of the packet is cut off at the eye end and the nurse holds the catheter with forceps as it comes out of the packet. Some catheters are in a double packet and the inner one can be used for holding the catheter.

The urine is collected into a large sterile receiver or a sterile specimen jar the lid of which is replaced immediately. After removing the catheter gently the skin is dried with swabs. The patient's bed is remade so that she is comfortable.

The urine is measured and tested for abnormalities. If an uncontaminated specimen has been obtained the label on the jar is completed and the specimen is despatched with the laboratory request form as soon as possible.

Equipment is washed and sterilised or collected in bags for disposal.

SELF-RETAINING CATHETERS are those which remain in the bladder for bladder drainage or washouts. One type commonly used is the Foley's catheter which has a cuff around the catheter below the eye end. This can be inflated with water (20 millilitres) through a tube attached to the side and the distended cuff prevents the catheter from becoming displaced.

BLADDER DRAINAGE takes place from the self-retaining catheter into a closed plastic bag which can be suspended from the side of the bed or a sterile bottle with a rubber bung and glass tubing (Lane's bottle). The urine can be measured and observed as it drains. Sometimes a spigot is left in the end of the catheter and this is released at regular intervals so that the bladder can be emptied. On these occasions it is necessary for the nurse to wash her hands first, and then to use a sterile spigot to replace that which has been removed, so that infection is minimised.

BLADDER IRRIGATION. On some occasions the surgeon may consider it necessary to irrigate or wash out the bladder, e.g. to remove blood clots after prostatectomy. One litre of sterile lotion is prepared as prescribed at a temperature of 37°C. The equipment is sterile and includes:

(a) disposable plastic syringe;

or (b) Canny Ryall syringe—60-ml capacity.

It is important to introduce moderate amounts such as 60 ml, then allow this to return into a sterile receiver before more fluid is introduced into the bladder, as the capacity of this organ is reduced when it is inflamed or after operation. When no fluid is returned, stop introducing fluid and inform the ward sister or the doctor. Blockage in a self-retaining catheter is reported.

As soon as the necessity for bladder drainage is passed, the self-retaining catheter is removed and the patient is encouraged to pass urine normally.

CHAPTER 37 | THE NERVOUS SYSTEM

The organs of the body require oxygen and nourishment so that they may carry out their functions, but it is also necessary that there should be some means by which they can work together in an organised manner. This control and co-operation is achieved by the:

(i) *Nervous system* in which messages or impulses travel like tiny electric currents betwen the brain and the other organs along nerve-pathways.

(ii) *Endocrine system*, where the glandular organs produce or secrete in very small amounts special substances called *hormones*. These pass directly into the blood stream and reach the organs in their blood supply.

THE NERVOUS SYSTEM consists of the brain and the spinal cord which together form the central nervous system and the nerves which extend from them to the surface of the body. The neurons are cells of the nervous system which have branches arriving at and leaving the cell. These vary in length and through them impulses pass from cell to cell.

The long branches are protected by a fatty covering and appear as *white matter* in the brain and spinal cord. Bundles of these long branches outside the brain and spinal cord form nerve fibres and these are grouped together as nerves which pass to and from the limbs. Most of them are thick like white thread but the largest nerve is the thickness of the little finger. This is the sciatic nerve which supplies the lower limb.

The nerve cells when examined anatomically appear grey and groups of them are referred to as *grey matter*. Grey and white matter are present in the brain and spinal cord. Nerve cells die unless they have a continual supply of oxygen. When they are destroyed in injury or disease they cannot grow again, but when nerves are damaged in injury healing can take place if the ends can be sutured by the surgeon within a short time of the accident.

The BRAIN (Fig. 48) is situated within the skull for protection as it is a soft and delicate tissue. The grey matter on the surface is arranged in folds (convolutions) to give greater surface area for the large number of brain cells in the outside surface (cortex). Beneath the cortex is white matter. Some collections of nerve cells are situated near the centre of the brain.

The brain is in three parts:
the *main brain* (cerebrum),
the *posterior brain* (cerebellum), *and*
the *brain stem* (which includes the medulla).

The *cerebrum* is in two halves joined at the lower centre portion. In the cerebral cortex are the centres for sensations of touch in the skin, pressure in the joints and muscles, vision, hearing, taste and smell, and the centres for movement and speech. There are also areas about whose functions little is known. Amongst these are intelligence, memory, imagination, will power, and activities of the mind like thinking and reasoning. Some

characteristics of the person as an individual depend on his or her normal
brain functions.

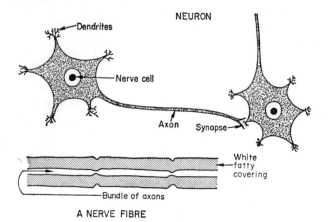

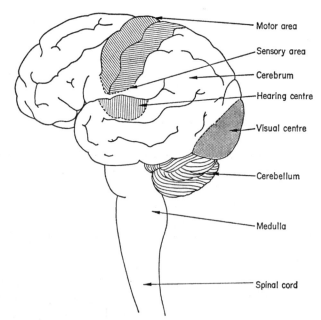

Figure 48. The brain.

Below and behind the cerebrum is the *cerebellum*, in which is the
centre for balance (equilibrium), and from here there is some control of
skeletal muscle tone and posture.

The *brain stem*, though small in size, contains nerve centres which are essential to life. These are concerned with:

1. Respiration.
2. Heartbeat.
3. Alteration in the size of the small arteries in skin and muscles.

Nervous tissue needs a continuous supply of sufficient oxygen. This is carried to the brain in the blood by arteries in the neck. De-oxygenated blood from the brain collects into veins which eventually enter the heart.

The brain stem continues downwards as the SPINAL CORD which is about 45 cms long and is protected by the spinal column. The nerve cells in the spinal cord are concerned with passing impulses to and from the brain and the muscles, joints and skin.

The brain and spinal cord are protected not only by the skull and spinal column, but are also surrounded by membranes, the *meninges.* Inside these membranes is *cerebro-spinal fluid* which is produced from blood plasma by special cells in small spaces (ventricles) at the centre of the brain. This fluid is colourless and transparent, and circulates round the brain and spinal cord acting *like a water cushion.*

Impulses pass from the motor (movement) area of the brain through the spinal cord to the muscles of the head, trunk and limbs. Outside the spinal cord they pass along MOTOR NERVES.

Impulses pass from the skin, joints and muscles to the spinal cord in SENSORY NERVES, and then to the sensory area of the cerebrum.

The central nervous system consists of the brain and spinal cord.

The peripheral nervous system consists of the motor and sensory nerves, and these are found leaving the brain (cranial nerves) or the spinal cord (spinal nerves).

The Cranial Nerves

There are twelve pairs of nerves entering and leaving the brain. Their functions include movements of the eyeballs, the eye-lids, the tongue and the face. The 1st pair of cranial nerves are from the nose (olfactory—sense of smell). The 2nd pair are from the eyes (optic—sense of sight or vision). The 8th pair are from the ears (auditory—sense of hearing). The 10th pair of nerves (the vagus, i.e. wandering nerves) supply most of the internal organs.

The Spinal Nerves

These are mixed nerves, *sensory* from the skin, joints, muscles and also *motor* to the muscles. They leave the spinal cord in pairs through the openings between the vertebrae of the spinal column. Some nerves in the region of the neck join together to form a plexus (network). From this plexus on each side of the neck arises the *phrenic nerve* which passes through the chest and supplies the *diaphragm*. When the two phrenic nerves are stimulated the diaphragm contracts and inspiration takes place.

A number of nerves leaving the lower end of the spinal cord also join together and from these arise the left and right sciatic nerves which supply the lower limbs.

Muscles of the chest and abdominal walls are activated by spinal nerves. The nerves entering the limbs branch into small nerves, and their names are usually taken from the region through which they pass or the bones which protect them, e.g. femoral nerve, radial nerve.

THE AUTONOMIC NERVOUS SYSTEM is that part of the nervous system by which muscle and glandular activity is accelerated (speeded up) or slowed down or inhibited (stopped). There are 2 parts of the system:

Sympathetic nerve supply which accelerates;

Parasympathetic nerve supply which slows down or inhibits activity.

Functions of the Nervous System

APPRECIATION of the individual's surroundings is possible by means of the nervous system including the sense organs, i.e. by seeing, hearing, smelling, tasting, touching and feeling pain, temperature and pressure. It is useful at this point to think about a person who is unfortunate not to have certain sense organs, e.g. a man who is blind. He enters a hospital ward for treatment for some medical or surgical condition and is unable to appreciate his surroundings by visual means. His other senses, e.g. hearing and touch, are probably more acute than normal, but the nurse needs to offer this patient special help so that he is able to be independent as soon as possible, is more content and also safe from possible danger.

LOCOMOTION, i.e. moving from one place to another, is accomplished by means of the nervous system and the voluntary muscles, the bones and the joints. This movement is brought into action in satisfying our needs, e.g. food, escape from danger, expression of emotion. Escape from danger necessitates speedy movement and this is brought about by REFLEX ACTION (see Fig. 49).

Example. If the hand touches a hot dish from the oven, impulses of temperature (heat) and pain pass through the nerves of the upper limb to the spinal cord, through a connecting nerve cell to a motor cell. The impulses then return along the motor fibres in the nerves to the muscles of the hand, which contract and the hand moves away from the hot dish. If the article were extremely hot, many muscles of the body would contract and the whole limb moves quickly backwards before the hand is damaged.

Other examples are blinking the eye-lids when a ball or a fly comes very quickly near to the eye, and coughing (forced expiration) when a crumb is inhaled.

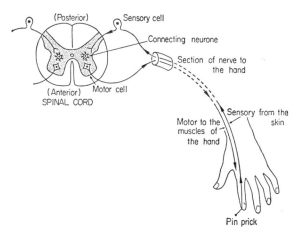

Figure 49. Reflex action.

More complicated reflex actions also occur in patterns as a basis for everyday actions like breathing, eating and walking. Some reflex actions can be controlled from the higher centres of the brain and the person resists the movement away from danger.

The *rate of activity* in heart muscle, any involuntary muscle of the alimentary tract, blood vessels, skin and the glands is controlled by two nerve supplies from the brain: one which *speeds up the rate*, and the other *steadies or slows it down* (or even stops it). In an emergency it is likely that muscle, heart and diaphragm activity are increased. The heart beats faster and more blood is pumped through at each beat, breathing is faster and deeper, the blood supply to the muscles is increased so they contract more quickly and effectively. At the same time activity in the gastro-intestinal tract will slow down, the salivary glands in the mouth produce less and the mouth will become dry. There is a sensation of nausea, and if the stomach is full after a meal a child may actually vomit. In the opposite way after a large meal most activity is in the digestive tract and the associated glands. The remainder of the body tends to be inactive and a short period of rest or relaxation is customary after a main meal.

The centres for reasoning, feeling, will-power, imagination and memory are in the brain.

BEHAVIOUR is the activity we observe in an individual and is closely concerned with the *nervous system, the emotions and mind.* Observation by the nurse of a patient's behaviour in illness assists her in understanding him and his needs, and also may contribute to the doctor's provision of a diagnosis.

Symptoms and Signs in Diseases of the Nervous System

PARALYSIS (PARESIS) is inability of the muscle to contract. It is due to interference with the passage of nerve impulses to the muscle.

SPASM of muscle is irregular increased contraction and occurs in tetanus (infection by tetanus bacilli), tetany (parathyroid hormone deficiency) and in meningitis.

TREMOR is uncontrollable shaking of the limbs, particularly the hands.

LOSS OF SENSATION means loss or reduction of vision, hearing, balance, smell, taste, touch, pressure sense, temperature and pain appreciation. The patient is not always aware of the sensory change and then it is detected in the doctor's examination. He may complain of pins and needles or numbness in the skin, indicating partial or complete loss in the touch sense of the skin or he drops articles for the same reason, he does not appreciate his food (loss of taste), loss of pain appreciation causes minor accidents, and walking is difficult when there is no sense of touch or pressure in the soles of the feet. He may have loss of vision or hearing.

VOMITING is a common symptom of cerebral irritation in children due to conditions such as meningitis.

HEADACHES are severe in meningitis and space-occupying lesions such as brain tumour, brain haemorrhage or oedema. It is useful to report exactly where the headache is from the patient's description.

PYREXIA is a symptom in infection, e.g. meningitis or brain abscess, but may be associated with disturbance of the heat-regulating centre in the centre of the brain due to head injuries and brain surgery.

The PULSE RATE rises in infection but may be slower than normal following brain damage.

UNEQUAL PUPILS of the eyes may indicate some complication, e.g. in head injury.

GAIT, i.e. manner of walking, may have altered in the course of the neurological disease.

LOSS OF CO-ORDINATION means the muscles and nervous system do not act together. The patient intends to touch his nose with his finger but his finger touches his cheek instead of his nose.

TWITCHINGS in muscles, such as those of the face, occur in uraemia and tetany, and sometimes are seen at the beginning of convulsions.

FITS (convulsions) may be due to cerebral irritation from different causes, e.g. infection, poisons, uraemia. They are characterised by muscle contractions, a period of muscle rigidity being followed by spasmodic contractions of all the major muscles in the body (see epilepsy).

UNCONSCIOUSNESS is a state of altered consciousness in which there are varying degrees briefly described as *sleep* from which he is easily aroused, *stupor* from which he is aroused with difficulty, and *coma* from which he cannot be aroused.

Following some diseases and injuries of the brain there may be PERSONALITY CHANGES due to alteration in cortical activity of the areas of the brain about which little is known. The patient's relatives and colleagues may be able to give most information regarding these.

Observations

These are useful as an indication of the patient's progress. Should a written report be required it is made immediately after the nurse leaves the bedside. The patient is not always able to give a great deal of information, particularly when he is drowsy or has difficulty with speech, and this is a reason for the nurse's careful observation.

Levels of consciousness are as follows:
1. Normal conversation.
2. Drowsy, with confused conversation.
3. Will answer simple questions only.
4. Will answer only yes or no.
5. Responds to painful stimuli, by movement.
6. Unrousable by any means.

Should a nurse be present when a patient has a fit, it is useful to observe the part of the body in which the attack began, and the length of time of the fit.

Investigations

LUMBAR PUNCTURE. The patient lies in a lateral position or sits on a stool so that his spine is well flexed. When he is ill, unconscious or restless the nurse supports him in the lateral position. The doctor injects a local anaesthetic, and then introduces the lumbar puncture needle into the sub-arachnoid space. The cerebro-spinal fluid flows from the needle and can be collected in sterile specimen jars which are labelled at the bedside and then despatched to the laboratories (biochemical and bacteriological) as soon as possible. If the pressure be abnormal, it is measured by attaching a glass tube to the needle. The fluid rises in this and a reading can be taken. After the procedure, the puncture is covered by a small dressing. The patient lies flat in bed and is undisturbed for about four hours. He is given drinks of fluid during this time.

SIMPLE X-RAY EXAMINATION of the head shows defects in the skull such as fracture. Information of other conditions may be obtained by radiography following the injection of air into the space, which contains cerebro-spinal fluid. This can be done during the procedure of lumbar puncture but the patient sits on a stool and the air rises into the ventricles which are spaces in the centre of the brain. On X-ray the air appears dense and shows abnormal positions of the ventricles.

A dye opaque to X-rays can be injected into the sub-arachnoid space in lumbar puncture and the X-ray film shows abnormalities of the spinal cord when these are present.

Very small holes (burr-holes) can be made in the skull, and the dye is introduced through a needle inserted through one of these. The ventricles are clearly outlined in the X-ray film.

Electrical impulses produced in the brain can be translated into a graph on a strip of paper. This is an ELECTRO-ENCEPHALOGRAM, a complicated procedure which aids in diagnosis of neurological diseases.

For THE CLINICAL EXAMINATION OF A PATIENT who may be suffering from a neurological disease the doctor will require some articles of equipment, for example:

Patella hammer with which to test *the reflex responses.*

Substances for testing *the sense of taste.* Sugar and salt are useful. They are presented in small screw-cap jars and are *not* labelled. A spoon and saucer are required.

Substances for testing *the sense of smell*, oil of peppermint, oil of cloves, are useful. These fluids are in small screw-cap jars, and not labelled.

Two copper rods, one in a jug of hot water to heat it, or two glass tubes with rubber bungs, one of which contains cold water and the other hot water. *Temperature sense* is tested with these.

A cotton-wool swab to test *the sense of touch.*

A small pin to test *the sense of pain.*

The length of circumference of a limb is measured with a tape measure. Wasting of muscles can be detected in this way.

One or two objects likely to be familiar to the patient and which can be held in the hand, such as a key or coin. These are used to test *the sense of fine touch.*

A blue skin-pencil with which the physician may mark out areas where there is sensory skin loss.

In addition to these, a torch will be required to test the function of the iris (the pupil of which should constrict in a bright light), a blood pressure machine, a stethoscope, an auriscope and tuning forks for examination of the ears and hearing, and an ophthalmoscope with which the doctor examines the retina of the eyes.

The patient's notes and X-ray are made available.

It is more comfortable for the patient to have visited the toilet before the examination begins, and the procedure is explained very briefly. The ward is warm and quiet, the windows closed and the screens drawn round the bed, which is stripped leaving the patient covered by a treatment sheet. It may be necessary for the patient to be undressed and he or she wears a brief garment over the pelvic area. The physician may wish to see him stand or walk, observing his posture or gait. During the examination the patient is covered with the treatment sheet as far as possible for he may become chilled during a lengthy examination.

When her assistance is required the nurse remains with him, but stays at the bedside throughout the procedure when the patient is a girl or a woman. After the procedure the patient is dressed and made comfortable; she may need a hot drink.

Medical and Surgical Conditions of the Nervous System

Damage to the brain is a complication of HEAD INJURIES, and the spinal cord may be involved in fracture or dislocation of the spine causing PARAPLEGIA.

Nerves in the limbs are occasionally severed in wounds caused by knives, broken glass, bullets or shrapnel. This type of injury may also be associated with a bone fracture. As these nerves contain both motor and sensory nerve fibres, the patient cannot contract a particular group of muscles to produce a movement and he loses the sense of touch and pain in an area of skin in the same limb. Repair of the nerve by suturing in surgical operation is most successful when it is performed soon after injury. The treatment is followed by physiotherapy in which the tone of the paralysed muscle is maintained and then improved and the patient undertakes a programme of exercises. While the nerve is not yet efficient the affected muscles are sometimes stimulated by small electric currents causing them to contract. Complete recovery may take some months, and patience and perseverance are required but it is very gratifying for the patient to return to his work with little or no disability.

The nurse is reminded that where there is temporary or permanent loss of sensation in the skin, the patient is unable to respond to painful stimuli and therefore does not move from discomfort or danger as he would do normally. There is then the possibility of injury from his surroundings such as pressure from splints and bandages and hot-water bottles.

In ELECTRIC SHOCK the high voltage of electricity passing through the patient into the ground or floor disorganises the passage of nerve impulses in the nervous system. Contraction of muscle is impossible, the patient falls to the ground, and respiration ceases because the diaphragm does not contract. In this emergency situation the electric current is switched off, but if it comes from a cable this is pushed away from the patient using a wooden stick or pole. Artificial respiration is begun immediately using mouth-to-mouth breathing or the Holgar Neilson method until assistance arrives. Being struck by lightning is a similar accident but in this case the electricity discharged from the atmosphere has passed through the patient and is absorbed in the ground. There is no danger of electricity being conducted to the person giving first-aid treatment on this occasion.

HYDROCEPHALUS is a congenital abnormality in which the fluid in the brain cannot drain away through the normal channels. The infant's head grows very large, preventing him from being able to sit up, and his mental and physical health is retarded. An artificial means of drainage can sometimes be made.

INFECTIONS of the meninges by meningococci, spread by droplet infection, is a form of MENINGITIS which has occurred in epidemics. For this reason a patient with this disease is isolated and the nurse wears a mask in addition to other precautions. Sulphonamides or penicillin are effective and the condition has become uncommon.

TUBERCULAR MENINGITIS is a severe form of tuberculosis but when treated early with a combination of drugs, e.g. streptomycin, P.A.S. and I.N.A.H. can be cured. Another type of meningitis is that caused by pus-producing organisms such as staphylococci or streptococci. These are introduced through a wound in head injury or from another part of the body in the blood.

The patient with meningitis has a raised temperature and quickly becomes ill with headache and a stiff neck. He dislikes the light and resents any interference, sometimes becoming restless. The cause is discovered by the examination of the cerebro-spinal fluid following lumbar puncture. He is nursed quietly in a darkened room. Retention of urine is avoided by giving him a bottle at 3- or 4-hourly intervals and his fluid intake is maintained at $2\frac{1}{2}$ litres a day. This is not easy when he is semi-conscious or delirious but important in preventing dehydration and avoiding the crystallisation of sulphonamides in the kidney tubules. He improves quickly with chemotherapy or antibiotics, and satisfactory nursing care prevents complications such as pressure sores, mouth infection, dehydration, lack of nutrition and spread of infection.

CEREBRAL ABSCESS is the result of infection spreading from an infected part somewhere in the body to the brain, e.g. mastoiditis, or follows head injury when infection enters through an open wound. The patient becomes very drowsy, and shows signs of infection. It is treated by antibiotics and drainage.

POLIOMYELITIS is a virus infection affecting the motor cells of the spinal cord and is spread by droplet infection. Some forms of the disease are characterised by paralysis in a group or groups of muscles. When the respiratory muscles are affected the patient's breathing is continued by a respirator. These machines are of two types:

(a) The patient's body lies inside the respirator and his chest is compressed by air pressing around him. Then as the air pressure falls the lungs expand. This process takes place 16 times a minute, *or*

(b) The patient's lungs are inflated by air coming from a machine. The air enters his chest through a tracheotomy tube.

Immunisation against this disease is available.

TUMOURS of different types sometimes form in the brain or spinal cord. Symptoms and signs of brain tumour may be due to intra-cranial pressure, and cause headache, interference with vision, vomiting, and raised cerebro-spinal fluid pressure. Removal of a tumour depends on its type and situation.

EPILEPSY is a condition characterised by fits. The cause is often unknown, but it is sometimes related to previous brain injury. Epileptiform fits may be observed in patients with head injury, brain tumour or uraemia, and in infants with fever but who have no special brain disease.

The fit may begin with an 'aura' in which the patient experiences a particular smell or taste, but often there is no warning. He falls to the ground unconscious and is found to be *rigid*, has difficulty in breathing, causing cyanosis. Then *convulsive movements* begin and during these he may bite his tongue or pass urine though this is not common. Following the attack, which lasts a few minutes, the patient is drowsy and may wish to go to sleep.

Injury is possible as he falls and it may be necessary to move him away from danger. The first-aider protects his head by placing a rolled-up coat beneath it. His tie is loosened and spectacles, if these be worn, removed.

Dentures are not easily recognised but if these are in the mouth and appear at all loose they should be removed when possible.

The lateral position is the most suitable if it is convenient. At the beginning of an attack or immediately the convulsive stage begins a rolled-up handkerchief or, in the ward, a 4-inch bandage is placed between the teeth to prevent him from biting his tongue. Injury to head and lower limbs in the convulsive movements is prevented by moving him away from a wall or furniture. After an attack the patient is allowed to sleep if possible. The nurse observes a patient in the ward for an hour or two as his behaviour may be unusual or unreliable until he has completely recovered.

When a cause for epilepsy becomes known, the appropriate treatment is given. Other cases of epilepsy are controlled by drugs such as phenobarbitone and epanutin. The patient is encouraged to lead, with the assistance of his relatives, a quiet and orderly life in as normal a way as possible. It is advisable that children attend an ordinary school. Some occupations are unsuitable, such as those which necessitate climbing heights or driving vehicles but he can be trained for several types of work. It is helpful for the patient to carry a card in wallet or handbag which states the treatment of most value should he have an epileptic fit. A nurse admitting a patient in emergency or for treatment of a general condition would report this patient's disability as she learns of it. His treatment by drugs will be continued by the doctor who takes charge of him.

Loss of consciousness for a few seconds occurs in a condition known as PETIT MAL. The patient may drop a cup or stop speaking for a moment but does not fall. These lapses are disconcerting to the patient but tend to become less frequent as he grows older.

A patient with PARKINSON'S DISEASE has severe trembling in the trunk and hands and stiffness of joints can result in jerky movements. It is a distressing and disabling condition, upsetting the patient a great deal. The nurse may notice a lack of facial expression and the patient sometimes appears not to want to be active. Drugs such as hyoscine and artane (a muscle antispasmodic) have been used. The intense tremor is relieved in a number of cases by a surgical operation.

DISSEMINATED SCLEROSIS is a disease which usually begins between 20 and 40 years of age, and its course shows as attacks between which the patient may appear quite well. Patches of degeneration occur in the brain and spinal cord and amongst a number of symptoms and signs the patient's speech becomes slurred and his limbs, particularly the legs, are weak and stiff. There is difficulty in bladder control. In the more severe cases the patient is disabled but benefits from physiotherapy which maintains muscle tone and joint movements so that he may be as active as possible. He is mentally alert and when naturally intelligent needs consideration not only in care of the skin and hair and nutrition, but also in preventing boredom and depression. This is an occasion when the nurse needs to understand that physical disability does not mean that mental disability is inevitable. In a long-term illness such as this may be, the nurse bears in mind the *person* who is the patient and considers all the methods that are available to lessen the effects of the disability.

In MYASTHENIA GRAVIS the patient, who is usually young, cannot contract her muscles properly. In severe cases the muscles of respiration may be affected and then she relies on a respirator for breathing and the nursing staff for her other basic needs.

The medical treatment for this disease is a drug, prostigmine, which causes the skeletal muscles to contract. Removal of the thymus has been found beneficial in some cases.

TRIGEMINAL NEURALGIA is intense pain in the side of the head due to inflammation of the 5th cranial nerve on that side. This acute condition causes the patient great distress. It is relieved by injections into a section of the nerve to reduce the pain or by division of the sensory nerves in surgical operation. Motor fibres of the nerve may be affected, so that he cannot blink to wash tears over the front of the eye or protect his eye against approaching foreign bodies. As an artificial protection he wears a transparent shield over the eye, which the nurse removes only when the patient washes, after which it is replaced at once.

Cranial Surgery

Special pre-operative preparation includes shaving of the head after the permission of the patient (or his relatives if he is unconscious or a minor) has been obtained. Electric clippers are used followed by shaving close to the scalp with a razor. The scalp is treated with skin antiseptic after washing thoroughly with soap or bacteriocidal detergent to remove the natural hair oils. Tube gauze cap or Netelast bandage is applied. This procedure may be repeated on the morning of operation.

After the operation, a crêpe bandage is applied to the head to prevent oedema under the scalp. The nurse reports any changes in consciousness, pulse rate and behaviour. Sutures are removed early, e.g. on the 4th day, and the scalp is massaged daily using, for example, a mixture of methylated spirit and nut oil to prevent a dry scalp. It is preferable for male patients not to wear a cap, but women like to have a cap. The patient resumes general activity as soon as possible, becoming independent and maintaining a high morale.

The Nursing Care of a Patient with Hemiplegia due to Cerebro-vascular Accident

This paralysis of one side of the body is the result of a clot of blood (cerebral embolism) or a haemorrhage (cerebral haemorrhage) pressing on motor tracts in the brain. Occasionally the speech centre is affected and then the patient has difficulty in making words; this is aphasia. The facial paralysis involves lips, tongue and cheek, and interferes with the way in which words are produced; this is aphonia. Difficulty in speaking causes distress and frustration in the patient. Immediately after the cerebral accident, there is the paralysis of the limbs, which are flaccid and limp. Later, a spastic condition arises and some groups of muscles in increased tone force several joints into flexion. Degrees of paralysis vary a great deal, from slight to disabling, and recovery can be variable in length of time. The patient may be unconscious on admission and then receives the appropriate care. Many patients are elderly and prone to develop bed-sores, broncho-pneumonia, cystitis, and in some instances become apathetic and do not seem able to make much effort.

The lateral position is suitable for the patient with hemiplegia but sufficient support should be provided for the head and shoulders so that the patient is sitting almost upright. His position is changed at two-hourly intervals day and night. Continual bending of the neck, lumbar-spine, elbows, wrists, hips and knees is avoided. Pressure areas, e.g. the heels, are protected by small pads or pillows beneath the angles. A thin pillow is placed to separate the knees and prevent them from rubbing. A water-bed may be useful. The elbow and forearm of the paralysed upper limb are supported on a pillow and the hand grasps a thick cotton bandage or a soft ball to prevent flexion at the wrist. Later exercises will include squeezing the bandage or ball every half hour. The foot is supported by a padded foot-board or a light plaster splint to prevent foot drop. A bed-cradle protects the legs from the weight of the bed-clothes, and a flannelette sheet covers the legs and feet which may feel cold as they are inactive (hot-water bottles are inadvisable: this patient may not have sensory skin loss but he cannot move from danger).

When the affected eye cannot close, oily drops are instilled three times a day. These are prescribed by the doctor.

A continual small flow of saliva from the mouth is mopped away. Special care is taken with the patient's appearance and personal hygiene; this adds to his morale and shows the nurse's respect for the patient's dignity during this accident called 'a stroke'.

When feeding is difficult, a naso-oesophageal tube is passed. Patience is required in feeding the patient who cannot drink easily. He is given soft foods but eats slowly. As soon as possible he feeds himself, using the unaffected hand, and a large bib-like diet cloth is useful.

Bladder function presents a problem. Retention of urine is common when the illness begins and catheterisation may be necessary with bladder drainage for a time. Then a bottle or bed-pan is given to the patient at frequent intervals until emptying of the bladder takes place normally. Adequate fluid intake improves bladder and bowel action. Glycerine suppositories and aperients relieve constipation. The stools are observed when severe constipation in an elderly patient is a possibility so that this situation may be avoided.

The joints are exercised when the patient has recovered from the acute phase. Movement in the affected limb is encouraged when the patient can manage these. The patient is lifted into a chair for an hour twice a day, and uses the commode when she can support herself sufficiently. He or she is encouraged to take some interest in everyday matters. A middle-aged person may have interests of his own which can be made use of in hospital, e.g. music by radio or tape-recorder.

The subjects of importance in an elderly patient's life are his or her family and friends, pets, a garden and household affairs. The nurse can speak to her about these, and a personal 'belonging' like a photograph is placed where she can see it. Visitors are important both in helping the patient by giving news and feeding her with small pieces of fruit or flavoured drinks, and in maintaining the contact which gives the patient a sense of security between the onset of illness and returning home again.

THE PRINCIPLES OF TREATMENT are:

1. General nursing care during the acute illness.

2. Promotion of activity and independence as far as possible. There may be some residual paralysis and the patient and his relatives adapt themselves to this disability which may be slurring of the speech or dragging one foot. Walking aids are often useful. Furniture can be placed conveniently in a room so that the patient can move from one piece of furniture to another and so become more mobile.

Overdose of Drugs

The diagnosis of patients admitted after having taken an overdose of tablets depends on the clinical examination of the patient and the identification of the tablets.

Poisoning by some drugs produces effects in the nervous system. *Strychnine* overdose results in convulsions. Following excess of *opium* or *morphia* the patient is in coma, the pupils are pin-point. The most frequent admissions to hospital following poisoning are those from

barbiturate or salicylate (aspirin) overdose, and usually the drug has
been self-administered. Both conditions are serious.

Barbiturate poisoning. The patient is drowsy with slow, slurred speech
or mental confusion. Coma results from an excessive amount of the drug
circulating in the blood stream. The limbs are limp, breathing is slow
and shallow, the blood pressure is low.

If the patient is conscious, first-aid treatment is to make him vomit by
giving large amounts of warm water to drink or by placing two fingers in
the back of his throat. In hospital the contents of the patient's stomach
are aspirated by passing a wide-bore tube into the stomach and withdraw-
ing the contents with a 50-ml syringe. The result from this is saved; an
analysis of the stomach contents together with that of any tablets found
by the patient's body will reveal the identity of the swallowed drug.

Following the aspiration, the stomach will be washed out, using 5 litres
of tepid water (27°C) or sometimes a solution of sodium bicarbonate or
saline. Tablets can remain in the stomach for 24 hours or more. The
patient needs to be observed carefully for a period of time following the
incident. If his condition is serious or likely to cause concern he may be
nursed in an Intensive Care Unit.

Oxygen is administered and a stimulant such as amphetamine sulphate
which is effective in these cases. The patient requires the general nursing
care of an unconscious patient. It is important that 3 litres of fluid are
administered each day by intravenous infusion so that the drug which
was absorbed will be excreted by the kidneys.

Salicylate poisoning. The effects of an overdose of aspirin take some
time to appear. They include ringing in the ears, flushing of the face and
deep respirations. The patient is often restless. An emetic or stomach
washout is given at once. An alkaline solution is administered intravenously or sodium bicarbonate by mouth to counteract the effect of
acidosis in the blood.

These emergencies may follow severe or temporary depression, and are
a sign of possible mental illness which requires treatment. A psychiatrist
may be asked to see the patient, and any details of the patient's previous
physical and mental health related to this would be helpful in a report—
for example:

(a) has the patient attempted such an action before?
(b) has the patient been exposed to an emotional crisis recently?

A small number of patients with acute depression may attempt to
injure themselves after they are admitted to hospital. Some supervision
is necessary and precautions taken so that they cannot accumulate drugs
in a bag or box in a locker. These patients need the nurse's understanding

and it is important to treat them in the same way as any ill person who requires medical and nursing care. Some young people are admitted to hospital in this way. They are likely to be emotional and do not realise the danger to which they have been exposed, but respond to the calm, orderly 'absence from fuss' atmosphere in the ward.

A patient with *acute alcoholism* is brought into hospital because it is suspected or known that he has injuries. If he is unconscious it is difficult to know whether this is due to head injuries or excessive alcohol. For this reason the patient is admitted for 12 to 24 hours' observation, at the end of which time signs of skull fracture or brain damage would be obvious and not confused with those of the original condition. The alcoholic patient who walks into the Casualty Department is usually noisy and aggressive. He resents interference and will react violently to painful stimuli. The medical officer may, therefore, consider it wise to postpone any but urgent treatment until the next morning. Vomiting is a natural response to the situation and will relieve the condition more quickly than any treatment. In his confused state and unfamiliar surroundings micturition is a problem, and the male nurse or attendant will accompany him to the toilet. Relief from bladder distension following increased fluid intake leaves him more comfortable and usually more amenable. It is best then for him to lie down until he has recovered, but he remains under observation as he may continue to be restless. His injuries are reviewed the next day, and if his condition is satisfactory he is discharged by the Medical Officer.

A patient admitted to hospital having taken an overdose of drugs (the drug may have been swallowed or injected) may be a drug addict. He is nursed in the same way as any other patient who is ill. The nurse may find him uncommunicative. If the patient was known to a psychiatrist, then this specialist would be called to see him. These patients are in a general hospital only a short time, and treatment or care continues as needed under supervision of the patients' own medical practitioner or specialist.

Violence in a patient on admission to the Accident–Emergency department may be due to drugs or alcohol. Skilled management is required and the student or pupil nurse should not expect to be left to manage such a patient.

CHAPTER 38 | SIGHT

The individual is aware of material objects around him through the sense organs, the eyes, ears, tongue, nose and skin. The eyes are part of the

o

visual apparatus which includes also the nerves passing from the eyes to the brain (the optic nerves) and the visual areas in the occipital lobes of the brain; the function of the visual apparatus is *sight*, i.e. *vision*. Objects which are seen must be of sufficient size and within a limited distance.

The Visual Apparatus

The two eyes are the sense organs of vision. In man they are situated in the front of the head facing forwards. The limited visual range of the eyes is increased by the action of the eye muscles and the joints in the neck which enables the head to rotate from side to side and move upwards and downwards. It is possible also to rotate the spinal column, and objects at either side and behind can be seen by contracting the appropriate voluntary muscles of the eyes, neck and back.

Structure of the Eye

This organ is spherical in shape and, except for the front or window of the eye, is enclosed in white fibrous tissue. This is the SCLERA; it is tough and light rays cannot penetrate it. Continuous with the sclera and forming the window at the front is the CORNEA which is transparent, and bulges slightly forwards. Beneath the sclera is the CHOROID, which is dark in colour and therefore does not admit light rays. The blood vessels to the different parts of the eye are found as a network in this tissue. At the front of the eye attached to the choroid is a ring of involuntary muscle from which extend fine ligaments holding the LENS in position. The lens is a transparent, circular, and elastic body situated behind the PUPIL; it is the only part of the eye which has the ability to change its shape (i.e. it can become thinner or thicker), and it focuses rays of light which enter through the cornea, on to the nerve tissue of the eye. Beneath the choroid is the RETINA which is nervous tissue and contains the nerve endings of sight. In the centre of it is a very sensitive area, the yellow spot. The retina is continuous with the optic nerve, leaving from the back of the eye. Where the nerve begins in the retina is the blind spot, and no impulses occur here. In the space between the lens and the cornea is a watery fluid, and the shape of the main eye-ball, behind the lens is maintained by jellylike fluid contained within it. In front of the lens and projecting over it from the choroid is the IRIS, which is coloured, and being composed of involuntary muscle fibres lying in circular and longitudinal directions can alter its shape. In the centre of the iris is an opening, the PUPIL. When the circular fibres contract, the pupil becomes smaller or constricts; this occurs normally in a bright light but is also

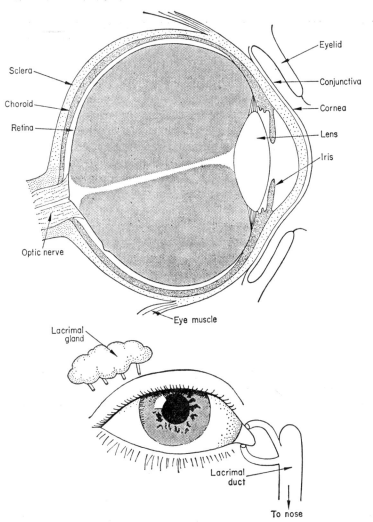

Figure 50. The eye.

seen as a sign in opium or morphia poisoning. When the longitudinal fibres contract, the pupil enlarges or dilates. This happens when the lighting is dim, and also as a result of stimulation of the sympathetic nervous system during an emergency. The main function of the iris is to regulate the amount of light entering the lens.

The function of the retina is to receive images of external objects. The cells include the rods which record objects in night vision; vitamin A in the diet is necessary for their function and to prevent night blindness. Other cells are the cones which record colour and objects in day vision.

FOR VISION TO TAKE PLACE light is essential. There should be no opaque substance between the object and the eye. The light rays fall on objects and then are reflected through the cornea, and focused by the lens on to the retina. Resulting nerve impulses are passed through the optic nerve to the visual areas in the occipital lobes of the cerebrum, where the picture is received. As the result of past experience the brain can give an interpretation of the picture, and it then has some meaning. Because there are two eyes in the front of the head, the brain receives two slightly different views of the object, and when these two views are combined together in the brain, there is an impression of depth and distance in the image received.

The ACCESSORY ORGANS OF THE EYE. The *eyebrows* are thickened ridges of skin, covered by short hairs, at the lower border of the brow. They protect the eyes from too vivid light and from sweat which forms on the forehead. The *eyelids* are two movable folds in front of the eye. The exterior surface is skin and the interior is *conjunctiva*, a membrane which continues over the front of the eye. Between the skin and the conjunctiva in the upper lid is a plate of cartilage, the tarsal plate. The functions of the eyelids is to protect the eyes from too bright light and dust and also to spread secretions (the tears) over the front of the eye. Protection of the eye is assisted by the eye-lashes, which grow like hairs on the borders of the eyelids and are nourished by sebaceous or oil glands.

Round the eye is a circular muscle and this can be contracted to 'close up the eye'. This is useful to protect the eye against sudden bright light and approaching foreign bodies.

The LACHRYMAL APPARATUS. A gland at the upper and outer angle of the orbit secretes the tears, and tiny ducts from this convey the tears to the conjunctiva lining the upper eyelid. TEARS are composed mainly of water and sodium chloride, hence their 'salty' taste, but they also contain a mild antiseptic substance, which helps to keep the eye free from infection. The eyelids spread the secretion over the front of the eyes to keep the cornea moist. It evaporates or passes through the lachrymal ducts into the nose.

Excess secretion is produced in emotion, in inflammation of the eye and when foreign bodies enter the eye. The *orbit* is a bony cavity in which the eye is situated for protection and consists of parts of seven skull and facial bones. Posteriorly in it is an opening for the passage of the optic nerve. The eyeball is supported in the orbit by tissues and a pad of fat.

Movements of the eye result from contraction and relaxation of muscles attached between the eye and the orbit in which it is situated. Normally the muscles of both eyes act in close co-operation and with precision so that the two eyes move in the same direction simultaneously, otherwise two different images are received in the brain. This is double vision, or *diplopia*.

ACCOMMODATION is the ability of the eye to focus the images of objects at different distances onto the retina. It concerns the lens, the involuntary muscle encircling it and the fluids within the eye.

Abnormalities in the Shape of the Eye
When the eye is too short from cornea to the back of the eye, the focus falls behind the retina; this is *farsightedness* or hypermetropia. If the eye is too long in the same direction, the focus falls in front of the retina; this is *nearsightedness* or myopia. Irregularities in the shape of the eyeball may produce some differences in the clarity of the image on the retina and this is *astigmatism*. The image in these different situations can be focused on to the retina by the addition of a lens specially made from glass or plastic to be placed in front of the eye. This lens is placed in a frame to fit on the head, i.e. spectacles. It is possible for the lens to be prepared by expert technicians to fit exactly over the cornea so that spectacles are unnecessary. This is a contact lens. It is expensive and requires special care such as keeping it free from injury and dust when not in use, and some patience is necessary in learning how to insert and wear it, but they are convenient and preferable to a number of people.

The nurse admitting a patient may find this person uses spectacles, and they are necessary for her to have in hospital otherwise she is incapacitated. Some elderly patients are less confused when they wear their spectacles and of course accidents are less likely to occur. Should the nurse meet a patient with a contact lens which is to be removed by the nurse, she will find a small rubber suction rod in the contact lens case. This is pressed lightly on to the centre of the lens while the eyelids are separated, and then withdrawn from the eye holding the lens. The lens is stored in a tiny box provided for this purpose.

Care of the Eyes in Health

PREVENTION OF INJURY. The eyes can be protected from intense sunlight, reflected light from snow and sand, heat from furnaces, by wearing dark glasses. Metal eye-shades, or goggles are worn by workers in industry when fragments of metal are likely to be ejected from material or machine. Goggles are worn by drivers of open, fast-moving vehicles when dust in the eyes can cause an interruption in concentration. Some games played by children are dangerous, e.g. arrows and darts, and they are dissuaded from running about with pointed scissors and knives in their hands.

PREVENTION OF INFECTION. Simple rules of hygiene are necessary; personal cleanliness, together with a clean environment, e.g. clothing and towels, and touching the eyes with the hands as little as possible. Injury of any kind, however slight, may predispose infection. Fortunately with improvements in hygiene infection is uncommon and when it does occur is treated satisfactorily with medications—prepared as eye-drops or ointments so there is less opportunity for spread of infection to other people.

LIGHTING is important to the health of the eyes, as inadequate illumination for close work leads to eye-strain, particularly if there be some slight imperfection in vision. The voluntary and involuntary muscles of the eye work less arduously when the person is out of doors. Many people find looking at distances a relaxation when compared with concentration at close range. Looking at objects which vary in distance from the eyes exercises the eye muscles.

Children need some observation at school with regard to their vision, for they may have difficulty and do not realise it. Their school reports may be disappointing because they cannot see the blackboard or read their books. Abnormalities such as squint are dealt with early, so that the unaffected eye is not overstrained, and the sight of the affected eye may not deteriorate.

Care of the Eyes during Illness

The patient who uses spectacles should have these to wear unless he is too ill. Any discharge from the eyes is mopped away and the lids are kept clean. The nurse is careful that bed-clothes do not brush against the patient's face during bed-making for he may not be able to close his eyes quickly and the conjunctiva may be damaged. If he cannot close the eyes properly during partial paralysis of the face as in exophthalmos (protrusion of the eyeballs), the nurse bathes the eyes frequently or instils oily drops such as liquid paraffin. Occasionally the eyes require protection by a perforated shield (Cartella type). When the reflex of 'blinking' which prevents damage to the eyes from dust and grit is absent and the lids cannot close, the cornea is protected from injury and drying by a shield. Injury or ulceration of the cornea may lead to blindness as the scar tissue prevents light rays from reaching the lens.

Nursing Patients with Eye Conditions

The possibility of losing one's sight will cause most people to experience great fear, and these patients need special help and understanding. Elderly patients with their eyes covered temporarily and after eye operations are obliged to lie still and possibly flat in bed. This and their isolation from relatives, friends and familiar surroundings may produce disorientation especially at night. They need frequent reassurance and confidence.

Disturbance of vision means some loss of independence to the patient; ways and means are found to prevent this as far as possible. It is helpful if he can know the geography of the room or ward, then his bed and the furniture are not moved from their original location. Similarly his personal articles are near to hand, and always returned to their places. Articles are not left on the floor where they may cause him to stumble. Feeding may be a problem at first. A plate with a raised edge and a spoon is useful and a large diet cloth cut like a bib-apron will prevent any soiling of the sheet which would distress the patient.

The nurse caring for this patient is very gentle. The eye is extremely sensitive to pain and pressure so the lightest of dressings are used with very little handling. Lotions are used at exactly 36°C (98°F) as the eye is also sensitive to temperature. Strict asepsis is necessary to prevent infection and if both eyes are treated, these procedures are regarded entirely separately for infection from one eye can be transmitted to the other. The nurse is quiet, making no sharp noises near to the bed to startle the patient. Neither does she permit the bed to be knocked or jarred. She does not, however, come to the bedside *too* quietly so that he is completely unaware of her approach, but speaks as she arrives and warns him also when she is about to move to the opposite side of the bed. He will recognise her by her footstep and voice and she speaks to him by name. Involuntary movement by the patient after an eye operation may cause damage to the delicate tissues.

It is necessary for the nurse to realise that a patient with both eyes bandaged is temporarily blind, and needs assistance in walking from one place to another. When one eye is bandaged or useless, the patient has for a little time some difficulty in judging distances and may have a few minor difficulties like placing a tumbler on the locker or lighting a cigarette and some patience and tact will be needed. It is courteous to stand by the patient at the side of his unaffected eye, so that he can converse without turning his head to an uncomfortable position.

Following removal of an eye damaged by injury or disease, there is some disfigurement and this has been overcome by the introduction of artificial eyes. These resemble a curved shell and are made by expert technicians so that they match in colour the original eye, and they fit the front of the orbital space. The normal movements of the eye are not possible, but the head movements are used to give the remaining eye more scope, and it is sometimes extremely difficult to know that the person has an artificial eye.

Symptoms and Signs

The patient may be experiencing *difficulty in seeing objects near to him,* or *those some distance away.* The former is common after middle-age. There may be *blurring of vision* or double vision, i.e. *diplopia,* or a patient may say he can see *haloes round bright lights.* In some conditions of an eye there is *partial loss of vision;* this is not always noticed as the other eye compensates. There may be *sudden loss of vision.*

Irritation occurs in inflammatory conditions of the conjunctiva or eyelid margin, and there may be a water discharge. When there is secondary infection, or in a direct infection, the discharge becomes purulent, and may be profuse when the condition is untreated. Haemorrhages are not common but may occur over the sclera as a result of injury to the base of the skull or to the eye itself.

Pain on one side of the head (neuralgia) and in the eye on the same side, when the patient is ill with abdominal pain and vomiting should be reported at once as this may be an acute condition of the eye requiring urgent treatment.

Pupils are unequal or do not react to light when there is damage or disease in the central nervous system.

Observations and Investigations

Reading average-sized print in good lighting at less than 30 cms may be observed in a person when there is some unrecognised visual difficulty. A test using letters in print or symbols is carried out during examination. Similarly minor accidents or mistakes can be an indication of inadequate vision.

The conjunctiva is frequently inspected during the clinical examination of a patient with a suspected anaemia in which case the membrane is very pale.

In diseases of the nervous system the muscles of the eyeball and round the eye may be paralysed and the doctor tests their movements. When the iris is paralysed, the pupil does not constrict as a bright light is brought near to it. If there is a discharge from the eye a swab is taken so that the bacteriologist can determine the type of infection. Prior to operation, the surgeon may request the bacteriological examination of a swab from the conjunctiva or lachrymal duct. If there is any infection present this is dealt with before the operation is performed.

The eye is examined by the doctor using an ophthalmoscope, in which a very small light is produced from a battery in the handle of the instrument, and the retina is viewed through the pupil of the eye. A darkened room is an advantage for this examination. Visual fields can also be tested, and give some indication of the area of the retina which is not functioning correctly.

Diseases and Conditions of the Eye

INJURIES (i) *Superficial, foreign bodies*, e.g. grit, insects. The grit may leave a small abrasion after removal.

(ii) *Penetrating foreign bodies*, e.g. fragments of metal which are embedded in the eye. The removal of these means skilled treatment in the ophthalmic department, and these injuries are extremely serious. They can usually be prevented by using protective goggles or eye-shields while exposed to the danger.

(iii) *Foreign bodies which penetrate and are then withdrawn*, e.g. arrows and darts. These are serious injuries.

(iv) *Corneal abrasions or lacerations*, e.g. branches or twigs swinging back across the face. These may not be deep abrasions but as the resulting ulcers heal, scars remain. When these extend over the cornea, total or partial blindness results.

(v) *Burns* involving eyelids and conjunctiva from fire or from corrosive fluids—acids or alkalies. First-aid treatment of the latter by immersing the face in a bowl of water and blinking rapidly or by flushing the eye with plenty of tepid water is *URGENT* to prevent progressive damage. These patients should always be referred to an Ophthalmic Hospital or Department.

(vi) Contusion—bruising (black eye). Cold compresses are applied to reduce the swelling. If the eye itself shows bleeding, medical attention is sought. X-ray examination is advisable in severe cases because of the possibility of orbital fracture.

(vii) Total damage to the eye in gunshot wounds, facial injuries.

INFECTIONS are less common in this country than in tropical countries where they are the cause of much blindness, e.g. trachoma.

STYE or hordeolum is the infection of an eyelash follicle. The stye at the inner or outer angle of the eyelid produces swelling out of all proportion to the actual boil. Application of heat by steam bathing reduces

o*

the pain, and the stye is localised, then discharges. Removal of the eye-
lash is sometimes necessary. General hygiene is observed during the
treatment of this condition. When styes occur the urine is tested for
glucose, as an underlying general condition may be present, diabetes
mellitus. Eyestrain predisposes rubbing the eyes, and tiny abrasions
caused in this way can be infected resulting in a series of styes.

BLEPHARITIS is a condition characterised by redness and 'itching' of the
eyelids and in severe cases crusts form along the lash roots. The lashes
may fall out or grow inwards irritating the eye. It is caused by unhygienic
conditions including pediculus capitus infestation, but most commonly by
dandruff.

The underlying causes are treated. Local treatment consists of cleansing the lids of all crusts and the doctor prescribes the application of an
antibiotic ointment.

CONJUNCTIVITIS is inflammation of the conjunctiva due to injury from
dust, foreign bodies or burns, or infection by pathogenic bacteria.
This membrane is susceptible to infection by pneumococci, gonococci,
staphylococci and streptococci, so steps are taken to prevent these, especially where babies are being cared for; before attending to a baby's eyes
the hands are washed and dried. A pregnant woman with gonorrhoea is
treated to prevent the baby being born through a birth canal containing
gonoccocal discharge. The resulting gonococcal infection of the infant's
conjunctiva may result in blindness. When an infection is possible or suspected, treatment by eye-drops is ordered by the doctor, to prevent development of the condition. The nurse reports any undue watery discharge
from the eye. Inflammation of the conjunctiva or the eyelids can be due
to hypersensitivity (or allergy) to substances with which the person comes
in contact. These are difficult to trace and are possibly connected with
the patient's special work or some medication used locally. The nurse in
hospital observes any reaction to the drug or chemical during his treatment, e.g. watery discharges, reddening of the eyelids or discomfort.

CATARACT is opacity of the lens; the light rays cannot pass through it.
The condition may be congenital, or due to a penetrating injury; it also
occurs in diabetes mellitus. The most common type is in people over 50
years of age and then both eyes are often affected, though opacification
may be more advanced in one eye than the other. In babies, the lens is
broken up by a needle and the particles are absorbed. But in older
patients the lens is extracted under local anaesthetic. The patient requires
a lens for vision and the extracted opaque lens is replaced by a lens in the
form of spectacles. Should the other eye be normal, the spectacles contain plain glass in front of the good eye.

GLAUCOMA. The tension within the eyeball is raised above normal; the drainage of any excess fluid inside the eye is obstructed. The hardness of the eyeball causes pressure on the optic nerve and will prevent the normal function of vision. It may arise suddenly and for no apparent cause, with pain in or around the eye and sometimes accompanied by severe vomiting and some abdominal pain. He may have seen coloured haloes round lights. Treatment is urgent in the form of eye-drops ordered by the doctor and sometimes a small section of the iris is removed to relieve the tension. It is important that the eye-drops are administered at the specified times and regardless of other nursing treatment. The chronic type of glaucoma is slow in its onset and the patient may not be aware of the condition before it is well advanced. There is aching in the eyes, misty vision and the patient sees haloes round the lights. It occurs in some cases of diabetes mellitus. The treatment is by eye-drops ordered by the doctor, or a puncture at the junction of the cornea-sclera under local anaesthetic, or the drainage of the fluid is achieved by operation.

STRABISMUS OR SQUINT. There is a deviation from the normal straight direction of the eye when looking at an object. In convergent squint the eye turns inwards. (This type is commoner.) In divergent squint, the eye turns outwards. The affected eye becomes progressively weaker. It occurs in young children and can be cured by special treatment in eye exercises by an orthoptist in a clinic. Glasses may be needed to correct long-sight and these would relieve the squint. Surgery is occasionally required in which appropriate eye muscles are shortened. Strabismus may be seen in medical and surgical conditions when the nerves to the eye-muscle, i.e. 3rd, 4th, or 6th cranial nerves are damaged, e.g. in brain tumours or injury.

Nursing Procedures

INSTILLATION OF DROPS. The prescription sheet is required and the name of the drug and dose, also the name of the patient are checked. The nurse stands behind the patient so that his head can be supported with the face looking upwards. She explains what she is about to do. A sterile pipette is used to draw up the required drops, the nurse holding with a swab the lower lid down against the cheek. With the other hand she directs the required number of drops into the lower conjunctival sac, allows the eye to close *gently* and mops away any fluid on the cheek. Any alteration in size of pupil, etc. is observed.

APPLICATION OF OINTMENTS. This is usually in a small tube reserved for one patient and is applied direct from the tube. Otherwise a glass rod is used. The lower lid is held down, the end of the tube or the sterile glass rod dipped in the ointment is drawn gently in and along the conjunctival sac. The *sides* of this rod are used rather than the end.

To EVERT THE UPPER LID in order to inspect the upper conjunctival sac or remove a superficial foreign body. The patient's co-operation is obtained; he looks down; a small rod is applied to the top of the tarsal plate in the upper lid. The lid is grasped at the eye-lash edge, pulled up and out and over. The whole lid will turn backwards like a hinge and the conjunctival sac can be viewed easily. With experience, the upper lid can be everted using a finger over the tarsal plate.

APPLICATION OF STEAM TO THE EYES. The patient frequently carries out this treatment after instruction from the nurse. He sits protected by a towel at a table on which is placed a large bowl containing 1 litre of boiling water. He is given a wooden spoon, the bowl of which is padded with white wool and a piece of bandage. The spoon bowl is dipped in the boiling water, the head is held over the bowl, and the spoon brought to within 3 cms *from the eye* so that the steam rises from the spoon on to the front of the eye. As the steam disappears, the spoon is dipped again into the hot water and the procedure repeated until there is no steam, about six minutes. The eye is dried with a sterile swab. It can be repeated every four hours. The spoon is stripped of the wool afterwards and boiled five minutes to prevent cross infection.

IRRIGATION OF EYES. Strict hygiene is observed. The procedure is explained to the patient and he is protected by a waterproof cape and a towel. The lotion is usually plain boiled water or normal saline and prepared at a temperature of precisely 38°C (100°F). It flows from an undine, which is a thin glass vessel with a spout and an opening through which the lotion is poured in, and over which a finger-tip can be placed to interrupt the flow.

The nurse stands behind the patient supporting his head and he looks upwards to the ceiling. He holds a receiver below the eye against the cheek, if he is able, otherwise another nurse does this. The nurse opens the eyelids, the upper lid against the brow and the lower against the bone of the cheek. She allows a little of the lotion to flow over his cheek so that he is reassured and knows when the irrigation is about to begin. The undine is held so that the spout is about one inch from the eye and the fluid flows over the eye from within outwards. This is the opposite direction from the natural flow of the tears and the reason for this is that some of the fluid from the front of the eye passing into the lachrymal duct at the inner corner of the eye may infect it. So the flow of the fluid is reversed and passes over the cheek into the receiver. After irrigation the eyelids are mopped dry and the patient made comfortable.

When SWABBING THE EYES the nurse washes and dries her hands first. Each swab, often of folded lint, is well moistened with warm boiled water, drawn *gently* over the eyelids from the inner corner to the outer corner of the eye, then discarded. When the lids are clean, the conjunctival sac may need to be swabbed. The skin of the eyelids is dried. Each eye is treated quite separately to prevent any risk of one becoming infected from the other.

Eye Bandages

Single eye with a single turn round the head above the ears then two turns over the head, down over the affected eye and under the ear, pinned at the front of the forehead.

Double eye: a single turn round the head above the ears, then one turn over the head, down over one eye-pad, under the ear to the other side of the head, but now up over the eye-pad and over the head. A fixing turn and repeat once more.

Special eye-bandages are made from three or four thicknesses of fine cotton material and are tied on by tapes.

EYE-SHADES are made from two thicknesses of dark green or brown paper tied on the head with tape. Some are manufactured from plastic and secured by fine elastic.

Drugs

Eyedrops. Atropine $\frac{1}{2}$ to 1%. Dilates the pupil and has a slow action.
Homatropine 1 to 2%. Dilates the pupil and has a quick action.
Eserine sulphate $\frac{1}{4}$ to 1%. Constricts the pupil.
Pilocarpine intrase $\frac{1}{4}$ to 1%. Constricts the pupil.
Local Anaesthetics. Cocaine 2 to 4% before the operation as eye-drops.
(N.B.: this is a Dangerous Drug.)
Antiseptic. Silver nitrate $\frac{1}{4}$ to $\frac{1}{2}$% as eye-drops, *or*
Silver-protein, commonly called Protargol 5%.
Treatment. Albucid (5 to 30% Sulphacetamide) as eye-drops.
Penicillin and other antibiotics.
Fluorescein is a stain used for the diagnosis of corneal abrasions. A drop is instilled in the eye followed by several drops of distilled water to wash away the excess. The abrasion shows up bright green under a light as from a torch.

Rehabilitation of the Blind Person

There is a Register of Blind Persons in this country so that they may receive aids to rehabilitation. Children attend special schools, where they are educated in general subjects by appropriately trained and experienced teachers who have a vocational interest in these children. The pupils learn to read in Braille, can become adept in verbal examinations and typewriting. Ball games are not practical but swimming is a much enjoyed sport. They learn particular professions and trades in which the senses of touch and hearing play a great part, e.g. physiotherapy, crafts and telephone operation, and they become greatly skilled. Workshops for the Blind have been organised so that they can become financially independent. Adults who become blind frequently find it necessary to change their employment and are encouraged to attend classes for new types of work. Some, however, can continue with their previous occupations with some adjustments, though this may take a little time and a great deal of patience. As a rule they dislike obvious sympathy, and appreciate opportunities to be independent, but some aid is necessary like a helping hand across a busy road, or a few words of explanation when most people can see what is happening. The blind person may use a white walking-stick to warn motorists of his disabilities, and there are special training centres for dogs for the blind. With such an animal the individual gains a great deal of personal independence in travelling about, and enjoys the companionship also. Books in Braille and on gramophone records, also radio programmes help those who are not mobile. There is a special weekly grant of money to all adult blind persons.

CHAPTER 39 | EAR, NOSE AND THROAT

Hearing

The hearing or auditory apparatus enables *sounds* in the environment to be received and appreciated. *Sound* is a series of vibrations or waves occurring in the atmosphere, and variations in sound are the result of differences in the vibrations:

   pitch depends on the frequency of vibrations;
   intensity depends on the size of the vibrations;
   quality depends on the combination of vibrations.

Vibrations are transmitted through solid materials like steel frameworks of buildings, the metal of a bell, the bones of the skull. Sounds of a very high or very low pitch cannot be heard by human beings, but a dog for instance can hear high-pitched sounds of which his master is not aware.

Structure and Function of the Ear

The *external ear* is in two parts,
(i) *the pinna* which lies outside the skull and is formed from cartilage and muscle and covered by skin;
(ii) *the external canal* one inch in length, curved in the adult, but with a single curve in the infant. The walls are formed from cartilage and part of the temporal bone, and the canal is lined with skin with hairs. The glands joined to the hair follicles produce wax.

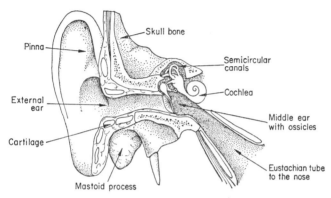

Figure 51. The ear.

The pinna collects the sound waves which fall on it and directs them into the external canal which passes them along to the ear-drum. This is a thin layer of fibrous tissue stretched across the canal, separating the external ear from the middle ear. On the outside is skin and on the inside mucous membrane. As the sound-waves reach the drum it vibrates

Behind the drum is the middle ear, a box-like cavity within the centre of the temporal bone. It is lined with mucous membrane and contains air which enters by the *Eustachian tube* from the nose. By this means the pressure of air on both sides of the drum (tympanic membrane) is made equal, otherwise the drum would not vibrate satisfactorily and the appreciation of sound would be lessened.

Across the MIDDLE EAR are slung three tiny bones called ossicles which are joined by ligaments. This arrangement of small bones between the drum and the inner ear causes the vibrations to be increased.

The INTERNAL EAR is a membranous cavity which contains a clear fluid. Between the membrane and the bone which contains it is more fluid. This fluid circulates the three subdivisions of the inner ear, the *cochlea*, the *vestibule* and *semicircular canals*. The *cochlea* is a membranous cavity in a snail-shaped hollow in the temporal bone of the skull, and within it are the nerve endings of hearing. This nerve ends in the AUDITORY AREA OF THE BRAIN which is in the temporal lobe.

The *mastoid process* is a bony projection from the temporal bone and is situated behind the ear.

Hearing

Sound waves travel along the external hearing canal reaching the ear-drum. The resulting vibrations are transmitted over the middle ear by the ossicles, and cause movement in the fluid in the cochlea. This pulling and relaxing on the nerve endings of the 8th cranial nerve of hearing causes impulses to pass to the auditory area of the brain where the impression of sound is received and interpreted.

Sense of Balance

The Semicircular Canals

These have no connection with hearing, but in disturbances of the hearing apparatus the function of the semicircular canals may be affected because of their close anatomical positions.

The structures are three canals at right angles to each other, containing fluid. One end of each canal is enlarged and this contains nerve endings of balance. The canals give information about the position of the head in space and transmit this through the 8th cranial nerve to the brain. When the head comes into an unnatural position in space, certain muscles contract to correct the position of the body and prevent injury. For example, when the person stumbles over an obstacle in his path, his head moves suddenly forwards and downwards, the fluid in the semi-circular canals exerts its pressure on certain nerve endings. Impulses pass to the cerebellum, which can control muscle tone and action, and muscles of the neck and back and legs contract. The spine straightens, the head rises upwards and backwards into a normal position once more, and the person has recovered from his stumble. In a less dramatic degree, this mechanism of balance or equilibrium is necessary for all the activities by which we move about. Disturbance of the semicircular canals leads to dizziness (vertigo), and vomiting (in sea-sickness there is a connection between the mechanism of balance and the vomiting centre of the brain). When damage to the temporal bone by fracture occurs there is a possibility that the sense of balance is lost, and when the head is tilted the person falls over on to the ground.

Care of the Hearing Apparatus in Health

CLEANLINESS of the pinna and external canal needs some care as there are several crevices in the pinna and a cleft behind it. Moisture is harmful as the skin will break down and is easily infected. After cleaning the skin with soap and water it must be dried thoroughly. A baby's skin is delicate and can become very sore. Dust and dirt should be removed from the hearing canal by washing with soap and water, possibly using the corner of the towel. A nurse with skill may use an applicator dressed with wool, but rigid instruments of metal or wood can damage the skin. Infection can result from this. Sometimes wax collects to such an extent, aided by dust from the air, that hearing is interfered with. The doctor may syringe the ear to remove it. The wax may be softened by a few olive-oil drops first. Normally there is rarely any problem from wax.

INTENSE NOISE from some kinds of machinery over a period of time can cause deafness in the workers operating the machines. They are provided with ear-plugs to prevent the force of the vibrations from affecting the ear-drums and inner ear.

INFECTIONS of the nose and throat are a disadvantage, for these can track along the Eustachian tube to the middle ear, and an inflammation occur (otitis media). It is for this reason that care is taken not to expose babies and small children to throat infections, and a nurse with a suspected infection may be transferred from the ward.

Care of the Ears During Illness

As a patient lies in the lateral position the appropriate ear becomes a pressure area, and a sore can occur at the edge of the pinna. The *pressure* of the head against the bed and *damp skin* behind the pinna may lead to soreness here also, particularly in infants. Frequent changing of position, cleanliness and thorough, gentle drying of the skin will prevent this soreness and a very little olive or arachis oil, or a skin barrier cream, e.g. zinc cream and castor oil will prevent water absorption.

A patient who is accustomed to a *hearing aid* should have this made available while he is in hospital unless he is too ill to make use of it. Otherwise he is unable to communicate easily with staff, relatives and the other patients.

Signs and Symptoms Associated with the Hearing Apparatus

DEAFNESS may be complete or partial. A rough test is to hold a watch or speak in front of one ear while the patient looks ahead and cannot observe watch or speaker. If he hears a question he will give a reply. There may be differences between the hearing efficiency in both ears, so they are tested separately. Electric apparatus is used for such testing; this is an audiometer.

PAIN is called 'ear-ache' and is frequently intense as the organs are in a confined space within the temporal bone, consequently even a small amount of swelling causes intolerable discomfort. Infants move the head rapidly from side to side and cry incessantly in addition to other signs of ear infection. Ear-ache may be due to conditions other than those connected with the ear, and is pain referred from throat, teeth, tongue, or neck glands.

TENDERNESS may be localised to the skin within the hearing canal when there are small boils, or over the mastoid process when this is infected.

DISCHARGES from the ear.

    (a) watery fluid in eczema of the skin in the hearing canal;
    (b) pus due to infection of the canal or coming from a middle-ear abscess through a perforation in the ear-drum;
    (c) blood in injury, e.g. from a rough or sharp foreign body in the ear;
    (d) blood or a water fluid coming through a perforated drum after injury to the coverings of the brain and blood vessels in skull fractures.

GIDDINESS or vertigo, resulting from disturbances of the semicircular canals in the inner ear.

TINNITUS, i.e. ringing in the ears. This symptom is not always due to disease of the ear itself but is often due to intolerance or overdose of drugs (salicylates, e.g. aspirin, in particular).

Examination and Investigation

The doctor examines the ear using an *auriscope*, an instrument in which a tiny electric bulb is supplied from a battery in the handle and illuminates the auditory meatus. Alternatively a *head mirror* is worn and a light beam directed from a lamp behind the patient on to the mirror, and reflected from here on to the ear. In both methods, an *aural (ear) speculum* is required, size according to size of patient's ear, also a wax curette, a wool carrier with swabs and a tuning fork. It is an advantage if the room can be darkened. The patient sits on a stool or lies with his head comfortably on the pillow, so that the doctor or sister can examine the ear without difficulty. The curve of the ear is straightened out by holding the upper part of the pinna between the first two fingers or finger and thumb and pulling gently upwards and backwards.

A child whose ear is to be examined finds it very difficult to remain quite still in the most suitable position and he is apprehensive because he cannot see what the doctor is doing. To avoid any possible injury from instruments the nurse holds the child by sitting on a stool facing the doctor with the child in her lap. One hand and forearm are placed across the child's arms as he sits looking to one side so that the doctor can examine one ear. The nurse's other hand and forearm support his head against her chest. If he is likely to move his feet, his legs are secured between her knees. In this way he is held quite firmly. The bull's eye lamp is behind the nurse's left shoulder and the light from this is reflected from the doctor's head mirror on to the ear.

Hearing is tested with *tuning forks.* These vary in size and when struck produce sounds of different pitch. It is helpful if the room is quiet for this test.

An audiometer is also used to test hearing. The result of the test is shown as an *audiogram.*

Conditions of the Ear

DEAFNESS, complete or partial, is caused by abnormality of any part of the hearing apparatus.

- (a) the ear being covered, e.g. by a helmet, cap, dressing or bandage;
- (b) an obstruction in the meatus, e.g. wax, a foreign body, an earplug;
- (c) perforated drum;
- (d) acute infection of the middle ear;
- (e) the tube to the nose being blocked, e.g. by changing air pressures while in an aeroplane;
- (f) fixity of one of the ossicles to the window between the middle ear and the inner ear in otosclerosis;
- (g) injury or disease of the 8th cranial nerve of hearing;
- (h) injury or disease of the auditory centre in the temporal lobe of the brain.

The *pinna* when damaged frequently by blows becomes permanently swollen and distorted. Loss of the pinna is a congenital deformity, not so disturbing in a woman, whose hair would hide the disfigurement. Treatment is by plastic surgery.

In the HEARING CANAL infection of the hair follicles produces *boils* (furuncles). Although these are very small they cause intense pain, there is swelling and tenderness. Dry heat by a well-protected hot-water bottle, or a lamp, or glycerine and ichthyol drops relieve the pain. There may be a suppurative discharge and this is removed by mopping with swabs. The infection is controlled by antibiotics ordered by the doctor when the type of infection is known. When the furuncles recur frequently the urine is tested for glucose as they are occasionally associated with diabetes mellitus. Acute general infection of the tissues of the meatus is referred to as ACUTE EXTERNAL OTITIS and may result from slight injury, e.g. abrasions or scratches and subsequent infection due to lack of hygiene. In CHRONIC EXTERNAL OTITIS, the skin tends to break down and there is an offensive discharge. Any local conditions such as otitis media, foreign bodies in the meatus are treated and soothing ointments ordered to stop scratching. No water should be allowed to enter the meatus as this aggravates the condition. The skin is kept dry by the use of astringent drops prescribed by the doctor. The nurse observes any reaction of the skin in the canal or on the face following the use of aural drops, as a patient may be allergic to one of these drugs. Accumulation of wax in the ear is removed using instruments or syringing when the doctor orders this procedure.

Small foreign bodies are sometimes found in the ears of children and cause irritation, deafness and after some time an aural discharge. The doctor, using a hook, removes materials which would swell in water, and the remainder are removed by syringing the ear. The nurse holds the child as previously described but occasionally a general anaesthetic is considered necessary.

The Middle Ear

The drum may be ruptured in direct injury, e.g. a blow from the hand over the ear, or as a result of fractured base of skull, or from blast due to explosion. If blood or a watery fluid flows from the ear after head injuries, a clean pad is placed over the ear to prevent infection, and the patient lies on that affected side so that the discharge flows out of the ear and does not accumulate inside the head to cause pressure.

Infection of the middle ear is *otitis media*; it may be acute or chronic and usually pus is formed.

In ACUTE OTITIS MEDIA the patient is feverish and complains of pain. The drum bulges and eventually bursts; the abscess discharges into the canal as a blood-stained muco-purulent fluid. The release of pressure in the middle ear reduces the degree of pain and the patient is more comfortable. The meatus is mopped frequently with dry wool or ribbon gauze to prevent breaking down and infection of the skin. The surgeon performs myringotomy (incision of bulging ear-drum) while the patient is anaesthetised. This operation is less frequently required now as penicillin controls a large number of these infections.

Serious complications can result from *acute otitis media*, as this box-like cavity is in close proximity to the meninges, the brain, channels (or spaces) containing venous blood from the brain, the inner ear, and the facial nerve. The prompt use of antibiotics in the acute infection has removed a great deal of the danger.

ACUTE MASTOIDITIS may follow an abscess in the middle ear when the infection spreads to the mastoid bone and an abscess forms there. The patient is acutely ill with fever, pain in the ear, a discharge from the ear when the drum ruptures and deafness. Swelling behind the ear causes the pinna to stand out from the head and the area is very tender. Treatment is by antibiotics and, if this is unsuccessful, simple mastoidectomy is performed. The discharge ceases, the perforation heals and hearing returns to normal.

CHRONIC OTITIS MEDIA and CHRONIC MASTOIDITIS give rise to a chronic ear discharge and deafness. The bone tissue becomes infected. Conservative treatment includes cleaning the ear and removing the discharge and particles of dead skin. Antibiotic drops are instilled; Neomycin is suitable for this method of administration when ordered by the surgeon. Surgery, a radical mastoidectomy, includes removal of all infected bone, the ossicles and the drum. The hearing mechanism is reconstructed using skin graft to replace the drum and artificial polythene ossicles.

OTOSCLEROSIS is a disease which begins in young people, usually women, and leads to progressive deafness. One of the ossicles in the middle ear becomes fixed to the oval window leading to the inner ear and vibrations are not passed on. Surgery is performed so that the small bone can move, or the bone is removed and an artificial replacement made from polythene is inserted.

The Inner Ear

Inflammation of the inner ear has spread from the inner ear or mastoid bone. The patient will be partially deaf and complain of vertigo (dizziness) and vomiting. The infection is treated by antibiotics or surgery, depending on its cause, and the vertigo by drugs.

MÉNIÈRE'S DISEASE is characterised by acute attacks of vertigo with vomiting, lasting 2 to 3 hours; there is some deafness or tinnitus. The inner tube of the labyrinth is dilated and the excess fluid presses on nerve endings of balance. Treatment is by reduced fluid in the vestibule—salt-free diet, fluid restriction and a diuretic, or by surgery using a special procedure to reduce the sensitivity of the balance mechanism. Dramamine is given in acute attacks.

Nursing Techniques

Cleaning the External Auditory Meatus
As in all techniques, the procedure is first explained to the patient in simple terms to reassure him and gain his co-operation.

The nurse needs a satisfactory light to inspect the meatus before and after the procedure. Equipment includes swabs of fine good-quality wool with angulated aural forceps or wooden applicators. If the latter be used, each with its swab is discarded when the swab has been used once. The doctor may order a special lotion to be used, otherwise dry swabs are usually sufficient. Water is rarely used, as moisture inside the meatus lowers the resistance of the skin to infection. The patient lies or sits in such a position that the ear to be cleaned is easily accessible to the nurse. If he is inclined to be dizzy or is ill, the head is supported on a pillow as he lies comfortably on a couch or in bed. A child is held by another nurse if he is likely to be restless.

The nurse holds the upper part of the pinna and pulls gently upwards and backwards to straighten out the curve of the meatus and, should the patient be an infant, the lobe of the ear is held. She then inserts the swab held in forceps or an applicator gently into the meatus about one inch, moves it slowly to take up any discharge and then withdraws it. The swab is discarded at once into the used swab bag. The procedure is repeated until the meatus is clean. A lotion may have been prescribed for cleaning the meatus. Water is sometimes harmful as in chronic external otitis, but if used the ear is thoroughly dried afterwards.

When the purpose of the cleaning is to remove discharge from the ear, the doctor may request a gauze drain or wick to be left in the meatus. This is about 5 cms of half-inch ribbon gauze inserted one inch into the meatus using the aural forceps. A sterile dressing over the ear may be necessary to absorb the discharge which flows along the gauze wick. During infection it is necessary to keep the skin free from discharge, injury (as from unskilful handling with forceps) and dampness.

All equipment is sterilised following the procedure.

Should both ears require this treatment, it is regarded as two entirely separate techniques, otherwise there may be cross-infection from one ear to the other.

Instillation of Drops into the Ear
After the procedure has been explained to him, the patient lies with his head inclined to the side so that the ear into which the drops are to be instilled is uppermost. His clothes are protected by a towel placed across his shoulder, as some prescriptions are coloured liquids. The external

meatus is cleaned if necessary. The nurse again checks that the ear-drops are those prescribed by the doctor on the patient's case sheet. (She has checked once already as she took the drops from the drug cupboard.) Oil drops may have been warmed but antibiotic drugs, e.g. penicillin, are not exposed to any heat. A pipette is used to instil the drops into the ear. The patient raises his head after the procedure and the excess drops are mopped with a swab. If necessary a swab may be left at the opening of the meatus and *not* in the meatus.

Drugs in the form of a powder may be applied to the external meatus by an insufflator (or powder spray), or if this is not available blown into the ear through a piece of stiff paper rolled into a cone.

BANDAGING THE EAR consists of turns round the head using a roller cotton bandage $2\frac{1}{2}$ inches in width. First a fixing turn is made beginning at the centre forehead. The bandage needs to be particularly firm at the lower centre forehead, then turns to cover the dressing from below upwards and towards the centre forehead. The bandage also needs to be particularly firm at the lower part of the dressing otherwise discharge may come down beneath it.

The other ear is left completely uncovered so that the patient can hear. The eye is not covered or irritated by the bandage, and to prevent this a tape may be tied round the turns at the upper outer aspect of the eye. A fastening pin is placed at the centre forehead to avoid discomfort when the patient lies on his side.

Rehabilitation of the Deaf

DEGREES OF DEAFNESS may be expressed as follows:

1. *Total deafness.* This is rare. The child does not begin to talk at the normal age. He attends a special school and learns to lip-read.

2. *Severe deafness.* The child has some hearing but it is insufficient for him to learn to speak as children usually do. Such a child would grow up deaf and dumb, but now he attends a school for the deaf and is taught to speak by specially trained teachers who use a machine called an auditory trainer. He learns to lip-read, and hearing aids also provide assistance.

3. *Partial deafness.* The child with this degree of deafness attends a special class in an ordinary school and is taught by a teacher experienced in dealing with deaf children. Hearing aids are used.

Hearing Aids
When there is no discharge from the ear the shaped mould fits in the ear, otherwise it is placed behind the ear. The mould is attached by a thin

cable to a transistor which is carried in a pocket or hangs from a hook or is attached to a spectacle frame. Vibrations are magnified by the apparatus, providing a greatly increased stimulus to the auditory nerve.

Deaf people miss a great deal in their daily lives which others take for granted. Social activities are difficult because they often depend on conversations, instructions, music, etc. These people tend to become uncommunicative and withdraw into themselves.

It is important to recognise early that a child is deaf so that he can be given aid before learning to speak. If he or she has not begun to talk at two years of age, the medical practitioner will test his or her hearing. When there is a family history of deafness, or it is known that the mother had German measles (rubella) in pregnancy, or the child was very jaundiced at birth or had birth injury, special note is made of this child's development in speaking. A Health Visitor can give advice on these occasions regarding a visit to the doctor.

Treatment of any underlying cause is given and rehabilitation is by means of hearing aids and classes in auditory training and lip reading.

Guidance is given to parents, and the child is educated in a school for the deaf or a partially deaf unit in a school, or he wears a hearing aid and attends ordinary school. He will be trained for occupations in which acute hearing is not essential.

Deafness Acquired Later in Life
The cause of deafness is treated if possible, for example by:
  (a) Tonsillectomy and removal of adenoids, *or*
  (b) Mastoidectomy, *or*
  (c) Reconstructive surgery, as in removal of the ossicle and its replacement by an artificial type.
Hearing aids are provided. Sometimes the person needs to be reassured that wearing a hearing aid is not disreputable but like spectacles a useful asset. He or she may need some training for a different kind of occupation.

When a patient is deaf in one ear only, it is courteous for the nurse to stand on his other side so that he may hear more easily. There is nothing to be gained by raising one's voice in speaking to a partially deaf person, and a normal manner of speech is most likely to be heard. The nurse however can help the patient by having her face in full view of the patient and using her lips more than usual as she speaks the words slowly.

The Nose and Pharynx

The nose (Fig. 52) is formed from two nasal bones joined to the maxillary bones of the face and cartilage. A septum of bone and cartilage divides the cavity into two nostrils. Attached to the maxillary bones are the scroll-shaped turbinate bones which make the inner surface of the nose irregular. The nose is lined with a mucous membrane except near the opening nostrils where there is skin with some short hairs. On the septum are a number of blood vessels which bleed when damaged. In the roof of the nose are the nerve endings of smell. Ducts from the maxillary sinuses and the frontal sinuses open into either side of the nasal cavity between the turbinate bones. Posteriorly the nose opens into the naso-pharynx where the adenoids are situated.

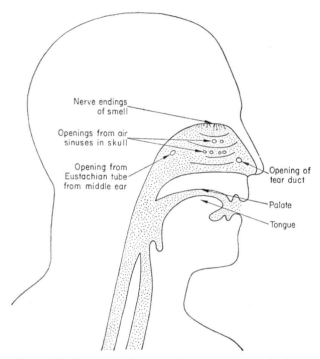

Figure 52. The nose showing the openings on the lateral surface of each nostril.

As air is drawn in through the nose during inspiration it is warmed as it passes over the mucous membrane and the dust in it is removed by the hairs and mucus in the nostrils.

The sense of smell is very sensitive but soon becomes fatigued so that a person may not be conscious of a certain odour a few minutes after being exposed to it. The nose in the adult needs little attention but an infant's nostrils may require some cleaning with damp wool to prevent blockage particularly when he regurgitates a little milk through his nose.

Care of the Nose in Illness

When there is some obstruction in the nose a patient breathes through his mouth, which then becomes dry, with a risk of mouth infection. The mouth should be treated frequently if the obstruction cannot be removed. Dry mucous membrane in the nose is uncomfortable, and can later feel very sore. A cream application is useful, e.g. Nivea cream applied with a piece of soft muslin or paper tissue so that the membrane is not damaged.

A profuse nasal discharge is mopped away with disposable swabs or paper wipes. 'Blowing the nose' should be avoided as far as possible because discharge may be blown into the sinuses causing infection. The increased flow of mucus in the common cold often affects the sense of smell, and as a result there is less pleasure in eating. Used paper handkerchiefs are collected in a bag and burned.

Symptoms and Signs

HEADACHES can be a symptom of many general diseases, but in some cases are caused by inflammation of the sinuses.

NASAL OBSTRUCTION may occur in one or both nostrils, and in the naso-pharynx, where the adenoids are situated. The patient says he 'cannot breathe properly'.

LOSS OF SENSE OF SMELL. The patient may say he cannot taste his food. The tongue appreciates salt, sweet, bitter and sour tastes but the flavour of food arises mainly from its smell.

EPISTAXIS, i.e. bleeding from the nose, occurs where the blood vessels are close to the surface of the mucous membrane on the septum. It is sometimes associated with a general condition, e.g. raised blood pressure.

DISCHARGES from the nose depend on the type of infection. In catarrhal conditions (forms of which are allergic responses to certain viruses or other stimulating factors) there is a profuse mucus discharge: Pus is produced in infection of the sinuses. Mucus or muco-purulent discharges may dry on the surface of the mucous membrane and perhaps with dust particles causing CRUSTS which leave a sore, perhaps bleeding, surface when removed.

TENDERNESS over the bone structure of the nose usually indicates injury, possibly fracture. It occurs over the maxillary sinuses when these are infected and the patient may speak with no resonance in his voice.

Examination of the Nose

The method is similar to that when the ear is examined, but the patient faces the doctor and the head is tilted backwards slightly. A nasal speculum is used to dilate the nostril and the beam of light is directed between the blades of the speculum on to the interior of the nose. Nasal forceps and swabs may be needed for cleaning the nostrils.

Investigations

A *Nasal Swab* is taken when a bacteriological examination is required. This is done in diseases of the nose and sinuses and when a healthy person is suspected of being a 'carrier'. This would be confirmed by a report showing staphylococci or streptococci.

Transillumination. The patient stands or sits in a small darkened room and a torch is switched on inside his mouth. Infected sinuses appear darker than normal.

Radiography. The nose may be X-rayed and show possible fractures, and the sinuses to confirm a diagnosis of infection, tumour or injury.

Conditions of the Nose

FRACTURES are common resulting from fights or children being struck by hard objects which are thrown or swung against them. If possible they are reduced immediately after injury by raising the part of the bone which has been depressed. In three to four hours swelling appears. When there is difficulty with breathing or considerable change in the appearance of the nose, the patient may be admitted later for further reduction of the fracture under general anaesthetic and a splint is applied.

FOREIGN OBJECTS sometimes find their way into the noses of children between two and five years of age and are usually on one side only. If placing a finger over the other nostril and blowing quickly down the affected side does not dislodge the article, the child should be seen by a doctor. The nurse holds the patient securely while the doctor passes a blunt probe behind the object and moves it forward. If this is unsuccessful, a general anaesthetic will be required. A small foreign object which remains in the nose causes a purulent discharge.

A DEFLECTED SEPTUM is a septum which is bent to one side, frequently the result of injury. It acts as a partial obstruction to the escape of mucus secretions and sepsis often follows. If causing symptoms, the operation (submucous resection of septum) is carried out under local or general anaesthetic. Afterwards, the patient is nursed sitting up in bed as there are packs in each nostril for a short time. After the removal of these there is a nasal discharge for some days which is mopped away with clean swabs. Steam inhalations help the patient to breathe easily and prevent drying of the secretions.

NASAL POLYPI are projections of swollen mucous membrane. They are the result of infection but also cause infection. When a polypus is damaged, bleeding can be severe. They are usually removed by an instrument with a wire loop.

EPISTAXIS is bleeding from the nose and may be due to:

1. Injury such as a blow from a fist or a ball.
2. A nasal infection like the common cold.
3. A foreign object in a child's nose.
4. In raised blood pressure when the bleeding acts as a safety valve.
5. It may be associated with a general disease, e.g. leukaemia or drugs in anti-coagulant therapy. Epistaxis may also be associated with the onset of an infectious fever.

Treatment of the patient during mild epistaxis. The patient is reassured, sits in a chair or in bed with the head slightly forward. A bowl or an absorbent cloth is held beneath the nose. He is instructed to breathe in and out through his mouth so that any risk of inhaling blood is avoided and to give an opportunity for blood to clot in the nose. Pressure may be placed on either side of the nose below the nasal bones with the finger and thumb; this is not always successful, and occasionally the blood merely trickles down the naso-pharynx into the mouth and is expectorated.

An ice-cold application may be placed over the bridge of the nose and it is thought by some people that this treatment applied to the base of the neck is useful. The patient may feel cold and shivery and a blanket or rug may be wrapped round his thighs and legs.

If the bleeding continues, the patient is seen by a doctor, who may pack the nostril using inch-wide ribbon gauze handled by nasal forceps. This cotton material aids clotting but the blood dries on the gauze and when the pack is removed there may be further bleeding. For this reason it is usual to soak the gauze in a liquid with an oily base or glycerine and perhaps antiseptics. The doctor requires a head mirror with a lamp and a nasal speculum. The pack is removed in one or two days. An alternative to the nasal pack is a small rubber balloon which is blown up inside the nose and presses on the bleeding point.

If the haemorrhage has continued for some time or the patient is already ill and feels faint, he should be laid flat with his head on a protected pillow, his nose pointing downwards so that the blood flows out and cannot be inhaled.

Any general condition causing the haemorrhage will be treated.

INFECTIONS

Boils in the nose (furuncles) are treated by application of heat, usually by bathing the nose in hot water. They are extremely painful until the pus is discharged and the patient may require a mild analgesic. There may be some contributory cause for these hair follicle infections and investigations may be carried out, e.g. bacteriological examination of a nasal swab and testing the urine for glucose.

The *common cold* is a virus infection of the upper respiratory tract including the nose and throat. It causes little more than some discomfort in most people, but can be serious in young infants and those who are already ill or who are about to have a general anaesthetic. The virus is spread by droplet infection and this transmission can be prevented by the infected person avoiding other people and, when this cannot be avoided, wearing a mask. A cold is of short duration—about four days—but uncomfortable, with headache, malaise, slight pyrexia, first a dryness in the nose and throat, then a profuse discharge of mucus. There is no known cure for the disease and the symptoms are treated as they arise. Artificial immunisation has not so far been considered practical.

SINUSITIS is usually the complication of a cold, but also arises if an abscess at the base of an upper tooth bursts into the maxillary antrum (air space or sinus).

ACUTE SINUSITIS. There is tenderness over the sinus and swelling of local tissue such as the cheek or round the eye. Pyrexia, headache and malaise can be quite severe.

In most cases, drainage of the abscess in the sinus is difficult. Ephedrine nose drops or sprays cause the mucous membrane to shrink and this treatment is followed by steam inhalations, using a deep household jug. Antibiotics may be prescribed.

In *chronic sinusitis*, the lining of the sinuses becomes thickened and produces a muco-purulent discharge; this is called nasal catarrh. There is headache at some time during the day. The most commonly infected sinus is the maxillary antrum and in treatment this is washed out. The nostril is anaesthetised using cocaine applied to the mucous membrane on an applicator. Fifteen to twenty minutes later the surgeon introduces a metal tube (cannula) from inside the nose into the lower part of the antrum which is then irrigated using normal saline solution at 38°C (100°F) through a Higginson's syringe. The fluid returns through the nose into a receiver held by the patient while he holds his head slightly forward. The surgeon will require nasal speculum, head mirror and lamp. The skin round the nose is dried at the end of the procedure. The fluid is inspected.

When the chronic infection persists it may be considered necessary to make a more permanent opening into the lower part of the antrum from the nose; this operation is ANTROSTOMY. A more extensive operation includes removing the infected mucous membrane from the sinus through the mouth and at the same time antrostomy is performed. Antrum wash-outs are performed each day and then less often until the discharge ceases. A short curved antrum cannula is used.

TUMOUR in a sinus is usually malignant and can be excised if it is discovered early; otherwise radiotherapy is arranged.

The Pharynx

This is a tube of muscle 15 cms long lined with simple epithelium. Anteriorly it opens into the nose and mouth, and below it is continuous with the oesophagus, but also opens at this point into the larynx. On the posterior wall of the *naso-pharynx* are the *adenoids* which sometimes swell in childhood and interfere with breathing through the nose. The Eustachian tubes to the middle ears begin in the naso-pharynx. In the *ora-pharynx* are the *tonsils* at either side of the throat. These assist in preventing infection from entering the lungs but can themselves become infected. The posterior wall of the pharynx is sensitive and when this is stimulated the body reacts by vomiting or 'retching' (this is a reflex or automatic action). The epiglottis is a flap of cartilage which closes over the larynx during swallowing and prevents food from passing into the air-passages instead of the oesophagus.

IN HEALTH, mouth breathing is discouraged as the mouth and tonsils become dry and possibly infected. Sudden movements or unexpected inhalation during eating may cause an unchewed piece of food to fall backwards from the mouth into the pharynx or larynx. This can be the cause of asphyxia unless the object is removed at once.

IN ILLNESS it is important to keep the pharynx clean and clear from obstruction. This is particularly stressed in the care of the unconscious patient as the reflex actions of coughing and swallowing are both absent. If food or liquid (or any object such as a wool swab) were allowed to enter the throat it would be inhaled and cause either complete or partial asphyxia, or later on a lung infection. In recovery from anaesthesia, vomit is a hazard for this reason. In deep coma the patient produces normal secretions from the lungs which cannot be swallowed and these are removed by placing him in the lateral position and allowing them to flow out of his mouth and by using suction with a catheter.

The tongue is a thick muscle attached to the floor of the mouth. In the unconscious patient the tongue muscle relaxes and it sinks into the pharynx if the patient lies flat on his back. This can produce instant and complete asphyxia. This patient is therefore placed on his side, supported by a pillow at his back if necessary, and with his mouth directed downwards. A pillow under his head and neck prevents twisting at the neck. Pushing the angles of the lower jaw gently forward will assist in bringing the tongue to the front of the mouth.

As the pharynx is a muscular tube, exercise by swallowing assists in keeping the throat healthy. This is another reason for giving a patient *frequent* feeds of fluid or food when he is allowed these. Sucking sweets or lozenges and gargling are also exercises. After tonsillectomy such exercise in the throat assists in preventing infection.

Symptoms and Signs

DYSPNOEA, DISTRESS and CYANOSIS are signs of asphyxia, which should be relieved quickly.

NASAL SPEECH and MOUTH BREATHING are noticed in a child with enlarged adenoids and other conditions such as polyps.

PAIN is a symptom in severe infection of the tonsils, and the throat is *sore* in a less severe infection. There may be a discharge of pus from infected tonsils.

LOSS OF VOICE or HOARSENESS OF VOICE are related to conditions of the larynx including the vocal cords. In whooping cough the pharynx contracts and the characteristic sound 'whoop' is made as the infant breathes in.

Hoarseness of voice is an early sign in carcinoma of larynx.

DYSPHAGIA is pain or difficulty in swallowing. This is sometimes associated with an iron deficiency anaemia which may be followed by a complication in the oesophagus.

Examination of the Throat

This is frequently included in the general examination of a patient as a sore throat is a fairly common sign in a general infection. The doctor requires a *head mirror and lamp* or a *throat torch*. A *tongue depressor* is used to press down the tongue. If the patient says 'Ah...' the tongue flattens. As only the tonsils and the posterior wall of the pharynx can be seen at this point, he may wish to examine the pharynx further and then will use a small round *mirror* fixed to a metal handle. To prevent this from clouding over in the throat it is first warmed and dried by heating over a *Methylated spirit lamp*, then dried with a medical tissue. The surgeon tests the heat of the mirror on his hand to make sure it is not too warm before inserting it into the mouth. Laryngeal mirrors are larger than post-nasal mirrors. When using these the surgeon may grasp the tongue with a gauze square to flatten it.

Investigations

A *throat swab* may be requested for *bacteriological examination*. The swab is fixed on the end of an applicator and is sterilised in a glass tube, sealed with a cork which acts as a holder for the swab applicator. The nurse requires some satisfactory lighting on the patient's mouth and throat and a tongue depressor. If the patient can help by flattening his tongue she can hold a throat torch, otherwise a lamp is necessary. The nurse sits or stands opposite to the patient, she withdraws the swab applicator from its tube and introduces the swab into the mouth without allowing it to touch anything. Then she draws the swab once firmly over the tonsil area, draws out the swab and re-inserts it into the tube, again without contaminating it. It is labelled with the name etc., and despatched to the laboratory with the request form.

The nurse should take care to avoid touching the back of the throat with the wool swab or the patient will 'retch' or vomit.

Conditions of the Throat

ENLARGEMENT OF ADENOIDS is normal in children, but if they cause obstruction or subsequent infection they are removed with the tonsils.

ACUTE TONSILLITIS is an acute infection lasting a few days. The patient is usually in bed a short time with fever. This is treated and aspirin in a solution relieves pain in the throat. It is difficult to swallow food but fluids are necessary. Syrups and hot drinks with honey are comforting but milk and lemon drinks are usually unpleasant.

In a few cases an abscess forms behind the tonsil (quinsey). This is very painful, and the patient cannot open his mouth or swallow, so his saliva collects below his tongue or trickles out. The abscess is incised under a local anaesthetic and the pus escapes through the mouth. Frequent warm mouth washes are given. The tonsils may be removed at a later date.

TONSILLECTOMY. This operation is performed when there are repeated attacks of tonsillitis, or a quinsy, or middle ear diseases (transmitted from the throat through the Eustachian tubes), or occasionally in some generalised infections.

The patient usually has a general anaesthetic and the blood vessels are tied off as the tonsils are removed. If the adenoids are removed at the same time, the vessels cannot be tied off in the same way and there will be some bleeding.

After the operation the patient lies supported in a lateral position so that he cannot roll on to his back with the head facing slightly downwards. He is not left while he is unconscious, and when recovered can sit up in bed. Pallor, rising pulse rate and restlessness are signs of bleeding. The patient may swallow blood when he is semi-conscious; in this case the nurse can see the movements in the throat. Advice would be sought immediately.

A FOREIGN OBJECT IN THE THROAT is sometimes removed by forceps as the surgeon views it through a mirror. Larger irregular objects, e.g. mutton bone, in the oesophagus are removed through the oesophagoscope. Perforation of the oesophagus is a complication and the patient is extremely ill. Open safety pins are very difficult to remove; there is a special instrument which will close the pin first.

In an ACUTE INFLAMMATION OF THE LARYNX, TRACHEA AND BRONCHI, there is stridor when the patient breathes. He is short of breath and cyanosed. To loosen the mucus so that he can breathe more easily, a steam tent is erected or he has inhalations of a respiratory detergent such as Alivaire. Antibiotics are also prescribed. Acute laryngo-tracheo-bronchitis in an infant can cause respiratory obstruction and intubation or tracheostomy is then necessary in addition to the previous treatment.

In *less acute infections*, steam may be administered by Nelson's Inhaler or the household jug. When the temperature is raised the patient is nursed in bed. The patient rests his voice in laryngitis by not talking.

In the early stages of MALIGNANT GROWTH of larynx the voice is hoarse. The disease is diagnosed by biopsy examination, and treated by radiotherapy or occasionally by removal of the larynx. A permanent tracheostomy is necessary in the latter case. Because the vocal cords are now absent the patient cannot talk in the normal way, but he is taught by a speech therapist to speak by forcing air from the stomach into the mouth where his lips, teeth and cheeks attempt to form the words.

In the operation of TRACHEOSTOMY, the surgeon make a 'window' in the trachea. TRACHEOTOMY is a simple incision made quickly to save life in emergency.

Reasons for operation are:

1. Obstruction in the air passages above the trachea, e.g. foreign objects, oedema from burns and scalds of throat, diphtheria, malignant growths in the larynx, surgical removal of larynx.

2. If the patient cannot swallow saliva it collects in the pharynx and is inhaled into the trachea. This occurs in head injuries, poliomyelitis, tetanus, injuries to mouth and larynx.

3. In acute and severe dyspnoea (difficulty in breathing).

The operation is frequently performed under local anaesthetic. A sandbag

P

is placed under the shoulders and the head is tilted back slightly. An incision is made at the base of the neck and then across or along the trachea. A little cocaine hydrochloride may be injected into the trachea so that the patient does not cough at this stage. Blood vessels are ligatured. With the patient's head in the normal position the incision into the trachea is made and the tracheostomy tube inserted. He returns to the ward and sits up in bed, his colour much improved.

To prevent the tube becoming blocked with mucus, it must be cleaned frequently.

(a) If it is a silver inner and outer tube, the outer tube is fixed by tapes tied round the neck by reef knots and is *not* removed by the nurse. The inner tube may be removed, cleaned with sodium bicarbonate solution and a brush or ribbon gauze, sterilised and replaced. The surgeon changes the outer tube about once a week.

(b) When a single tube is used, it is cleaned by passing a sterile catheter attached to a suction machine down in the tube and about 5 cms beyond the end of it. It is withdrawn as soon as the mucus is removed. A few millilitres of normal saline are sometimes injected into the tube to prevent the mucus from becoming too thick.

Should a tube come out, the nurse inserts the dilators just inside the wound until the doctor or sister can re-insert another sterile tube. Satisfactory lighting is necessary.

An emergency basic tracheostomy set, sterilised in sealed packets or box (C.S.S.D.), is always on the ward. With it are various tracheostomy tubes also sterilised in sealed packets and ready for use.

CHAPTER 40 | THE MOUTH

Food enters the mouth, which is the beginning of the alimentary tract This cavity is formed by the upper jaw (maxilla) and the lower jaw (mandible). In these bones grow the teeth. The roof of the mouth is the hard palate and attached to this bone at the back of the mouth is the soft palate of muscle tissue. In the floor of the mouth is the tongue and on either side of the posterior part of the mouth are the tonsils. The lips close the oral cavity at the front. Epithelium lines the mouth and this is kept moist by secretions from the salivary glands and mucus glands. The mouth opens into the pharynx, a muscular tube which also opens into the nose and by the Eustachian tube to the middle ear. From the pharynx also pass the oesophagus to the digestive tract and the larynx to the respiratory tract.

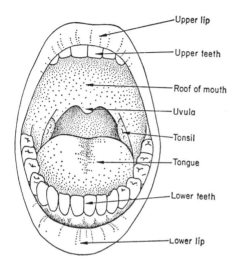

Figure 53. The open mouth.

The *tongue* is composed of striped muscle covered with epithelium which contains taste buds. It is attached to the mandible and a small fragile bone at the top of the throat called the hyoid bone.

The Functions of the Tongue

1. The tongue pushes food between the teeth for mastication.
2. The taste buds, tiny swellings on the surface of the tongue, contain the nerve endings for the sense of taste (bitter, sweet, salt and sour).
3. It is used in speaking.

The first TEETH are twenty in number and begin to appear at about six months of age, the two lower central teeth usually erupting first followed by the two upper central teeth. They are all present normally when the child is two years old, and are called deciduous teeth because they fall out as the child grows older. There are thirty-two permanent teeth (Fig. 54) and these begin to erupt at about the sixth year, pushing out the earlier teeth as they develop. Most of them are present by the twelfth year except the wisdom teeth. These can appear at any time after 18 years, but in a number of people one or more of them do not erupt.

CHART OF THE DECIDUOUS TEETH

Upper right									Upper left
E	D	C	B	A	A	B	C	D	E
E	D	C	B	A	A	B	C	D	E
Lower right									Lower left

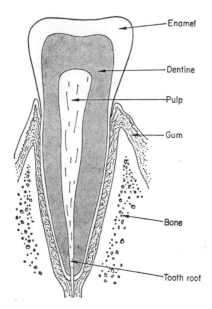

Figure 54. A tooth.

CHART OF THE PERMANENT TEETH

Upper right															Upper left
8	7	6	5	4	3	2	1	1	2	3	4	5	6	7	8
8	7	6	5	4	3	2	1	1	2	3	4	5	6	7	8
Lower right															Lower left

1 and 2 incisors used for biting.
3   canine. Animals use these for tearing food.
4 and 5 pre-molars.
6 and 7 molars used for grinding food.
8   wisdom teeth (molars).

The front teeth bite the food, the tongue pushes it between the molars where it is mixed with saliva and ground up into a soft mass suitable for swallowing. There is some digestion of cooked starches. The teeth are supported in the alveolar bone. The gums surround the neck of each tooth, so that the root of the tooth is not exposed.

The *tonsils* are lymphoid tissue and remove some infection entering the mouth.

There are three pairs of *salivary glands*, the largest of these being the *parotid glands* which lie in front of the ear above the angle of the jaw. The channels (ducts) from these open near the molars in the upper jaw while the ducts from the other salivary glands under the mandible and under the tongue open into the floor of the mouth. Tartar tends to collect on the teeth near these openings, i.e. outside the first molar and inside the lower incisors. It is removed by the dentist.

SALIVA is the liquid produced by the salivary glands. It contains water, mucus and ptyalin, a substance which acts on cooked starches in food when this is chewed.

Care of the Mouth in Health

Development of the jaws depends to some extent on *exercise*, and foods which need to be chewed are useful in the diet from the time the first teeth develop. Chewing also encourages the flow of *saliva* from the salivary glands. Saliva keeps the tissue lining the mouth healthy, and aids speech.

The teeth, like bone, require *calcium and vitamin D* for their development and these two foodstuffs are for this reason essential in the diet of pregnant and lactating women and growing children. Teeth can be harmed by the presence of sugar continually in the mouth, for example when eating sweets and biscuits, and dental decay (caries) may occur. Excess and continual eating of these foods is therefore avoided. Adequate regular meals are advised, and the end of a meal includes a piece of raw apple, carrot, or celery to chew, otherwise the mouth is cleaned with a toothbrush or rinsed with clear water. After the last meal of the day the teeth and gums are brushed to remove particles of food.

Unhealthy gums may shrink and expose the roots of the teeth, and the bone holding them is affected so that they become loose. To prevent this, the gums are brushed frequently with a soft brush unless they bleed easily. Small, thin toothpicks can be used to remove particles of food from between the teeth and massage the gums. Dental salt brushed or massaged over the gums cleanses and tones up the surface tissue.

Regular visits to the dentist, for example at six-monthly intervals, to receive advice and treatment are advisable in maintaining the health of the mouth.

Dentures replace extracted teeth, should fit well and be efficient for biting, chewing and speaking. They are cleaned twice a day using a brush.

Care of the Mouth in Illness

The production of saliva is most important in keeping the mouth healthy, and for this the patient needs adequate fluid intake by mouth or by other routes. Fruit juices, especially lemon, added to water stimulate the flow of saliva. Even though a patient cannot eat and swallow food, he may be able to chew a little fruit like raw apple, peeled grapes or a piece of pineapple and then expectorate it into a bowl. Chewing gum is another method of increasing the flow of saliva into the mouth.

In fever, or when the patient breathes through his mouth or his fluid intake is not sufficient, the mouth becomes dry. It is uncomfortable, the patient cannot speak easily and his food and drinks are unappetising because his sense of taste is lessened. Mucus and food particles collect at the back of the tongue on the hard palate, on the teeth and inside the cheeks as 'sordes'. Infection of the mouth is possible and this may have serious consequences if the infection spreads to a parotid gland, causing parotitis, or to the lungs, causing pneumonia. The main object in the care of the mouth is to keep it clean and moist.

1. Frequent rinsing of the mouth with a mouthwash is refreshing and keeps it moist.

2. Brushing the teeth and gums using a medium or soft toothbrush, toothpaste or powder, followed by a mouthwash, can be performed by the patient when he is well enough. If he is incapacitated, e.g. with bandaged or paralysed hands, the nurse can brush his teeth for him, allowing the fluid to flow out of his mouth into a bowl. This method of cleaning the mouth is unsuitable for patients who cannot swallow, have paralysis or infections of the throat or who are unconscious.

Electric toothbrushes are now available. There is a handle which contains the battery. Each patient has his own brushhead.

3. The mouth can be cleaned using dental squares damped with cleansing lotions and attached to swab-holding clip forceps. It is essential to use the clip forceps in which the squares can be held firmly when the patient is unconscious as he has no cough reflex and a loose wisp of cotton in the mouth can be inhaled. A torch is useful when inspecting the mouth and a wooden tongue depressor employed when viewing or cleaning inside the cheeks and the back of the tongue. White vaseline applied

thinly to the lips prevents them from becoming dry, sore or cracked. When the patient cannot hold his mouth open, a mouth gag is held between the molars.

4. Mouth irrigation is necessary after operations on the mouth or special treatment, e.g. radium insertion into the tongue, or while the lower jaw is wired to the upper jaw to immobilise fractures. 500 ml. of lotion such as glycothymoline 1 in 4 is prepared at 38°C and small amounts of this are injected into the mouth using an irrigation syringe or a Higginson's syringe with a metal tube or cannula attached to it. The patient lies on his side and as the fluid is injected into one side of the mouth it flows out at the other lower side into a receiver. This is not a safe procedure when the patient is unconscious.

Care of the Mouth and Teeth

Reasons for Keeping the Mouth and Teeth in a Healthy Condition
The appetite and enjoyment in eating food are improved. Digestion is aided by adequate production of saliva, which is the natural liquid in the mouth, and the mixing of this with the food during chewing. Discomfort in the mouth discourages the person from chewing food.

Certain conditions are less likely to occur in a healthy mouth such as halitosis (unpleasant breath), gingivitis (inflammation of the gums), carious (decayed) teeth.

The mouth is a cavity which opens into the digestive tract and the lungs. Ducts from the salivary glands open into the mouth. Infection of the mouth can result in infection in these parts of the body.

The Patient's Mouth and Teeth
In illness, particularly fevers, the mouth becomes dry and unpleasant. This occurs also when the patient in respiratory distress breathes through his mouth as in pneumonia or congestive heart failure. Dryness of the mouth prevents the appreciation of taste. Loss of the sense of taste removes pleasure in eating food. Speech is altered as the mouth becomes very dry, and a harsh croak will replace intelligible words when the mouth is neglected. The patient with a sore mouth cannot tolerate food in the mouth.

One complication of an infected mouth is the inhalation by the patient of infectious material. This may result in lung infection. Inflammation of the parotid salivary glands is called parotitis and this may also complicate an infected mouth.

Care of Patient's Mouth and Teeth

The principle of this treatment is to keep the mouth moist and clean.

Whenever possible the patient cleans his own teeth. Mouth cleaning is done twice a day at least, i.e. morning and evening, and after all meals if possible.

(a) If the patient can go to the bathroom he cleans his mouth there, but it is helpful for the nurse to make sure this has been done. Some health education may be necessary if the patient has not been in the habit of caring for his mouth and teeth.

(b) The patient in bed who is able to brush his teeth and gums needs the following articles:

    Beaker containing mouthwash.

    Toothbrush with medium or soft bristles.

    Tooth powder or paste.

    Bowl or receiver.

    Face towel.

(c) If he is unable to clean his teeth then this is done by the nurse. An electric toothbrush may be available.

Cleaning the mouth of an ill patient who is conscious but unable to brush his teeth and gums or have them brushed by the nurse.

The nurse explains to the patient what she about to do and places his *face towel* below his chin. His co-operation is essential so that he opens his mouth as necessary. A *torch* is useful when inspecting the mouth and a *tongue depressor* can be employed to view the inside of the cheeks and the back of the tongue. With clean hands the nurse attaches dental squares damped with *cleansing lotions* to *swab-holding* or *clip forceps*. The squares can be damped by rolling them in a towel, pouring water over the towel then wringing it out. The squares are removed and are ready for use. Suitable lotions include *sodium bicarbonate* 1 teaspoonful to 600 mls water which dissolves mucus, and *glycothymoline* 1 in 8.

Some routine in cleaning the mouth is useful.

(a) The tongue is cleaned first with strokes from side to side, making sure the back of the tongue is clean. (Swabbing the tongue from front to back may cause the patient to retch or vomit.)

(b) Then the upper teeth, inner and outer surfaces of the upper jaw.

(c) Then the lower teeth, inner and outer surfaces of the lower jaw.

(d) Inside the cheeks. Food collects here.

(e) The roof of the mouth, and the floor if necessary.

A little glycerine and lemon in the mouth may assist in keeping it moist but is uncomfortable in a sore throat. White vaseline or lanoline can be applied thinly to the lips to prevent them from becoming dry, sore and cracked.

The nurse may assist the patient in using a mouthwash when she has cleaned his mouth with squares. This is more refreshing for him and helps towards keeping the mouth moist besides providing him with a little activity and feeling of independence. It is unwise, however, for him to use a mouthwash if he has difficulty with breathing or any paralysis of the throat.

The Cleaning of the Mouth of a Patient who is Unconscious or Mentally Confused

A mouth gag may be required to open the patient's mouth. It is placed between the molars or back teeth. Dental squares are held firmly in swab-holding or clip forceps. The mouthwash is not used.

After treating the mouth equipment is disinfected or placed in a bag for disposal.

Mouth toilet is carried out every two or four hours, before and after meals, for these patients:

(a) very ill or unconscious patients;

(b) those with high fever;

(c) those who have fluid diets, or are being fed by tube or who cannot have food by mouth;

(d) those with infections of, or operations on the mouth.

Care of Dentures

Dentures are cleaned with the patient's toothbrush and toothpaste or a special denture brush and are rinsed in cold water. When a patient is not able to wear his dentures, they are kept in a labelled container in his locker.

Patients who are unconscious or about to have a general anaesthetic do not have dentures in the mouth as the denture may obstruct the throat. The nurse will find that the patient's lower dentures are removed easily; the upper denture is attached to the roof of the mouth by suction and to release it, the nurse can press upwards on the back of the plate; this removes the suction and the dentures can be taken out. Plates which support one or two teeth are fragile and require careful handling as indeed do all dentures.

Unless there is a definite reason for the patient not wearing his dentures, the nurse should enable him to have them, for they are important in his appearance, speech, taking food and general self-respect.

Crowned Teeth

The crown of the tooth has been damaged. The tooth is filed down to a suitable shape and size. A crown is made to fit the base and appear as the original tooth, and this is fixed in position using an adhesive. During a general anaesthetic, part of the equipment is placed in the mouth and special care is required when there are crowned teeth. On the patient's

P*

notes should be noted clearly N.B. CROWNED TEETH, so that medical and nursing staff are aware of the situation.

Observations of the Mouth

The mouth may be dry and the tongue brown and coated. In some cases there is an offensive smell. The gums may bleed and inflammation is sometimes associated with extreme tenderness of the gums. The teeth may be unhealthy or decayed and occasionally broken, discoloured or absent. White patches inside the cheeks occur in thrush, which is an infectious condition, sometimes seen in the mouths of infants. The tonsils may be red, swollen, inflamed.

The condition of the mouth is related to many general diseases and its examination is therefore included in a general examination of the patient. The mouth is dry when there is dehydration, the tongue is brown and coated in some acute abdominal illnesses, the tongue is flat and red in pernicious anaemia. Koplik spots are seen inside the cheeks in measles. Bleeding of the gums sometimes accompanies a disease of the blood. Ulcers in the mouth may follow some minor damage to the epithelium, for example from dry toast or the common cold, but more severe forms result from infection in the mouth and throat or malignant growths, e.g. on the tongue.

Examination and Investigations

The procedure is the same as for the examination of the throat as described on page 435.

There are many methods of investigation.

X-rays of the teeth and their supporting bone, demonstrating conditions affecting the alveolar bone and any retained roots of teeth. Fractures involving the maxilla and mandible are shown in X-ray photographs.

Blood investigations are carried out when there has been excessive haemorrhage, following extraction of teeth or when a disease of the blood is suspected associated with bleeding from the gums. When abnormal tissue is observed in the mouth the surgeon removes a small amount for examination under the microscope. This is a *biopsy*. Should infection in the mouth be suspected, a swab of the infectious material is sent to the bacteriological laboratory so that the infecting organism may be identified. At the same time tests are made by which it will be known whether the bacteria are penicillin sensitive. If this is found the patient's treatment includes penicillin injections. Otherwise *sensitivity tests* are made with other antibiotics to ascertain which will be most useful.

Aspiration of abscess in the mouth is carried out by the doctor with a sterile needle and syringe, and the fluid obtained is collected in a sterile container to be examined later in the laboratory.

Medical and Surgical Conditions of the Teeth

DENTAL CARIES results in cavities in the teeth. 'Filling the teeth', i.e. conservation of teeth, is performed by the dental surgeon. The cavities are cleaned by drilling and then they are filled with a substance which sets very hard, after which the filling is polished. Unless the pulp of the tooth is affected there is no pain, though the drill vibration may cause a little discomfort, and a local anaesthetic is rarely needed. Deeper cavities may penetrate to the pulp and the inflammation causes toothache.

TEETH EXTRACTION is carried out under local anaesthetic. If there is infection some type of general anaesthetic is administered and the patient's consent for this is obtained. More complicated teeth, e.g. unerupted wisdoms, may be removed by a surgical operation. During this operation a tube is passed through the mouth into the trachea and the anaesthetic is administered with oxygen by this endotracheal tube. This prevents the inhalation of blood.

Inflammation of the pulp following dental caries may cause an ABSCESS at the apex of the tooth which tracks through the bone and causes swelling in the soft tissue of the face. Bacteria and toxins may enter the patient's blood stream and these can be a cause of disease elsewhere in the body. Usually the infection is controlled before the tooth is removed or at the time of its removal. Appropriate antibiotics are prescribed for administration by intramuscular injection.

An antrum (air space in a bone of the cheek) may be infected from upper molar teeth.

GINGIVITIS is inflammation of the gum, in some cases due to lack of oral hygiene. In one severe form there is acute ulceration accompanied by intense swelling of the face; this is called *Vincent's angina*.

HAEMORRHAGE occurs following an extraction. Extensive haemorrhage is controlled by pressure over the bleeding point in the form of a firm pad, e.g. a roll of bandage. This is placed so that it projects above the level of the teeth on either side of the bleeding point. The patient bites on the pad, which is then pressed on to the bleeding point. If the bleeding continues the socket is sutured by the surgeon.

Bleeding after a tooth extraction is excessive in a patient with *haemophilia*, a disease in which the blood lacks a blood-clotting factor. The patient has blood and plasma infusions before and after the operation.

CARCINOMA is a disease of the mouth which begins at the side of the tongue, sometimes after continuous pipe-smoking or by irritation by broken or carious teeth, or occasionally on the floor of the mouth when there have been inadequate or poor dentures. The type of carcinoma which begins in an antrum causes a swelling in the mouth.

There are many forms of treatment including surgery and radiotherapy and treatment is successful if the condition is observed and diagnosed early.

FRACTURES involving the jaws are due to direct violence, for example, when a motor car occupant is thrown forward on to the windscreen when the vehicle stops suddenly, or a blow on the face.

Treatment of Fracture of the Mandible (lower jaw)

This injury may be complicated by fractured bone penetrating into a tooth socket, and there is a wound into the mouth. This is a compound fracture and infection is possible.

The tongue is not firmly anchored in the mouth when the mandible to which it is attached is fractured. It may obstruct the air-passages, particularly if the patient lies on his back and the jaw is unsupported.

The injury is extremely painful and the patient suffers from some degree of shock.

Treatment is by reduction of the fracture under general anaesthetic. Fixation (immobilisation) is by fastening the teeth of the lower jaw to those of the upper jaw either by metal splints or by 'eyelet wiring'. In the latter, metal caps are cemented to the crowns of the teeth. Hooks in the crown splints opposite to each other are tied together or secured by rubber bands. Sometimes the fractured ends of bone are wired together internally (interosseus wiring).

With regard to displacements of the maxilla (upper jaw), when reduction has been completed the fractured bone is fixed by means of wires or rods to a plaster head cap.

The patient being treated by one of these methods cannot open his mouth and is therefore prevented from eating or speaking. His nutrition is maintained by the provision of a diet containing the normal amount of foods but in a liquid or semi-liquid form. Most of the menu for the general patients can be reduced to pulp by using an electric mixing machine. A gap is allowed between the jaws by removal of a tooth if necessary and the patient is fed or feeds himself through this opening either by a tube or preferably from a narrow spoon. Some patience is required by the patient as taking a meal may be a lengthy procedure but usually he becomes skilful in the procedure. Clear water is given at the end of the meal and utensils must be scrupulously clean. The mouth is irrigated after each meal or every four hours.

The patient finds the inability to eat and talk frustrating and becomes easily depressed. It is likely he is concerned about the results of the injury. If he can meet another patient who has been in a similiar situation and made a satisfactory recovery, the patient will be more confident and optimistic. He is encouraged to get up and walk in the ward when his general condition allows this, and is encouraged to become as independent as possible in the circumstances.

Occupational therapy helps the patient by providing some physical activity and an interest which does not necessitate speaking.

OPERATIONS ON THE JAW include removal of inflamed gum margins round the teeth, and removal of unerupted wisdom teeth. The surgeon may request the application of heat pads to the face before he incises an abscess.

Following these operations there may be haemorrhage or oedema and treatment includes the application of icebags to the face.

CHAPTER 41 | REGULATION OF BODY TEMPERATURE

In spite of varying temperatures in the environment, as when bathing in a cold sea or working near furnaces in an iron foundry, the temperature of the body remains at a fairly constant level of 37°C. *This temperature represents a balance between heat produced by the body and heat lost from the body*, and the balance is controlled (like a thermostat in a central heating system) by the heat-regulating centre at the base of the brain. Blood transports heat round the body, again like a central heating system in which hot water circulating through pipes warms the air in different rooms.

When the temperature of the air round the body falls, nerve endings in the skin are stimulated and impulses pass to the heat-regulating centre in the brain. Following this the body mechanisms which produce heat become more active. On the other hand, when the body is producing heat in excess the heat-regulating centre causes the mechanisms for cooling the body to come into action.

Heat is produced in the body as a result of *metabolism in the tissue cells*, i.e. the conversion of foodstuffs and oxygen into carbon dioxide, water and urea to provide cell energy. The faster the rate of metabolism the more heat is produced. (This happens in thyrotoxicosis and infections.)

Active organs like the *heart, diaphragm and liver* produce heat continually. During exercise *contraction of skeletal muscles* releases a great deal of heat in the body.

When the body is exposed to cold and is stimulated to produce more heat, it responds by '*shivering*'; this is uncontrolled contraction of skeletal muscles in an effort to produce heat. Otherwise the person may stamp his feet or fling his arms out and then across his chest—this is also muscle action. Children playing energetic games do not feel the cold. The patient in bed is inactive and does not tolerate a lower temperature as well as the nurse who is busy in the ward. The least active of people, like a newly born infant or an elderly man or woman, produce much less heat than an energetic healthy child or adult, and therefore need more protection against cold.

Heat loss occurs from the surface of the skin by:

radiation when heat rays leaving the body pass through the air and fall on to another object. The body loses heat, and the air and the object become warm.

conduction when heat passes between objects in contact with each other. A person lying on the cold ground loses heat rapidly.

convection in which heat rises from the warm skin, air currents are formed and heat passes in this movement of air to other objects.

These methods are assisted by blood being brought to the surface of the skin by dilation of the arterioles; the skin becomes flushed when the person is hot and more heat is then lost through the skin.

The *evaporation of sweat* from the skin is the method by which most heat loss occurs. As the water changes into water vapour (i.e. a fluid into a gas) heat is absorbed from the object on which this takes place. Sweat is secreted by glands in the skin and about 600 ml is produced each day without the person being aware of it. This is known as *insensible sweating*. During active exercise the amount of sweat secreted (stimulated from the heat-regulating centre) can increase to 3000 ml (3 litres) in one hour, and the patient is conscious of sweating. This is known as *visible sweating*.

The rate at which sweating takes place is increased by a greater flow of blood to the skin and by movement of cool dry air over the surface of the body. When the air surrounding the body contains water vapour to excess, sweating becomes more difficult and no sweating can take place when the air is saturated with water. If the air is warm (over 27°C), and saturated (humid), then *heat stroke* may occur. The heat-regulating centre is out of order and the body temperature rises with that of the environment. The situation is serious and demands immediate treatment.

Heat is lost from the body also in the exhaled breath during respiration and a little in urine and faeces.

When the temperature of the environment is very low, heat loss is prevented in a number of ways.

The smooth muscle fibres in the skin contract, causing the hairs to stand upright; this is 'goose flesh' and it is an effort to keep the warmed air near to the body.

The smooth muscle in the walls of the arterioles contracts, preventing blood passing into the skin where its heat would be lost through the skin. The individual is pale and his skin is cold.

He lies 'curled up' to conserve heat so that as little body surface as possible is exposed to cold air, particularly in the axillae and groins where blood vessels are immediately below the skin.

Clothing prevents loss of heat and the most efficient garments from this point of view are those which entrap warm air round the body, such as wool, furs and cellular materials. Leather is warm because it shields the body from moving cold air. Plastics and rubber do this very competently too, but they are waterproof and water vapour collects inside garments of these materials, preventing evaporation of sweat from the skin. The wearer begins to feel extremely hot and uncomfortable.

When the temperature of the environment is very high, loss of heat from the body is hastened by:

(i) removal of close-fitting garments to allow exposure of the skin to cool air;

(ii) lying relaxed with the limbs slightly separated from the trunk so that cool air circulates over as much skin as possible;

(iii) increased ventilation by opening windows or using a fan;

(iv) extra cold or iced water to drink, increasing *cool* blood in circulation;

(v) alternatively, encouraging more blood to circulate through the skin and increase sweating by giving hot drinks of tea or lemon. Alcohol has a similar effect and the 'warming' effect is largely temporary. Some foods like mustard and curries also encourage sweating;

(vi) sponging the skin with water; a thin film of moisture left on the skin to evaporate cools the body quickly (as does profuse sweating);

(vii) bathing in the cool sea, or in treatment a cold wet pack (p. 453).

Reduction of Temperature

PYREXIA is a raised body temperature 37°C to 40°C (98·8°F to 103°F). The causes include inflammation and infection of tissues, and the patient feels hot and uncomfortable with headache, thirst and slight delirium at night.

Simple Methods of Cooling the Patient

Heavy bed-clothes are removed.

Thinner night-wear is used by the patient.

Windows may be opened or electric fans are placed by the bed.

A bed cradle is placed directly over the patient.

It may be possible to use a balcony room which is cooler than the main ward.

The patient is protected from direct sunlight by sun-blinds or a sun-shade.

Extra fluids are given, especially iced drinks with fruit juice, such as orange and lemon.

A cold compress on the forehead. This is a single layer of thin cotton material lightly wrung out in cold water.

Simple sponging of the skin.

HYPERPYREXIA is 41°C or a temperature raised above this.

The causes include:

(a) INFECTIONS, e.g. lobar pneumonia, malaria, septicaemia, typhoid fever.

(b) HEAT STROKE in which the heat-regulating centre of the brain fails. This follows the exposure of the body to raised temperature and humidity accompanied by lack of ventilation. The body is no longer cooled when evaporation of sweat from the skin ceases.

(c) HEAD INJURIES AND CRANIAL SURGERY, when the base of the brain is involved and the heat-regulating centre does not function correctly. Appropriate *simple methods* of cooling the body are used, and treatments ordered by the doctor may include *tepid sponging*, or *cold wet packs*.

Nursing Treatments to Reduce the Temperature

SIMPLE SPONGING OF THE SKIN means sponging the patient's face, then his body in sections, the upper limbs, lower limbs and trunk, using warm water and two sponges or flannels, one for the face and the other for the body. The skin is mopped dry with a towel, not rubbed to cause friction which would increase warmth in the body. Soap is unnecessary as the skin is clean. The time necessary for carrying out the procedure should be only ten to fifteen minutes, and the patient is made comfortable afterwards with clean bed and personal linen. A little eau de cologne or skin talcum powder applied to the body is also cooling and refreshing. Insomnia caused by pyrexia can often be relieved by this simple treatment and the patient immediately falls asleep. The night nurse will observe this when the feverish patient is sponged and made comfortable early in the morning, and then he sleeps until breakfast time.

TEPID SPONGING. The patient is suffering from an infection or a disturbance of the heat-regulating centre and his temperature is between 38·4°C and 40·6°C. His condition may change rapidly and the nurse observes the colour of his skin and his general behaviour throughout the procedure.

The doctor or sister indicates what the body temperature should be on completion of the tepid sponging. This is usually 1·6°C below his present temperature; for example, if his temperature is now 40°C this is expected to fall to 38·4°C but not below that level. To reduce the temperature during generalised infection suddenly to normal predisposes a state of collapse.

The patient's body will be sponged over with tepid water 27°C so that a thin film of water is left on the skin to evaporate, thereby taking heat from the surface of the body. He is undressed and lies between sheets. His face is sponged and dried. A piece of disposable towel lightly wrung out in water and placed on the forehead is cooling. Six plastic sponges or disposable flannels are used and four of these are moistened thoroughly in the tepid water and placed in the axillae and groins where blood vessels are close to the skin. The limbs in rotation are sponged, using about 8 or 10 long strokes away from the trunk and water is left on the skin to evaporate. The sponge becomes warm and so is then placed in a bowl of cold 15°C water to cool it before being immersed again in tepid water. Ice may be needed to cool the water sufficiently. The chest, abdomen and back are treated also. The sponges in the axillae and groins are changed when they become warmed. The patient's temperature is taken and as soon as it is 1°C below the previous temperature, the nurse stops sponging as the level will continue to fall further for a few minutes. She mops excess water from the skin and makes the patient comfortable, changing bed-linen and renewing personal clothes. The temperature is taken 10 minutes after the procedure and this is recorded on the temperature chart, with a reference to 'tepid sponging'.

The treatment lasts 20 to 30 minutes. Should the patient become very pale and cold and lies weakly in bed, sponging is stopped immediately. Blankets are put over the patient and he is warmed gradually. Later he may have a warm drink but stimulants like alcohol are peripheral dilators and should be avoided. The doctor or sister is informed, and will be told the patient's temperature. Tepid sponging can be carried out twice a day and is particularly useful in the evening so that the patient has more restful sleep. When the heat-regulating centre is disturbed this treatment may be ordered every four hours.

COLD WET PACK. When the patient's temperature is extremely high, above 40°C, more drastic treatment is necessary. This is usually in head injuries or heat stroke and the object is to reduce the temperature to between normal and 38°C. The mattress is well protected by waterproof covers and is covered by a sheet. The patient is undressed and lies on this covered by a second sheet. This latter during the procedure is replaced by a sheet wrung out in cold water 15°C, and this is placed closely against the skin over as large an area as possible. An electric fan or the draught from a window will hasten the evaporation of water from the surface of the body with its cooling effect. Rectal temperatures are taken and recorded; these are more accurate than mouth temperatures and convenient when the patient is unconscious. The treatment may be continued indefinitely until the need has passed, changing the sheets at least once a day. Should the sheets dry quickly, they are kept moist by replacing them or spraying with water. A greater cooling effect is obtained by placing large cubes of ice near the body but *not* touching it to cause pressure.

Basic nursing care is continued throughout. This treatment is also used to reduce the temperature in a patient with head injuries and brain damage to sub-normal, i.e. hypothermia, so that his metabolism is slower. A 'subnormal' thermometer which records to 30°C is required to assess the patient's rectal temperature.

A simpler method of cooling a patient is to cover the patient in his nightclothes by two large cradles. Over these is placed a sheet turned back at the top and bottom of the bed, to allow a current of air to pass through the cradles over the patient. A fan at the bottom of the bed will increase the draught.

This treatment can be continued until the patient shows signs of improvement.

Hypothermia

In this state the body temperature is below normal, 24°C to 35°C and this occurs when the body produces little heat and is exposed to cold.

During hypothermia the rate of metabolism is lowered, and the brain requires less oxygen. This fact is made use of in short operations on the heart and major blood vessels of the heart, when the blood supply to the brain is reduced during the operation. The actual operation on the heart on these occasions takes about six minutes.

To produce hypothermia in these operative cases, the patient is placed in a cold bath or pack after being anaesthetised. The effect is increased by drugs such as CHLORPROMAZINE.

The patient with head injuries may be treated by application of a cold wet pack which will cause his temperature to fall to 32°C, and his need for oxygen and foodstuffs will become less. This is an advantage while he is deeply unconscious and the brain is suffering from the effects of the injury. It is in progress from one to three weeks.

Accidental Hypothermia

Young infants and elderly men and women who are exposed to cold in severe winter conditions without adequate clothing, shelter and indoor heating, react by becoming drowsy, then stuperose and finally comatose. The temperature is below normal and may be as low as 24°C; a special rectal thermometer for recording low temperature is necessary to confirm it. The babies are rigid and cold to touch, and in advanced cases oedema is present. In both age groups the situation is serious. The elderly person living alone may have been in this condition for some time.

The infant in accidental hypothermia is admitted to hospital, undressed and placed in an incubator at 20°C. *It is important that the body temperature is raised slowly.* The temperature within the incubator is raised to 32°C, during three to four days. He remains in the incubator two or three more days, and can then be brought into the nursery or ward where the temperature is 20°C. Oesophageal feeding is in progress beginning with 1 teaspoon of sugar in 150 ml of water, and increasing to his normal diet in seven to ten days. The usual basic nursing is continued throughout.

An elderly patient is admitted into bed in a ward temperature of 19°C and covered by one sheet and one blanket. He is not given warm fluids. *It is important not to warm the patient too quickly.* Rectal temperatures are recorded hourly, and the treatment continues until the temperature has risen to a level between 32°C to 35°C. General basic nursing care of the patient is resumed and the temperature will continue to rise until it is normal.

CHAPTER 42 | THE ENDOCRINE GLANDS

The organisation of and co-operation between the body's function is brought about in two ways:
   (a) through the nervous system;
   (b) by special substances in the blood called *hormones*.

HORMONES are produced by ductless glands which form the *endocrine system* (Fig. 55), and the substances pass directly into the blood stream. Their general function is the co-ordination and balance between the various cell activities in the body. They act either directly on tissue, or through other glands, or upon the nervous system.

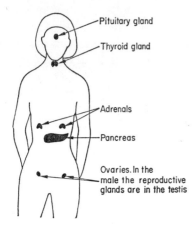

Pituitary gland

Thyroid gland

Adrenals

Pancreas

Ovaries. In the male the reproductive glands are in the testis

Figure 55. The endocrine organs.

The **pituitary gland** is about the size of a pea, situated at the base of the brain and attached to it by a stem. It develops as two parts with different functions. The *anterior lobe* secretes a number of hormones, one of which controls growth, and others which influence the thyroid gland, the adrenal glands and the sex glands.

Oversecretion of the growth hormone, e.g. due to a tumour in childhood, leads to *gigantism*, the child though tall is physically weak. If this over-secretion occurs in an adult the bones of the hands and feet and the lower jaw enlarge in thickness and in length, and the skin also becomes thickened. This is *acromegaly*.

Undersecretion of the anterior pituitary hormones leads to multiple hormone deficiencies elsewhere in the body and is called Simmonds' disease

The *posterior lobe* of the pituitary gland secretes a hormone which prevents the passing of much urine (the antidiuretic hormone). It pro-duces other hormones which cause contraction of other unstriped muscle, e.g. intestine.

Damage of the posterior lobe of the pituitary, usually by a tumour, results in a lack of the antidiuretic hormone and causes the disease

Diabetes Insipidus. To compensate for the high output of fluid in urine, the patient drinks vast quantities of water. Treatment is by hormone drugs or surgical removal.

A pituitary tumour may be removed by the surgeon either through the skull or through the roof of the nose. Occasionally the tumour is made inactive by radiotherapy.

In the treatment following the operation or radiotherapy, hormones, normally produced by the pituitary or stimulated by them, are replaced by appropriate drugs, e.g. cortisone, thyroid extract, sex hormones.

The **adrenal glands,** two in number, are situated above the kidneys but have nothing to do with these organs. Each gland is composed of two parts acting independently of each other; the outer part is the CORTEX, and the inner part is the MEDULLA.

The ADRENAL CORTEX produces hormones called *steroids.* These hormones have various functions.

    1. Control the use of salt (sodium chloride) in the body.

    2. Influence the use of sugar in the body.

    3. Encourage bone and muscle growth.

    4. Reduce sensitivity (allergic) reactions and interfere with tissue reaction to infection.

    5. Increase energy output, and help to prevent muscle fatigue.

Hormones produced by the adrenal cortex are essential to life.

DISORDERS OF THE ADRENAL CORTEX

Undersecretion of the Cortex Hormones

Atrophy (wasting) of the glands can occur suddenly and for no known reason, producing a condition known as Addison's disease. The patient becomes extremely weak, suffers from cramps in the legs and his blood pressure is very low. Brown pigmentation is observed in the skin and the mucous membrane of the mouth. Attacks or crises occur with extreme weakness, abdominal pain, vomiting and dehydration. The disease when diagnosed is treated by cortisone. Extra salt is often given by mouth. Intravenous infusion of saline relieves the dehydration and lack of salt.

Oversecretion of the Cortico-steroids

This is due to a tumour or overgrowth of the adrenal cortex. The patient becomes obese, particularly in the face and trunk, but there is muscle wasting, and the blood pressure may be raised.

Cortisone, a steroid or adrenal hormone, is administered as tablets by mouth or by injection. It is prescribed in a variety of diseases such as rheumatoid arthritis, acute leukaemia, in severe status asthmaticus, ulcerative colitis, and in allergic reactions. Cortisone is also necessary as treatment when there is a deficiency in the production of adrenal or pituitary hormones.

There are side-effects to the administration of this drug.

The side-effects include oedema and care of the skin, the face becomes moon-shaped, the blood pressure may be raised or sugar passed in the urine.

The nurse observes the patient's general appearance, and tests his urine. The blood pressure and electrolyte balance in the blood are checked by the doctor.

The patient who takes cortisone at home is given instructions on a card which also contains details of the patient's name, his general practitioner, and the hospital which he attends, and of the drug dosage— steroid treatment must not be stopped suddenly. He keeps a reserve supply and should be seen immediately by a doctor in sudden illness or accident.

Hydrocortisone, prednisone, prednisolone and fludrocortisone are other steroid drugs and are used as treatment on similar occasions.

The ADRENAL MEDULLA produces two hormones, adrenaline and nor-adrenaline, both of which stimulate the body to survive in an emergency. *The Effects of Adrenaline in the Body are:*
   (a) the heartbeat becomes faster and more forcible;
   (b) blood pressure rises;
   (c) the face becomes pale;
   (d) respiration is deeper and quicker;
   (e) carbohydrates supplied from the liver are increased, and the
       blood sugar rises.

The main effect of nor-adrenaline is to raise the blood pressure. Adrenal medulla is not essential to life.

ADRENALECTOMY is sometimes performed for patients with secondary growths from carcinoma.

Uses of ADRENALINE *(synthetic) as a Treatment*
Synthetic means that the drug is made in a laboratory. Adrenaline is destroyed in the stomach and therefore is given by injection into the subcutaneous tissue, or into muscle. The absorption and effect are rapid. In acute attacks of bronchial asthma, an injection of adrenaline dilates the bronchioles by causing the smooth muscle in these to relax. The patient breathes out more easily. In skin rashes due to hypersensitivity (allergic reactions), e.g. URTICARIA, adrenaline causes constriction of the blood vessels in the skin and thus reduces the oedema or swelling.

Adrenaline is used also in connection with local anaesthetics, e.g.

cocaine on mucous membranes, as it assists in keeping the local anaesthetic to the prescribed area.

NOR-ADRENALINE (also synthetic) is used in treatment of various forms of shock when the blood pressure is extremely low. It is administered in a slow intravenous infusion with normal saline. Observation of the patient during the procedure is important, the rate of blood pressure may vary considerably and the contents and rate of flow in the infusion are altered accordingly by the doctor.

The THYROID GLAND is formed of two parts joined by a short narrow band. It is situated below the thyroid cartilage of the larynx in the lower part of the neck. A hormone *Thyroxine* is produced which contains iodine, and this is the only use to which iodine is put in the body. When the blood level of thyroxine falls an anterior pituitary hormone stimulates the thyroid to produce more thyroxine. The thyroid hormone controls cell processes in the body and influences the normal growth and development in young children.

OBSERVATIONS in patients with suspected thyroid disorders include his weight, the skin, pulse rate, temperature, and general behaviour—which may vary between intense excitability and lethargy.

The patient's relatives can give useful information when the patient himself has not noticed any change and the medical and nursing staffs have not previously known the patient. Sometimes photographs assist, and are also useful in checking future progress.

CLINICAL INVESTIGATIONS
Basal metabolic rate is the rate at which activity in the cells takes place when the body is at rest. The test is carried out in a special quiet room, and the patient has not recently been active or excited. It is a skilled procedure, requiring care in management, and other tests now being used are:

1. Measurement of the level of circulating thyroid hormone in the blood.
2. Radioactive uptake.

Radioactive iodine uptake. The only part of the body which uses iodine is the thyroid gland. When a small amount of radioactive iodine is taken by the patient by mouth, it reaches the thyroid gland. The speed with which it is picked up and used by the gland shows the activity of the gland.

DISORDERS OF THE THYROID GLAND
Undersecretion of the Thyroxine can be present in the very young infant although it is not common. The child does not develop normally. He

would become a dwarf, mentally and physically slow, with a thick tongue protruding from his mouth which causes saliva to escape. This condition is known as *cretinism* and is treated with thyroid extract as soon as it is diagnosed. If treated very early, the child can develop to an average physical and mental level, but the treatment must be continued throughout life.

At middle age the thyroid gland secretion may become reduced and the person (more commonly a woman) becomes heavy and obese, her hair is thin, and her face appears puffy. She is lethargic and consequently is careless of her general appearance. This condition of *myxoedema* is successfully treated with thyroid tablets, but the medicines will be required permanently.

Iodine deficiency in the diet occurs in places far from the sea because most of the available iodine is obtained from sea foods, i.e. sea fish, and vegetables and plants grown near to the sea. The thyroid gland tries to overcome this deficiency of iodine by growing larger, and the person has a *goitre* which appears as an increasing swelling in the lower part of the neck. The main problem is of pressure on structures in the neck and unsightliness of the goitre. In England this condition occurred in Derbyshire and became known as 'Derbyshire Neck'. To prevent this deficiency, a small amount of iodine is included in some table salts, so no one taking this type of salt with food is likely to develop a goitre.

During adolescence the endocrine glands take a little time to attain a true balance of secretions, and during this time a slight enlargement of the thyroid may be seen.

Oversecretion of the thyroid gland causes *Thyrotoxicosis* and this condition occurs in both men and women. The metabolic rate is raised. The patient is hot, the skin moist or sweating, so she wears thin night-clothes for comfort and it is obvious that she has lost weight. She sits up in bed appearing anxious and apprehensive, and this picture is more striking when the eyes protrude and give the face a staring expression. This protrusion of the eyes is *exophthalmos,* and the white of the eye can be seen surrounding the iris. Sometimes she cannot close her eyes completely at night and in this extreme situation care must be exercised in keeping the exposed cornea moist to prevent corneal ulceration.

In untreated cases, the patient's temperature is raised, and the pulse rate is fast even while sleeping. Even though she is losing weight her appetite is large, for she is burning up food quickly. This is an illustration of advanced thyrotoxicosis which can affect the heart, eventually causing atrial fibrillation (a disorganisation of the heart muscle contraction) and heart failure. Occasionally the excitability becomes uncontrollable and special nursing is required. At the present time, a patient presenting early symptoms is examined and a basal metabolic rate assessed.

The treatment varies according to the patient. It may be prescribed in the form of drugs. *Neomercasyl* or *Thiouracil* is a drug which reduces the production of thyroxine. Administration needs to be continued and the dose is carefully assessed. Radioactive iodine is sometimes used in the treatment of women after the child-bearing age and particularly when there are signs of heart failure.

Surgery may be suggested as an alternative and operation is PARTIAL THYROIDECTOMY. The preparation of the patient is not complicated but there are certain observations to be made during the first 24 hours *following the operation*. If the patient has difficulty in breathing and becomes rather cyanosed, there is pressure on the trachea, usually from a *blood clot* under the wound. To prevent *asphyxia* the doctor is called and he will remove the clot by opening the wound. If blood escapes from the wound it will collect under the back of the neck, and dressings should be inspected here.

A quick rise in temperature with a rapid pulse and uncontrolled excitement indicate that there is a temporary excess of thyroxine in the blood. This is not often seen but is always serious. Treatment is by sedation and hypothermia. This is a 'thyroid crisis'.

Spasm of the muscles in the hands or perhaps twitching of the face is *tetany* and shows a sudden lowering in the calcium level of the blood. This occurs when part of the parathyroids have been removed with the thyroid tissue in which they are embedded. The doctor will probably give calcium gluconate by intravenous injection to correct this.

A hoarse voice or loss of voice follows disturbances of the laryngeal nerves which pass up from the chest close by the thyroid gland.

The patient is reviewed at a later date to ensure that the remaining thyroid tissue secretes sufficient hormone for the body's needs.

The **parathyroid glands,** of which there are four in number, are attached to the thyroid gland, but there is no connection between them. They secrete a hormone *parathormone* which controls the use of calcium in the body.

Disorders of the Parathyroid Gland

A reduction of parathormone in the blood produces tetany, which is spasm in the muscles noticed first as twitchings of the face and contraction of muscles in hands and forearms so that they are drawn up to the chest. It is painful. Calcium gluconate is given by intravenous injection.

Excess parathormone production is rare and results in a rise in the level of calcium in the blood. Calcium is withdrawn from the bones, which become soft and bend easily. The skeleton is distorted and the patient cannot be as active as a normal person.

The **Islets of Langerhans in the pancreas** are collections of small cells lying between the other secretory cells in this abdominal organ. They produce a hormone INSULIN, which has a major role in the use of carbohydrate in the body cells and controls the storage of glucose as glycogen. Normally, when the blood sugar rises, more insulin is secreted so that the excess sugar is used up and the blood sugar returns to its normal amount.

Other hormones are concerned in the level of sugar in the blood: anterior pituitary hormone, adrenaline and cortisone.

OBSERVATIONS include testing urine for glucose, noting the patient's weight, condition of his skin, eyes, and general health.

Clinical Investigation

The doctor collects 20 millilitres of blood from a vein and this is shaken in a bottle containing some crystals to prevent clotting. The amount of blood sugar is calculated in the laboratory. Fasting blood sugar estimation is made from a blood sample taken in the early morning.

Disorders of Insulin Production

Diabetes Mellitus is usually of unknown cause and although it can be corrected by administration of insulin, it should not be thought of as insulin deficiency. Occasionally it can be due to disease of the pancreas.

Oversecretion of the Islets of Langerhans is caused by a tumour of these cells and is rare. It produces low blood sugar and gives rise to attacks of faintness and giddiness. These attacks are relieved by sugar or food by mouth. The condition is cured by removal of the tumour.

The Sex Hormones

The testis in the male and the ovary in the female produce hormones.

Testosterone. The male sex hormone is responsible for the male secondary sex characteristics, the deep voice, growth of beard, muscle and bone enlargement and the development of the sex organs.

Methyl-Testosterone, a preparation of male sex hormones, is sometimes prescribed for patients with advanced carcinoma of the breast. It relieves the symptoms of pain and ulceration, and slows down the spread to other parts of the body. It is also prescribed when there is an absence or deficiency of testicular secretion.

Female sex hormones secreted by the ovary are OESTROGENS and PRO-GESTERONE.

Oestrogens are responsible for the onset of puberty with the menstrual cycle, development of the breasts and sex organs, increase of subcutaneous fat and hair growth. These hormones are produced by the egg cell as it develops in the ovary, and in the first half of the menstrual cycle cause thickening of the lining tissue (endometrium) of the uterus.

There are many manufactured preparations of female sex hormone, the most commonly used being STILBOESTROL, which may be prescribed for one of the following reasons:

To stop breasts secreting milk when the mother cannot feed her baby: either it is not safe for her to feed the baby or she has lost the baby.

To relieve very severe menopausal symptoms. Normally no treatment is required for the headaches, hot flushes, insomnia or emotional upsets, but if these are so severe as to interfere with health, the doctor may prescribe oestrogens. The menopause tends to last longer with this treatment than in normal cases.

In inflammation of the vagina in elderly women, oestrogens are administered either by mouth or by local application in a cream.

Stilboestrol has been used in carcinoma of the prostate gland with some success. The action is probably the suppression of the male sex hormone which stimulates the malignant growth.

This drug has similarly been prescribed for elderly women with advanced carcinoma of the breast when surgery is not possible.

Progesterone is secreted by the tissue remaining when the ovum bursts from the ovary at ovulation midway through the menstrual cycle. This hormone causes further thickening and development of the endometrium, and it plays a part in the maintenance of the foetus during pregnancy.

The organs of reproduction in the male are the two TESTES, which are situated in a pouch of skin, the SCROTUM. They are suspended by the spermatic cords which pass through the inguinal canal into the abdominal cavity. Each testis consists of a large number of tubules which produce SPERMATOZOA.

SPERMATOZOA are the male reproductive cells. They are extremely small and are produced in large numbers during the reproductive phase of life beginning at early adolescence. Each cell has a long motile tail by which it can move in fluid.

Between the tubules in the testis are cells under the influence of a pituitary hormone. They secrete a hormone TESTOSTERONE. This hormone is necessary for the development of puberty and the normal male sex characteristics.

Both oestrogens and progesterone are much reduced during menstruation. In pregnancy they are produced in large quantities and are excreted in the urine. Immediately before childbirth the production of progesterone ceases.

At the menopause, usually betwen 45 and 55 years of age, these hormone productions gradually lessen. The skin becomes drier and the hair is thinner, the breast tissue and the sex organs shrink though the subcutaneous fat may remain throughout the body. When the physiological change is complete a woman can bear no more children. Following removal of *both ovaries* in operation the menopause will follow and the surgeon will explain this to the patient together with other details of the operation. Besides hormones produced in pregnancy, another is secreted by the placenta. This is known as the GONADOTROPIC hormone and it is excreted in the urine. In a pregnancy test, the urine is examined for this hormone.

The hormones secreted by the endocrine organs are present in the body in extremely small amounts, but have definite and sometimes intense effects on the individual's personality.

CHAPTER 43 | THE REPRODUCTIVE SYSTEM

Organs of Reproduction

The Male Reproductive Organs (Fig. 56)

The testes develop within the abdomen and shortly before birth come down into the scrotum. Occasionally this does not happen and an operation to correct this is sometimes performed before puberty when the glands should become active. Spermatozoa will not develop in the warm temperature of the body, and the normal situation of the testis is in the scrotal sac as an external organ.

A tube or duct leaves each testis and forms with blood vessels and nerves the spermatic cord, which passes into the abdomen. The duct is joined by another tube from a small sac in which a secretion is formed; it also acts as a reservoir for the germ cells. This fluid now containing spermatozoa is known as *semen*. The main duct passes through the prostate gland at the neck of the bladder and enters the urethra which is the channel passing through the penis.

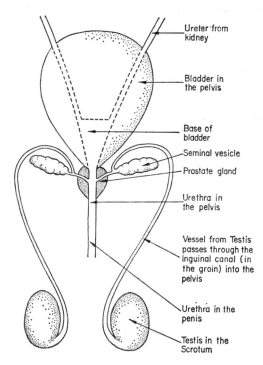

Figure 56. Male reproductive system.

The Female Reproductive Organs (Fig. 57)

Ova (egg cells) are produced in the two ovaries of the female. They are the largest cells produced by a human being and are discharged from the ovaries usually one each month during the reproductive phase of life beginning two or three years after puberty until menstruation stops. The time when menstruation ceases is known as the menopause and occurs most commonly at 45 to 55 years of age.

The OVARIES are situated in the pelvis and each ovary is shaped like an almond and is about the same size. It contains at birth a number of germ cells. At puberty, these are able to develop and mature, each becoming an ovum enclosed within a sac of fluid. This is an ovarian follicle and during its development secretes hormones called OESTROGENS which cause thickening of the lining of the uterus and influence the female sex characteristics.

The developing ovarian follicle appears on the surface of the ovary and then bursts. The ovum is discharged into the peritoneal cavity but is attracted to the fringed end of the uterine tube which leads to the uterus. Ovulation (the discharge of the ovum from the ovary) takes place approximately every 28 days during the reproductive phase of a woman's life.

There is a scar at the place where the ovum left the ovary and this

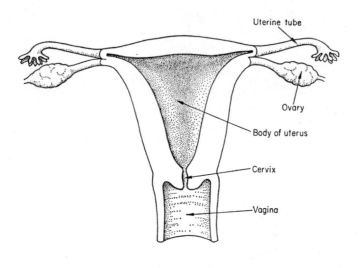

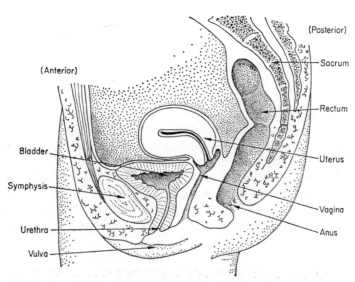

Figure 57. Female reproductive tract and pelvis.

produces another hormone PROGESTERONE which causes further thickening of the uterus lining tissue, making it suitable for the nourishment of the ovum should this have been fertilised by a male germ cell in the meantime. The ovum passes down one of the two uterine tubes to the uterus (womb). These tubes are made of unstriped muscle capable of contractions and are lined with special cells which assist the ovum to travel towards the uterus.

The UTERUS is situated in the pelvis. The bladder is in front of it and the rectum is behind it. It is a hollow organ of unstriped muscle, about 8 cms by 6 cms by 5 cms in size. The lining tissue is endometrium and the organ is covered from above by peritoneum. Behind the uterus the peritoneum forms a pocket, the Pouch of Douglas. It is supported in the pelvis by the pelvic diaphragm and by ligaments, and there is a lavish blood supply which will be needed in pregnancy.

The VAGINA is a canal from the uterus to the exterior of the body. It is about 10 cms in length, and the tissue in the walls lies in folds so that it can enlarge to allow a baby's head to be born through it. In the virgin a membrane called the hymen partly closes the lower part of the vagina. This enlarges after puberty and becomes soft; it stretches or is torn during sexual intercouse, and much more so during childbirth.

Before puberty the lining of the vagina is a thin tissue which is easily damaged or infected. During the reproductive age and due to the sex hormones this tissue becomes like the skin, and protects the tissues beneath from friction, injury and infection. After the menopause when the sex hormones cease the tissue returns to the very thin tissue. Mucus from the uterus and cervix keep the vaginal tissue healthy. Two glands (Bartholin Glands) at the lower end of the vagina maintain the moist surface of the vestibule and labia minora.

The VULVA are the parts surrounding and protecting the vaginal opening, which is between the thighs. The labia major are two folds of fatty tissue covered by skin and hairs. Within these are labia minora which are smaller and covered by mucous membrane. The latter enclose the vestibule into which the urethra opens in front of the vagina. At the anterior point of the vestibule is the clitoris, a sensitive small projection of tissue. The perineum, which is formed from skin and muscle, separates the vagina from the anal canal and rectum.

The MENSTRUAL CYCLE is under the control of hormones and this physiological activity in the female reproductive tract begins at puberty and ends at the menopause. Each menstrual cycle lasts about 28 days though the length of time varies slightly in individual women, and it begins with the first day of the menstrual loss. On the 14th day of the cycle, ovulation (the ovum leaving the ovary) takes place. When the ovum in the uterine tube is not fertilised it passes into the uterus, and, as there will be no further development of the cell, it is cast off from the body together with the superficial endometrium and some blood. This is the menstrual flow, occurring 14 to 15 days after ovulation, and lasting about 5 days.

Menstruation is a normal physiological occurrence in the female during the reproductive phase of life. The young female needs some explanation of the events, and older women do not always know the best way in which to do this when they themselves lack the words with which to understand and explain. A nurse in her work with girls and women should be prepared to give simple information to those who need it at a suitable time. Girls should know about menstruation before the cycle is likely to begin. Explanations may come from mothers, teachers, or their school colleagues, but a girl may be in hospital as a patient at this time. It is then the ward sister who may need to assume the responsibility and the nurses should observe and report any symptoms and signs of the onset of a menstrual period.

On the day before menstruation there may be a little headache, feeling of fullness in the breasts, and a slight nervous tension. Physiologically there is some water retention causing fullness in the breasts and in fact an increase in body weight. This is due to congestion in the pelvis as the uterus and blood vessels have become a little enlarged. There may be some constipation or difficulty with micturition and a general feeling of heaviness in the lower abdomen with some slight backache. By the end of adolescence there is comparatively little discomfort and that which does persist often has a simple physiological explanation.

Simple hygiene during menstruation. First a knowledge of what is happening in the body determines a healthy attitude. As with any excretion from the body it is necessary to maintain the cleanliness of the skin round the vaginal orifice. A warm bath every day is cleansing and comfortable and, if not available, hot water for washing is essential. Sanitary pads or tampons are used to absorb the menstrual flow. The former are replaced as frequently as necessary otherwise the blood dries, is unpleasant and causes skin irritation. When a tampon remains in the vagina, particularly towards the end of menstruation, it becomes dry and may be difficult to remove in addition to the possibility of causing abrasion in the stratified epithelium. These should be replaced frequently during menstruation.

Constipation is to be avoided as this increases the slight pelvic congestion already present. A normal amount of exercise is useful, for being sedentary during menstruation tends to increase the general discomfort.

Some women prefer to spend their leisure time in some occupation more restful and quiet than usual on the first day, but there is nothing harmful in swimming and games provided suitable protection is worn for comfort and cleanliness.

Because of the periodic loss, which includes blood, some women are inclined to suffer from a mild degree of anaemia.

Disorders of Menstruation

AMENORRHOEA is absence of menstruation. Absence of reproductive organs, an imperforate hymen or hormone disorders prevents menstruation from occurring in the normal way. Menstruation stops during pregnancy and while the mother feeds her baby. In adolescence emotional upsets including examinations, starting work, and a complete change in the way of living, can result in amenorrhoea lasting a few months. It also occurs in severe wasting diseases, though these are less common now, mental illnesses, disorders of the pituitary gland and follows radiotherapy to the pelvis. Infertility accompanies amennorhoea.

DYSMENORRHOEA is painful menstruation and there are a number of causes. It is seldom experienced after pregnancy. Exercises just before menstruation and as soon as possible afterwards relieve pelvic congestion, and constipation when present should be treated.

When dysmenorrhoea appears later, it is usually due to some disease and disappears when the disease is diagnosed and treated.

MENORRHAGIA. The menstrual loss is greater than normal or the period is longer than usual. In describing the degree of menorrhagia the patient will say how many days the periods last and possibly the number of sanitary pads she has needed to use. It occurs when there are fibroids of the uterus (benign tumours) or polypi (projections of tissue which sometimes break off leaving a bleeding point) and also in congestive conditions such as inflammation of the uterine tubes, and in prolapse of the uterus.

The cause when diagnosed is treated, and also the anaemia resulting from the blood loss.

METRORRHAGIA is bleeding from the vagina apart from menstrual periods and after the menopause. This form of bleeding can appear like a menstrual period and the patient may confuse it with menstruation, describing it as one of irregular or too frequent periods.

Causes include cervical and intra-uterine polypi and hormone disturturbances, but it is also a symptom of carcinoma of the uterus. For that reason any woman with irregular loss from the vagina, especially over 40 years of age, is advised to consult a doctor immediately. Then examina-

Q

tion and investigations are made to determine the cause of the bleeding, and appropriate treatment is carried out.

Reproduction

In human beings reproduction takes place by a union of a male germ cell (spermatozoon) with a female germ (ovum), usually in the uterine tube of the female. Large numbers of spermatozoa are deposited in the vagina during sexual intercourse and they can live for one or two days in the female genital tract. If there is an ovum in the uterine tube when the male germ cells have arrived there, having travelled through the cervix and body of the uterus, a spermatozoon penetrates the cell wall of the ovum and fusion takes place. This is CONCEPTION or fertilisation, and the life of the new human being begins at this moment.

The nucleus of the fertilised ovum contains substance from both parents and the new individual will inherit some characteristics from each parent. Sex is determined at the time of conception and depends on the type of male germ cell which fertilises the ovum.

Pregnancy

The fertilised ovum embeds itself in the uterine wall a few days after conception and continues to develop there. From a single cell which divides and subdivides, groups of cells later become organised into tissues and eventually in 280 to 300 days the fully developed foetus is born. While in the uterus it floats in a membraneous bag of fluid. The foetus obtains its oxygen and nourishment from the mother through the placenta, a mass of vascular tissue attached to the uterine wall and from which blood vessels pass to and from the foetus in its umbilical cord.

Signs and Symptoms of Pregnancy

During pregnancy menstruation ceases and in the first three months the woman frequently experiences for a short time a little nausea, sometimes with vomiting early in the mornings. There is a feeling of fulness and tingling in the breasts and frequency of micturition is fairly common. As the uterus enlarges the abdomen increases in size—at twelve weeks the upper border of the uterus is just above the symphysis pubis. Some women tend to gain weight.

Abdominal or vaginal examinations confirm pregnancy. The foetal heart may be heard through a stethoscope at 5 months and later the form of the foetus, especially the head, can be palpated through the abdominal wall. Towards the end of pregnancy the mother can sometimes feel the baby move.

When confirmation is required early in pregnancy, tests are carried out using the knowledge that during pregnancy excessive amounts of hormone are produced, and these can be detected in the woman's urine.

Ante-natal Care
As soon as she suspects she is pregnant, the woman visits her own doctor or attends an Ante-natal Clinic which is administered by the local authority through the Medical Officer of Health. The doctor carries out a general examination including heart and lungs, and takes a medical history. A vaginal examination is also made. The midwife tests her urine especially for glucose and albumen, she assesses the blood pressure and measures her weight. Specimens of blood are obtained for blood counts and haemoglobin, blood groups including Rhesus factor, and for a Wassermann reaction.

Apart from the technical information involved, the woman meets those who are likely to attend her during her confinement. The relationship between them begins at the first visit to the clinic or surgery and continues until after the baby is born. This gives her more confidence if problems or complications arise.

When required, she is given advice regarding health measures. These include diet, rest, exercise, clothes which are comfortable to wear, care of the breasts. If she is being admitted to hospital, arrangements for the care of those at home may be necessary, particularly when there are small children. When she will have her baby at home, she perhaps needs a home help. Maternity allowances are explained and forms completed. At a large clinic a medical social worker may be available to give advice on economic or domestic difficulties. Mothercraft classes are useful for those for whom this is a first pregnancy, and in some clinics there are fathercraft classes too. These are concerned primarily with the management of the infant, bathing, feeding, but also provide more opportunities for answering questions, creating confidence and strengthening the parent-doctor-midwife relationship. Management of breast feeding is explained to the mother-to-be. She attends relaxation classes so that during labour she is able to relax completely between the uterine contractions when requested by the midwife, thus removing a source of fatigue and tension.

During a first pregnancy the woman may be apprehensive as well as being pleasantly excited. She needs some reassurance and confidence. After several pregnancies the woman becomes very experienced, is not so apprehensive, but still appreciates consideration and understanding, for each pregnancy is in some way or other different from other pregnancies. Talks and films on childbirth have been used to foster confidence and knowledge in the parents-to-be, and a meeting of this kind is an opportunity for the father to be included in this relationship. During pregnancy it is usual for the woman to look and feel extremely well and she is placid and content, but late in pregnancy she becomes tired easily and physical effort is difficult. Her attention is concentrated on the unborn child, and the other members of the family may feel rather unimportant. It helps them considerably if they too can share in the attention for the baby-to-come, and the new member of the family when he arrives will have been accepted already.

During the ante-natal period it will be decided whether the baby should be born in hospital or at home. Priority for hospital beds is given to women having their first babies, to those for whom the birth may be difficult for medical reasons (this includes the infant as well as the mother), and the mothers of large families who live in conditions unsuitable for the delivery of a baby and the care of the mother afterwards. In many hospitals and maternity homes, the mother and baby are discharged home after two to five days when medical and hospital treatment is no longer needed, for this makes it possible for more women to have their babies in hospital. In a maternity hospital there may be a unit in which the mother is attended by her own general practitioner and midwife. The length of stay is normally 48 hours. The district midwives supervise these mothers and their babies, and they need some general care from relatives, friends or neighbours for about ten days after confinement.

During CHILDBIRTH the uterine muscle, aided by abdominal muscles and diaphragm, contracts and pushes the baby out through the dilated cervix and the vagina. The rhythmical contractions of the muscles cause the mother to have pains (hence the use of the word 'labour' to mean childbirth).

Three Stages of Labour
Stage 1. A slight loss of blood-stained mucus discharge (a 'show') may appear first. Then there are rhythmical abdominal pains becoming more frequent. During a pain the abdomen will become hard as the muscles contract. The bag of fluid in which the baby floats helps to *dilate the cervix* and the baby's head descends into the pelvis. The membranes rupture.

Stage 2. The head passes through the birth canal, appears at the vulva and is delivered, followed by the shoulders and the remainder of the trunk and limbs. Muscle contractions continue throughout.

Stage 3. After the baby is born, there are a few more uterine contractions and then the 'after-birth' is delivered. This consists of the placenta, its membranes and the umbilical cord. There is also a loss of blood.

The PUERPERIUM is the period of time following childbirth and is taken to be two weeks. The mother and infant are under the supervision of the midwife. Recuperation from the last weeks of pregnancy and labour takes place quickly and a normal healthy woman will be getting up on the third day and is active by the end of the week. Adjustment to the demands of the young baby, however, need to be met and it is usually about two weeks before she is carrying on all the duties in the care of family and home.

For a few days after the baby is born there is a discharge of blood from the vagina, and it is necessary for the vulva to be cleansed two or three times a day. When the woman needs to be in bed vulval swabbing is carried out as a clean procedure, and when she is able to go to the bath, washing well with soap and water will be adequate. In modern hospitals bidets are part of the sanitary equipment. After using the toilet the patient sits on the bidet facing the taps. The flush of water cleanses the vulva and anal areas which are then dried with absorbent paper. The direction of cleansing should be from the vulva towards the anal area. The bidet requires proper cleaning between patients' use. Baths and toilets, towels, bed-linen and clothing should be scrupulously clean, for infection is a possibility and though a rare occurrence now, preventive measures are still necessary. In hospital the nurse sterilises bed-pans after each use, washes her hands before attending to mother or infant, and disinfects the plastic-covered mattresses, etc. when each woman is discharged. At home the same principles apply though in a different way, and conscientious cleanliness and careful routine are employed.

The discharge will disappear and the uterus become smaller more quickly if the mother lies face downwards for an hour each day.

Diet, bladder and bowel action are normal. Any swelling in a leg, especially with pain, is reported. Occasionally the mother takes a little time to recover her usual behaviour, and needs special patience and understanding during the puerperium.

Care of the Infant at Birth

The infant is covered by a greasy substance when he is born and this is removed by bathing him or by using arachis oil. His eyes and nose are cleaned gently when necessary. He passes a little black faeces in the first day (meconium) and then the stools become normal. He is put to the breast as soon as it is convenient to the mother, and her first milk is thin and pale (this is colostrum). Breast-feeding is arranged every four hours unless he weighs under 7 pounds, when it may be every three hours. The breasts are used alternately or he feeds 10 minutes at each breast. Cleanliness is essential; warm water without soap is used and the nipples are dried well. While feeding, the infant has the nipple and the pigmented area round the nipple in the mouth otherwise the milk ducts are not being squeezed sufficiently to eject milk. There is also a risk of the nipple becoming cracked and this predisposes to infection and breast abscess. The infant will lose weight after birth but should have regained this within two weeks. He sleeps at this time about 20 hours a day.

Management of an Emergency Childbirth

Arrangements are made for a woman to have her baby in hospital or for the midwife to be with her at home. Occasionally, however, labour will begin earlier than expected or some unusual weather and road conditions prevent the mother, doctor or midwife from reaching their required destinations.

Should a nurse be called to help a woman in labour, she should send a message to a doctor or midwife without delay, as these are the people qualified to deal with the situation. The mother is reassured and possibly anxious relatives need some words of comfort also. As much privacy as possible is ensured, depending on the situation. Children are given into the care of a neighbour or older child, one person is chosen to assist in preparation for the childbirth and others are asked to collect articles and clothing for the infant, boil large amounts of water if no hot water is available in the house, and take messages. Some method of lighting may be necessary. Matches, an electric torch, a coin for gas or electric meter and another for the telephone can save much time and anxiety.

The woman in the first stage of labour is encouraged to walk about between the pains. It is helpful if she can pass urine at intervals to prevent retention of urine. She is given small amounts of nourishing fluid but not large meals difficult to digest as the doctor may wish to give a small anaesthetic to help her. If she has a 'show' or the membranes have ruptured a vulval pad or towel will be needed and this must be quite *clean* to prevent infection. Sponging of the hands and face and combing the hair are necessary for her general comfort when the pains continue for some time. In the meantime preparation is made for the actual birth:

1. Waterproof sheeting or thick paper under the sheet on a bed.
2. A bowl of hot water, clean flannel and towel for washing the vulva.
3. A packet of vulval or sanitary pads. (These may be available in the house in the confinement pack as issued from the Ante-natal Clinic.)
4. Clean night-clothes for the patient.
5. A clean overall for the nurse.
6. For the baby, a cot, cradle, box, drawer or basket is prepared by lining with a small blanket and a sheet over a pillow or mattress.

7. Two pieces of thick string or narrow tape and scissors to cut the string. Scissors to cut the cord must be clean and boiled if possible.

8. A towel in which to wrap the baby.

9. An old, thin handkerchief with which to wipe his eyes and clean his mouth.

10. A large dish or bowl in which to receive the placenta.

When the doctor or midwife arrives he or she will give instructions. If, however, the woman's painful contractions become more intense and more frequent and help has not yet arrived, the nurse undresses her and puts on a loose gown and she lies on the bed covered by a clean sheet and a blanket. The second stage will begin very soon if she has her bowels opened a little without being able to control them and it is important then to see she is lying down in a convenient place without delay. Adequate lighting is necessary.

In the second stage the membranes have ruptured and the pains change and become forceful. The baby in an emergency is usually born quickly, and then the mother immediately becomes less tense.

The baby lies on the bed and the first matter of importance is to maintain an air-way, for some of the fluid in which he floated may be in the air-passages. He can be held up firmly by the feet so that the fluid flows out of his mouth and mucus is wiped from the mouth and throat with a clean handkerchief on the little finger. By this time he has begun to cry and, especially if quickly and loudly, this a welcome sound. Excess mucus is wiped from the eyes, a brief examination is made to note sex and general condition. He is still attached to the mother by the umbilical cord. After a few minutes the arteries in the jelly-like cord have stopped pulsating and then the cord is tied very firmly in two places 15 cms and 20 cms from the baby. Avoid thin string or thread as these cut through the cord tissue and there may be some bleeding. The midwife or doctor who arrives will cut the cord between the ligatures. Otherwise the baby and placenta are wrapped in a large clean towel with the baby's head exposed and transported with the mother in the ambulance to the hospital.

The baby is wrapped in a towel so that his hands do not touch his face and then a flannelette sheet to keep him warm. He is laid on his side in a cot, clothes basket or in a large drawer. He must not be overheated so hot-water bottles are not used. Until qualified assistance arrives it is essential to observe frequently that the infant is breathing satisfactorily, a normal colour, and not bleeding from the umbilical cord.

Should his condition be considered not very satisfactory, for it may be a premature birth, a decision is made regarding baptism if the parents wish this. The Christian nurse can baptise the infant into the Christian

faith by sprinkling a little water on his forehead, making over it the sign
of the cross and saying: 'In the name of the Father, the Son and Holy
Ghost, I baptise thee...', giving him the name of a parent, or as the
parent wishes. Later the priest or minister will arrange a short ceremony
according to the family's religious denomination.

Should more than one child be born it is useful if the person managing
the situation can indicate with coloured pencil or pen on the foreheads of
the infants the order in which they were born. It is always customary to
record the time at which any birth takes place and later the father will
register the birth at the Register of Births and Deaths.

The afterbirth is delivered about 10 to 20 minutes after the infant. This
is collected in the bowl or dish, and is kept carefully for the doctor or
midwife's inspection. Should any part of the placenta or membrane be
retained, there is a possibility of haemorrhage.

Then the mother is washed, the bed-linen changed and she is made
comfortable. Although fatigued, she is happy in a deep, satisfying way.
She is given the baby to hold for a few minutes and the father comes in
to see them both together.

During a normal confinement at home the baby would have been
washed and dressed, and may be put to the breast to feed. Other children
come in to see their mother and the new arrival also, though this is not
convenient or suitable in hospital. A husband who wishes to be with his
wife during childbirth explains this to the doctor or midwife. His
presence can be a great comfort to the mother and being together at this
time is satisfying to them both. During an emergency he may have given
a great deal of assistance.

Problems which may arise in childbirth are haemorrhage, injury to the
perineum, and infection. Haemorrhage can be severe and occurs either at
the end of the first stage or as the placenta is separating. Medical attention is essential. If bleeding is severe in an emergency situation telephone
999 and say exactly what is happening, and give the address of the house
in which the emergency is. A 'Flying Squad' of obstetricians and midwives is available. Infection is prevented throughout the whole procedure
by strict cleanliness and attention to general hygiene, and is uncommon
now. Injury to the skin is prevented by skilled procedure and co-operation
between mother and her doctor or midwife. It is most likely to occur when
the baby is born quickly or is very large. Sutures are inserted when necessary by a doctor.

Problems of Fertility
There are variations in the fertility of different people, and married
couples sometimes seek advice from their medical practitioner regarding

subfertility or overfertility. Several of the problems are not yet solved but when a solution which is acceptable to both the partners is found, there is a general improvement in the health and happiness within the family circle.

Advice on problems of this kind is also given by doctors and their teams in centres of the Family Planning Association, an organisation outside the National Health Service. The aim of this organisation is to ensure that advice and information regarding the planning of families can be available for those who wish to take advantage of it. They would wish that 'every baby is a wanted baby'.

Literature regarding all aspects of family planning is available at the bookshop attached to their centre: 27/35 Mortimer Street, London, W.1.

Infertility

When clinical investigations are necessary the childless couple are referred to a special clinic attached to a hospital where they meet medical specialists. Tests are carried out to ensure that the male partner is not sterile, e.g. by a sperm count. The number of spermatozoa produced may be much smaller than normal and the cells not so active. There may be problems regarding sexual intercourse: the hymen in the female vagina occasionally does not stretch easily, emotional tension in the woman can prevent a satisfactory union. Tests are possible to show whether or not spermatozoa have been deposited in the vagina during sexual intercourse.

Ovulation in the female is assessed by the woman keeping a chart of temperatures (this rises often following ovulation), and it may be considered necessary for a specimen of endometrium to be obtained for microscopic examination to show whether the menstrual cycle is normal. This is endometrial biopsy, an almost painless procedure performed in the out-patient clinic.

The uterine tubes may be completely or partially closed; this is tested by tubal insufflation, in which a gas, carbon dioxide, is blown through the tube and a measure (manometer) attached to the insufflator indicates at which pressure the gas can pass through the tube.

In an X-ray (salpingogram) an opaque dye is injected into the tubes before X-ray. Laparoscopy is the examination of pelvic organs by viewing them through a metal tube which has been inserted through the abdominal wall. Illumination is by means of a tiny bulb at the end of the tube attached to a battery. The patient has a general anaesthetic.

Advice or treatment is suggested depending on the results of the investigations. If conception has not occurred within a few months the couple may consider the adoption of a child and this takes place with certain formalities through a Registered Adoption Society.

Q*

Drugs are being developed which may sometimes be prescribed for the female partner of a childless couple. The drug is known as a 'fertility drug' and is given under careful supervision. Occasionally the result is a multiple birth, i.e. more than one infant is born.

Overfertility

The married couple have a number of children while they are still young, and for health or economic reasons in the family it is inadvisable for the family to be enlarged at the present time. The attitude towards this depends very much on religious views, ethical standards, education from parents, ministers of religion, the press, radio, television, etc., and also relationships within the family circle. Methods of dealing with this problem include abstinence from sexual intercourse, use of the safe periods, i.e. the time when it is unlikely that the ovum will be in the uterine tube during the menstrual cycle, mechanical contraceptives used by the husband or wife to prevent spermatozoa from entering the cervix of the uterus, and chemical preparations used by the wife to inhibit the activity of the spermatozoa. Intra-uterine devices are small, plastic aids which remain in the uterus permanently. Oral contraceptive pills, which are hormone compounds preventing ovulation, are being used in some cases under the prescription of a doctor.

Advice on these methods is given by medical practitioners, or consultants in the Family Planning Association.

Where parents cannot care for a large number of children, some may be placed with foster parents by the local authority. National Family Allowances paid to the mother for children after the first child assist with the feeding and clothing of her children. Health visitors give advice, and social workers help by arranging for additional domestic or financial aid.

Complications of Pregnancy

ABORTION (this word has the same meaning as 'miscarriage'). This is the loss of the pregnancy from the uterus before the 28th week, and occurs most commonly at about the 12th week when the placenta is not yet firmly attached to the uterine wall. Among the causes, the most common is understood to be a malformed foetus. Some lack of development or hormonal balance in the woman's reproductive tract may also be responsible. A general disease like diabetes, nephritis or an acute infectious disease may predispose abortion, and a large tumour in the wall of the uterus prevents accommodation of the developing pregnancy. A sudden emotional upset can cause pregnancy to terminate before the 28th week.

In some cases of abortion the woman has had amenorrhoea for two or three months and then slight vaginal bleeding occurs. There is no severe definite pain. On examination pregnancy is confirmed but the cervix is closed. The treatment is mainly rest and reassurance. This is '*threatened*' *abortion*.

If, however, the bleeding is heavier and more continuous, and rhythmical pain is present, the *abortion becomes 'inevitable'*. The cervix is dilated and the products of conception begin to pass through the vagina. When these are passed complete a '*complete*' *abortion* has taken place. However, the membranes may rupture and the foetus is passed, leaving placenta tissue and membrane behind. This is an '*incomplete*' *abortion*. Haemorrhage may follow unless the uterus is completely emptied soon afterwards.

The woman is distressed by the early termination of the pregnancy and needs reassurance. To know whether the abortion is complete or not the doctor needs to see everything that has been passed from the vagina, so the nurse saves any vaginal loss on clothing, vulval pads, in a bed-pan etc. for him to inspect. The patient may be admitted to hospital and is treated by complete rest in bed with scrupulous hygiene in care of bed-linen, washing of the nurse's hands, and aseptic technique in nursing procedures to prevent infection entering into the uterus.

A drug may be ordered by the doctor to cause uterine muscle to contract, e.g. ergometrine, but unless the remainder of the products of conception is passed quickly, the patient is anaesthetised in the operating theatre and the uterus evacuated. If there has been blood loss this is replaced before, or immediately after, the operation. Antibiotics or chemotherapy are used when the abortion has occurred outside the hospital and there is a risk of infection.

Termination of pregnancy is considered when a further pregnancy or childbirth would be likely to endanger the mother's life. The decision is made in consultation with two doctors, the patient and her husband. Before 1967 it was illegal for this operation to be performed for any other reason, but since the Abortion Act became law in that year pregnancy can be terminated if it is likely to cause the woman mental or physical harm. The decision must be agreed upon by two doctors and performed by a gynaecologist in a registered hospital or clinic. A general anaesthetic is necessary and the operation is best carried out early in pregnancy.

Termination of pregnancy brought about by unskilled procedures in unhygienic conditions can result in serious complications, and the aim of the Abortion Act was to avoid this situation. The serious complications are haemorrhage, injury to internal structures like the uterus and the bladder, and infection which may result in the inability to bear a child in the future. The girl or woman with one of these complications would be admitted to hospital.

Sterilisation is in itself a minor operation but sufficient consideration must be given before it is performed as it is difficult to reverse in the woman, and not so far possible in the man.

The operation in the female entails destroying the Fallopian tubes. In the male the tubes which convey spermatozoa to the urethra are cut.

After sterilisation the man or woman cannot produce a child. Sexual intercourse can take place normally.

ECTOPIC GESTATION (pregnancy outside the uterus) is a complication of pregnancy. The fertilised ovum cannot move through the narrower portion of the uterine tube, and continues to develop within the tube. (The tube may be narrowed as a result of previous infection in the tube, which caused salpingitis.) When the ovum has become as large as the dimension of the tube, it either aborts from the end of the uterine tube into the peritoneal cavity accompanied by abdominal pain and some internal bleeding, or it bursts through the wall of the tube and bleeding occurs. Haemorrhage is usually severe and *tubal rupture* following ectopic pregnancy is a surgical emergency. The woman has abdominal pain on either the right or the left side of the abdomen, and becomes very pale and may faint. Her pulse rate is rapid and the volume is weak. On admission to hospital, she is anaesthetised in the operating theatre, the abdomen is opened, the uterine tube ligatured and removed (salpingectomy). Then a blood transfusion is given.

PRE-ECLAMPTIC TOXAEMIA is a serious complication of pregnancy. This is a term used to describe a collection of symptoms in late pregnancy which precedes *eclampsia* in which fits occur, and the pregnancy terminates before full term.

The symptoms are a *raised blood pressure* (this having been normal at the beginning of pregnancy), *oedema* and *albuminuria*. It is an advantage of skilled ante-natal care that these symptoms are observed early and appropriate treatment begins at once. The woman is admitted to hospital for complete bed-rest and close observation. In some cases the labour is induced so that the baby is born earlier than expected.

Women with *general medical conditions* require special medical supervision during pregnancy. These include heart disease, either congenital or following acute rheumatism, and pulmonary tuberculosis, which is less common now. Anaemia is common and most women are given iron throughout pregnancy. Inflammation in the pelvis of the kidney (pyelonephritis) can occur and also acute retention of urine. Previous kidney disease may predispose kidney stress. Hypertension is suspected when the blood pressure reading is raised. This worsens when she is active but improves following rest in bed.

Unless *syphilis* in the mother is treated before or during pregnancy, the child may be born with secondary syphilis. If she has untreated *gonorrhoea* with a vaginal discharge, the baby's eyes will be infected as he passes through the birth canal, and the severe infection will cause blindness unless treated immediately.

A *diabetic mother* needs special supervision as there is a tendency for her to have a large baby and there may be some risk to the baby before birth.

German measles is avoided during pregnancy for the virus can affect the foetus in the early stages. Very high temperatures in *infection* are also harmful. A vaccine is now available for girls before the child-bearing age.

SPECIAL OBSERVATIONS DURING PREGNANCY

Bleeding from the vagina does not occur normally during pregnancy. Towards the end of pregnancy it is serious.

Abdominal pain may be the onset of an acute obstetric condition such as abortion.

Swelling of the feet may be the result of too little rest, but if there is swelling of the hands and face as well, it may be an indication of serious complications such as pre-eclamptic toxaemia.

Gynaecology is the Study of Diseases of Women

SYMPTOMS AND SIGNS IN GYNAECOLOGICAL DISEASES

Backache is a common though vague complaint and may be accompanied by fatigue and feeling of general ill-health.

Vaginal discharges are various. *Menstrual flow* is a normal issue from the vagina, as also is a white sticky mucus discharge occurring for a day or two midway through the menstrual cycle. It is the secretion from the cervix and tends to be more profuse during adolescence and during emotional upsets. It is referred to as *leucorrhoea*. A blood loss from the vagina can be heavy as in incomplete abortion or slight as after injury or infection. Amounts should be reported carefully and the relationship with normal menstrual flow or the menopause noted. White curdy discharge occurs in monilia infection, and yellowish-white, frothy discharge in trichomonas infection. Pus-forming bacteria, such as staphylococci and gonococci, produce a *purulent discharge*.

Blood-stained discharge is *offensive* when there is a carcinoma of the cervix, and sometimes the purulent discharges also are particularly unpleasant for the patient.

A discharge coming into contact with the vulva can cause severe itching of the skin; this is *pruritus*.

When vaginal loss or discharge occurs during pregnancy, vulval pads are kept for inspection by the doctor as the type of loss may give some indication of the type of pregnancy complication should one be present. The high standard of cleanliness of the skin, vulval pads, linen required when there is a discharge from the vagina cannot be overstressed.

Stress-incontinence is the passing of urine involuntarily when the patient laughs, sneezes, coughs or makes a sudden movement. It is associated with prolapse of the uterus as is also a feeling of 'bearing down' as the uterus descends into the vagina.

Bleeding from the vagina may be excessive and the patient may collapse. It may be a small quantity as an irregular period or after the menopause. The patient may have symptoms and signs of internal bleeding which is not visible. Any bleeding from the vagina other than during menstruation should be reported to a doctor.

INVESTIGATIONS

Vaginal examination. This is a clean procedure except during childbirth, the puerperium and following abortion; then it is an aseptic technique.

The procedure is explained to the patient, the screens are drawn round the bed or couch. She should have passed urine recently. Adequate lighting is necessary in the form of an adjustable lamp.

The patient lies in the Sims' position (three-quarter prone position with upper leg drawn up). An alternative position is lying on her back with her head on two pillows, hips, knees and ankles flexed and feet separated and flat on the bed or couch. In either case she is protected from becoming cold by sheets and only the vulval area is exposed. The doctor wears a clean disposable glove, swabs the vulva with warm lotion, lubricates one or two fingers of the gloved hand with an antiseptic cream or jelly such as Chlorhexidine and inserts the finger or two fingers into the vagina to make the examination. Should the wall of the vagina require inspection, a Sims' or bi-valve speculum and a light will be necessary. Swabs of cervix or vagina may be taken for culture and microscopic examination. The patient is made comfortable, the diagnostic swabs are sent to the laboratory, and the doctor makes a report on the patient's records. The equipment is disinfected.

Dilatation of the cervix and curettage of the uterus is performed when a specimen of endometrium is required for examination. The patient is anaesthetised and is placed in the lithotomy position in which the lower limbs are flexed and supported by poles.

Culdoscopy is an alternative to laparotomy when an examination of the ovaries is required. The instrument used is a metal tube which is introduced through the posterior space of the vagina into the pouch of Douglas. A small electric bulb at the end of the tube illuminates the pelvic organs.

Insufflation of the uterine tube is the blowing of carbon dioxide through a cannula inserted into the cervical canal when the uterine tube is suspected of being completely or partially closed.

Gynaecological Conditions

DISPLACEMENTS OF THE UTERUS

Retroverted Uterus in which the uterus bends backwards from the vagina instead of forwards. In a minor degree it is fairly common and does not cause symptoms. In surgery the ligaments which support the uterus are tightened up so that the uterus is brought forward, otherwise a Hodge pessary is inserted into the upper part of the vagina by the doctor, and this pushes the body of the uterus towards the symphysis pubis.

Prolapse of the uterus. The pelvic floor is skeletal muscle and ligaments. When this floor becomes weakened it loses tone and stretches. The pelvic organs are not supported as they are normally, particularly the uterus, which sags downwards into the vagina. This is prolapse of the uterus and it occurs usually in a woman who has had a number of pregnancies. She complains of low backache and may have menorrhagia. the actual prolapse she describes as 'coming down'.

Treatment is by surgery. The ligaments are repaired by sutures which are inserted through an incision in the vagina; this is sutured by catgut. There are nylon sutures in the perineum. A vaginal pack is left in after operation and this is removed the next day. Occasionally catheterisation is needed when the patient has difficulty in passing urine. It is necessary for her to empty the bladder completely otherwise urinary infection will follow. Cleanliness and dryness of the perineal wound are important. These patients become mobile about the third day and go home on the tenth day.

When surgery is unsuitable (the woman wishes to have more children) or the patient is an elderly woman or suffers from a general illness the doctor will prescribe a plastic ring pessary which is inserted into the vagina by the doctor or the sister. Pessaries are changed when the patient visits the out-patient clinic for further examination.

The patient consults the doctor if the pessary becomes uncomfortable as it may have moved in position.

CYSTOCELE is the bulging of the bladder in the wall of the vagina as the uterus sags downwards. The patient passes a little urine whenever she coughs or sneezes or makes a sudden movement. This is called 'stress incontinence'. It causes the patient discomfort and inconvenience.

RECTOCELE is the bulging of the rectum into the wall of the vagina.

INFLAMMATIONS AND INFECTIONS IN THE FEMALE REPRODUCTIVE TRACT

Vulvitis, inflammation of the vulva, can be the result of lack of hygiene or the effect of vaginal discharges on the skin. Washing of the vulva with soap and water and drying well at frequent intervals, prevention of irritation by changing vulval pads which have absorbed discharges as soon as necessary are essential hygiene procedures. The doctor orders treatment for the cause of the discharges and this may include medicated pessaries.

Pruritus, a condition of the skin associated with severe irritation, may occur on the vulva, and is caused by a vaginal discharge but sometimes follows glycosuria in diabetes mellitus, and the urine is tested for glucose when a woman reports this condition. Occasionally there is no reason found.

Vaginitis occurs easily in girls and elderly women because the vaginal tissue is not then resistant to general organisms like staphylococci and streptococci and E. Coli. Foreign bodies are occasionally found in the vagina of a female child having caused a local inflammation. An elderly woman may not have visited the clinic, where a ring pessary for prolapse of the uterus would have been changed; in time the vagina becomes infected, producing an offensive purulent discharge. In this case removal of the pessary is necessary and the vaginitis is treated with vaginal irrigation and appropriate antibiotic therapy. The gynaecologist may consider oestrogen pessaries suitable treatment for the senile vaginitis.

Infection is possible during or following abortion and childbirth. This *sepsis* is avoided by the rules of domestic cleanliness, washing and drying of hands, the wearing of masks and aseptic techniques in attending to the patient. A woman admitted to hospital with such a sepsis is isolated from all other women in ante-natal, labour or post-natal wards. For this reason these patients enter a general hospital and not a maternity hospital.

Salpingitis is inflammation of the uterine tube or tubes. It is caused by infection from the vagina and uterus, e.g. gonorrhoea, or following abortion or childbirth. Infection may enter from the peritoneal cavity in which there may be some generalised infection, e.g. from the appendix, or by the blood stream, e.g. tuberculosis. The patient is ill with fever and has lower abdominal pain. There may be a vaginal discharge. The cause is treated when known, and medical and nursing treatment included for the infection. The condition may recur. Partial or complete closure of the uterine tubes is a complication and leads to sterility or ectopic pregnancy.

Gonorrhoea infection by gonococci is transmitted during sexual intercourse and can cause inflammation of the urethra as well as inflammation of the tissues of the uterus, uterine tubes and the peritoneum. There is a highly infectious purulent discharge from the uterus through the vagina. Sterility may follow the complication of salpingitis. Women who suspect they have gonorrhoea are encouraged to attend a special clinic where details of their illness are regarded as confidential and names need not be used but records are kept. Treatment is by large doses of penicillin and admission to hospital is not usually necessary. The organism causing the disease has shown signs of becoming resistant to penicillin. As with other infectious diseases it is important to prevent spread of the disease, and to trace contacts so that they may be treated also.

The conjunctiva of the eyes is susceptible to this infection, and one complication of gonorrhoea in the female is that when she gives birth to a baby and she has a gonococcal discharge in the vagina, the baby's eyes will become infected as he passes through the birth canal. The resulting conjunctivitis can cause blindness. It is prevented by treatment of gonorrhoea before and during pregnancy and in suspected cases, when the mother is suspected to be infected with gonorrhoea, eye-drops are instilled into the baby's eyes immediately after birth, as prescribed by the doctor.

Trichomonas is an organism which is able to move about in the vaginal secretion. It causes vaginitis and the discharge is yellowish white, frothy and intensely irritating to the skin. Treatment is by medicated pessaries or a vaginal cream prescribed by the doctor and it is continued throughout the menstrual period when the organisms are more active. Flagyl is an oral drug frequently prescribed for this condition.

Monilia, a fungus, also causes vaginitis and produces a white curdy discharge. This organism is in the air and can occur elsewhere in the body, e.g. the mouth (when it is known as 'thrush'), the intestines and the lungs. It is treated by Nystatin, an antibiotic effective in fungus infections.

TUMOURS. As in other parts of the body these are of two main types: (a) simple or benign, (b) malignant. The *simple tumours* include fibroids of the uterus, or more accurately fibro-myomas, for they arise in the uterine muscle tissue. There may be one large tumour and this is removed surgically, leaving the uterus intact, or a number of small round fibroids. When these cause menorrhagia, hysterectomy (removal of the uterus) is usually necessary. *Malignant tumours* of the uterus are either of the body or in the cervix. The former is more common in women who have not had children and can be removed in the early stages. Occasionally radium is used first, and the operation may be followed by deep X-ray therapy.

The cervix is very close in anatomical position to the ureters, the bladder and the rectum and these may be involved in early stages of carcinoma of the cervix. Treatment is by radium or surgical removal of the total uterus, upper part of the vagina, both uterine tubes, both ovaries and surrounding lymph nodes. This operation means to the patient that she will not menstruate, neither will she have any children, and there will be an early menopause because the ovaries have been removed. Hormone treatment is prescribed to offset these effects.

Diagnosis of the very early cases of carcinoma of cervix by cervical cytology is possible.

Women who are advised to have this examination are those in the reproductive phase of life and usually over 20 years of age.

Attendance at a clinic is arranged. A 'smear' of the cervix is taken. (There is no pain or discomfort in this procedure.) The result is examined by an expert. If cells are seen to be slightly different from normal these are removed in a simple operation. The test is repeated at intervals, e.g. 3 yearly.

The main sign in cancer of the uterus is vaginal bleeding between or after the periods, i.e. metrorrhagia. This irregular bleeding can be confused with erratic menstrual periods at the menopause. A woman with irregular vaginal bleeding or bleeding after the menopause is advised to see her general practitioner without delay. He refers her to a consultant surgeon and investigations and treatment in hospital follow immediately.

Other tumours in the reproductive tract include those of the ovary. These are variable, some are small cysts and easily removed and a few contain fluid and may become very large. Malignant cysts or tumours arise in some women, especially after the menopause, and give rise to pain and ascites.

New growth of the vulva is a malignant condition in elderly women beginning by an ulcer or white patches on the vulva. Vulvectomy is performed by the surgeon and the patient needs skilled nursing treatment but recovery is usually satisfactory.

THE NURSE'S APPROACH to patients with a gynaecological condition:

The patients include women of all ages, but girls before puberty are usually admitted to a children's hospital. Tact and consideration are necessary when nursing a girl or young adolescent in a gynaecological ward; she appreciates strict privacy, and may be embarrassed by the references to the various illnesses in the ward, so professional discussion is best reserved for sister's office. The woman who has had an abortion, or wanted children and not been able to have them may be reticent in this particular group of patients. Older women who, in their youth, were led to understand that gynaecological operations are extensive and disabling, need reassurance and to be persuaded to become mobile early after operation. The general atmosphere of the ward is cheerful and optimistic. The patients are appreciative of their treatment and the sympathetic understanding which the nurses can give each of them as individuals.

In carrying out the nursing techniques, an adequate knowledge of the anatomy and physiology of the reproductive system is necessary. Screens and curtains are used carefully to ensure the patient's complete privacy. She needs often to be reassured; this is accomplished by an explanation of the procedure together with the nurse's efficiency. The result will be the relaxation which is essential before any nursing procedure is begun. She will be more comfortable if she has recently used a bed-pan to pass urine.

The prevention of cross-infection is important and the nurse carries out appropriate methods of social cleanliness, sterilisation and disinfection. Manual dexterity is also required, for gentleness is a combination of consideration, muscle co-ordination and practice.

As in all bed-side techniques, the nurse is expected to make observations and report them intelligently. She may be required to make some record of the procedure.

Before operation the surgeon or a deputy explains to the patient what the operation entails, how it will relieve her symptoms and the ultimate result of the operation on her as a person, and she gives consent to the operation or treatment. It is useful for any medical practitioner when she attends for advice in the future to know which operations she has had. If the pupil nurse finds in her conversation that the patient does not know the name of the operation or what it means in clear, simple language, she informs the sister, who will explain to the patient or refer the matter to the surgeon.

In many cases relating to the future possibility of a married woman having or not having children, the operation is discussed with the husband as well as with the patient.

Nursing Techniques

CLEANSING OF THE VULVA is best carried out in the bath or by washing the area with soap and water and drying well during the daily bed-baths. This is a preliminary to vulval swabbing which is necessary before aseptic technique such as urethral catheterisation, and clean techniques like vaginal irrigation, and also when there is a vaginal discharge during the puerperium or in some forms of vaginitis.

Preparation and position of the patient is as for vaginal examination and adequate lighting is available. The nurse washes and dries her hands.

The swabs are held in sterile forceps or in the gloved hand when the procedure precedes an aseptic technique, otherwise they are held in the right hand, while the fingers of the left hand separate the labia. The parts of the vulva are swabbed in an anterior-to-posterior direction to prevent E. Coli infection from the anal sphincter and perineum.

The labia majora are swabbed alternately, followed by the labia minora and the vestibule, using each swab once only before it is discarded. The lotion used depends on the purpose of the procedure to follow, warm sterile water or a non-irritating antiseptic. It is important that the labia and the perineum should be left quite dry or the skin will become sore. A sterile vulval pad may be necessary. An observation may have been made, e.g. discharge from the urethra or vagina, lack of cleanliness, ulcers.

VAGINAL IRRIGATION. A funnel and a catheter No. 8 are used. Glycerine may be ordered as an alternative to a watery fluid, and about 60 ml will be prepared. This medication is hygroscopic and attracts the normal secretions. Debris and bacteria are discharged from the vagina with the glycerine so the ultimate result is a *cleansing of the vagina*. The patient needs a vulval pad.

VAGINAL PACKS are inserted with aseptic technique:
   (1) to sterilise the vaginal skin before operation;
   (2) to prevent infection from entering the uterus; *or*
   (3) to assist in controlling uterine haemorrhage.

Packs are rolls of sterile gauze 5 to 7 cms in width according to the reason for the procedure and 1 to 3 rolls may be prepared. They are used dry or medicated as ordered. Sponge-holding forceps, a speculum and adequate lighting are prepared. It is important that a record is made of the number of packs inserted so that, when they are to be removed in 24 hours, there is no risk of a pack being left in the vagina.

THE INSERTION OF MECHANICAL PESSARIES, which include the ring pessary for prolapse of the uterus and the Hodge pessary for retroverted uterus, is a skilled technique and carried out by the doctor. The pessary must be firmly in position and not cause friction or unwanted pressure. The patient returns for a review in three months' time, but reports in the meantime if there is pain, discomfort or discharge.

INSERTION OF MEDICATED TABLETS OR PESSARIES. The vulval area is washed and dried or swabbed, and a clean plastic glove is used to introduce the tablet or pessary $7\frac{1}{2}$ cm into the vagina.

The Breast

The breasts of the female begin to develop at puberty, being influenced by the female hormone activity which commences at that time. They are organs of glandular tissue supported by fat, and situated on the pectoralis muscles of the thorax. Ducts from the glands open on to the nipple, which is surrounded by skin slightly darker than that elsewhere.

After childbirth the glands secrete milk, which is extracted through the nipple by the infant sucking at the breast. The secretion of milk is stimulated by this sucking activity. Successful breast feeding continues for about five or six months until weaning, which begins at three to four months, is complete. It is part of the normal mother–infant relationship.

At middle age the glandular tissue disappears, and is replaced by fibrous tissue. The fatty tissue remains, and may even increase.

If the breasts are very well developed or enlarged in the lactating period some support is needed. This should be a brassiere of correct size. with the support beneath the breasts. Proper fitting is essential for comfort.

The breasts in the male do not develop. Occasionally in newly born infants the breasts are large and may even secrete a little milk. This is due to an excess of female hormone from the mother remaining in the infant's blood. It is of very short duration, and is not abnormal.

Diseases of the Breast

Acute mastitis is inflammation of the breast due to infection. It usually occurs during the time the mother is feeding her infant and may be the result of lack of hygiene or a cracked nipple. The breast is tender and tense with throbbing pain. The mother has a raised temperature and feels ill. She usually stops feeding the baby and there is treatment for localised infection. She is instructed regarding hygiene in care of the breasts during lactation. The baby will be given modified cow's milk feeds.

Simple (benign) tumours of the breast may consist of a large single tumour or several small ones. They are usually removed, though they need not cause anxiety.

Carcinoma of the breast occurs most frequently between the ages of 40 and 60 years. Because of the possibility of this disease, all single tumours of the breast are removed and the tissue is examined in the laboratory. After diagnosis the surgeon decides on the form of treatment and this may be:

(a) Removal of the breast, part of the pectoralis muscle and the local lymph nodes—this is radical mastectomy.

(b) Radical mastectomy either before or after radiotherapy treatment to local lymph nodes.

(c) Hormone treatment, e.g. by testosterone before the menopause, or stilboestrol after the menopause. Deep X-ray treatment is applied to the tumour if this cannot be removed.

Radical mastectomy. The patient loses fluid from the wound during this operation and replacement by intravenous infusion may be necessary. Fat and skin have been removed and the remaining edges of the skin are drawn together by sutures. Tissue fluid may collect beneath the wound and would cause tension but a small tube at the axillary end of the wound assists in draining this fluid. This process is assisted sometimes by the use of a suction motor. A firm mastectomy bandage prevents oedema and supports the wound.

Broncho-pneumonia in elderly women is prevented by breathing exercises and early movement.

To prevent stiffness in the upper limb on the side from which the breast was removed, the patient is encouraged to move that limb from 12 hours after operation. A suitable exercise is brushing the hair at the back of her head every hour in the day, using the affected arm.

Many women are distressed when they realise this operation is necessary because it will alter their appearance. They are reassured at the same time the operation is explained to them that a brassiere can be obtained for them which has a special filling on the affected side and allows normal movement for the arm and chest.

Diseases of the breast in the male are unusual but carcinoma has been known.

CHAPTER 44 | OTHER ASPECTS OF
NURSING SERVICE

There are many aspects of nursing in which it is possible to specialise after registration or enrolment as a nurse. During training some experience may have been gained in one or more of these fields. Each has its own technical skills, but most important of all is the way in which a nurse may have to adjust herself to a totally different physical and emotional environment from the general ward, if she is to give of her best and find satisfaction in the new sphere of work.

1 Operating Theatre

Experience in this department is optional for both students and pupils. For those who are allocated for theatre experience it can mean, initially at any rate, a certain amount of excitement and fear.

Some nurses find the lack of contact with conscious patients very hard to bear, although they may find compensation for this in the very close team-work that must exist between all members of the staff and the surgeons and anaesthetists. This team-work is vital if the department is to be a safe place for patients to receive treatment in and a calm tension-free place for the staff.

The fundamental techniques that have to be learned by all nurses working in theatres are:

Preparation of the theatres.

Preparation, sterilisation and storage of instruments.

Preparation and sterilisation of equipment.

Management of the theatre table.

Positions used in operations.

Preparation of the anaesthetic room.

Care of patients during anaesthesia.

A theatre nurse must be quick, quiet, methodical and absolutely reliable in relation to cleanliness and sterility of equipment. She must be on the alert all the time for the unusual occurrence, both outside and inside the theatre, and cultivate a sense of anticipation whilst attending those who are anaesthetising, operating or assisting the surgeon. The 'runner' in the operation team is the only means by which those who are 'scrubbed up' can obtain emergency supplies, and is as important as any other member of the theatre team in efficiency, conscientiousness and co-operation.

2 The Out-Patients' Department

It is in this department that the patient and his relatives may receive their first impression of the hospital and its staff. The manner in which they are greeted and directed to the appropriate clinic will influence all their future dealings with the hospital and probably all other hospitals also.

Fear and anxiety are reduced by simple kindnesses and ordinary courtesy. When sudden and unexpected illness, however slight, necessitates a a visit to a hospital which is unfamiliar to the patient and his relatives, patience and tact are essential in dealing with enquiries, and any necessary instructions are given slowly in a clear uncomplicated explanation which the patient can understand without effort.

Patients arrive by ambulance, car or on foot, and it is usually arranged that vehicles can draw up by the main door of the out-patients' department. Wheel chairs may be used for transporting those who arrive by ambulance into the reception hall.

The patient is greeted as he enters and is made welcome by the nurse. A receptionist may perform this duty in hospitals where there are several clinics in which the nurses remain to attend to the patients during consultation with the doctor. The patient presents the letter from his medical practitioner, and he is directed to the appropriate clinic where the nurse reassures him and puts him at his ease. She explains briefly but simply what is going to happen. He is shown where the toilet is. A specimen of urine may be required. He undresses in a private cubicle in preparation for the medical examination. Washable dressing-gowns or towel coats are provided. Some assistance in undressing may be required from the nurse or relative.

In the meantime his relative or friend waits in the reception hall, which is comfortable and furnished in a bright and cheerful manner. Magazines are provided for reading, and refreshments may be available at a canteen counter in or adjoining the department. The patient, however, is advised not to have anything to eat or drink before the consultation as the extent of the examination is not yet known, and occasionally an anaesthetic is necessary.

The nurse notes any relevant points made by the patient and his relatives concerning his past or present illnesses and sometimes his social and domestic background, as this information may assist the nurse in the management of situations which arise. Some items of information may be of importance to the doctor. This is particularly necessary when the patient is very young, very old, cannot speak easily or cannot be easily understood.

Observations to be made are similar to those of a patient on admission to the ward. The nurse may be required to take the patient's temperature and pulse, to examine urine and test it for glucose and protein, and measure the patient's weight and height. She prepares him for examination by the doctor, and when necessary for X-ray examination. The doctor's requirements are also attended to, so that the consultations proceed without delay.

At the end of the examination and investigation the consultant physician or surgeon explains his findings and opinion of the patient. The relatives may also see the consultant physician or surgeon, who then writes to the patient's own medical practitioner. Knowledge of the patient's diagnosis, etc. is confidential to the patient, his relatives and the hospital staff concerned in his treatment and care.

If it is necessary for a patient who has attended a clinic alone to be admitted to a ward in the hospital his relatives are informed at once. The clinic nurse accompanies him to the ward, and introduces him to the ward sister.

3 Accident Department

Patients arrive by ambulance, car or on foot. They are suffering from injuries or acute illness. Severity of condition varies greatly; some injuries are minor or the illness is without complication and easily treated, but in certain cases the patient is dangerously ill, requiring immediate treatment and sometimes resuscitation. Assessment of the patient's condition on arrival is extremely important, and a sister or experienced staff nurse will be the nurse on duty at the 'front door' of the accident department.

A calm atmosphere of confidence and efficiency is necessary in this part of the hospital, and the patient will be reassured by this as he arrives. If he has arrived on foot, he is given a chair so that he can sit down, but when he has been brought in on a stretcher or is ill, he lies on a couch. Cot-sides are attached to the casualty bed-trolley when the patient is restless or unconscious.

Relatives or friends who may have accompanied him are directed to the Registration Office or desk, where they give details for record purposes. It may be possible for them to have a hot or cold drink from a cafeteria or milk machine while the patient is being examined and treated.

A nurse remains with the patient. If he is able to walk he is shown where the toilet is as he may have been travelling for some time before admission. Otherwise he is offered a urinal. A specimen of urine may be required for examination and testing.

He is undressed on instructions from the sister in charge in preparation for a medical examination. Some patients such as those suffering from shock, severe internal injuries or burns are not undressed until they have received emergency treatment.

The clothes are placed in a bag to which is fastened a label with the patient's name and the date. Sister instructs where the bag will be stored, or whether the clothing, etc. can be taken away by relatives. In an emergency admission the patient may have money or valuables on his person. With his permission these are placed at once in a safe, either in the department or in the administrative offices, and he is given a receipt. Special care of the patient's property is required when he is unconscious or unknown. If the name of an unconscious patient be known an identification label is attached to him, e.g. round the wrist or ankle.

The nurse makes observations as of any patient on admission. She is prepared to take his temperature, pulse and respiration, test his urine, or prepare him for examination and emergency treatment. Oxygen therapy may be ordered, and occasionally she is required to carry out artificial respiration. The doctor or sister may need equipment which the nurse prepares for their immediate use.

In the meantime the relatives are told by a senior member of the staff what is going on, and perhaps they need to know the reason why they must wait in the department. When the patient is extremely ill and no relatives have arrived with him, they are informed by telegram or by the police. A priest or chaplain is also informed. Following serious accidents or attempted homicide the police may make investigations, and the sister in charge arranges this with them. There may be enquiries from the press reporters, and sister deals with these.

The casualty nurse needs always to be calm, quick and efficient. She should be generous in sympathy and service, and sometimes great courage and self-control are required of her.

4 District Nursing

Most families have had the experience of nursing a sick relative at home, and the hospital-trained nurse will understand how much improvisation and skill are needed to look after the patient competently. The demands on our District Nursing Service are increasing all the time as our patients are discharged home earlier, and more patients, such as children and old people, are kept at home under the care of their general practitioner in preference to hospital care.

Enrolled nurses are now being employed by many local health authorities to work with registered nurses in the District Nursing Service, which is a most important part of the National Health Service.

Apart from the skills of improvisation and the adaptation of hospital techniques to the home environment, the district nurse needs to be able to adapt herself to each home that she visits. In hospital, she is the hostess to her patients, receiving them with courtesy, nursing them with skill and kindness. On the district she becomes the invited guest in each home she visits, and her welcome and her nursing results will depend as much on her good manners as her professional skillls.

The Queen's Institute of District Nursing has set the pattern for teaching registered and enrolled nurses how to adapt their hospital nursing techniques to the home environment, and how to work under the supervision of general practitioners, and in co-operation with other health social workers.

The Queen's Institute awards certificates to nurses who complete a course of training, and pass a written and practical assessment.

Nurses who work on the district find great satisfaction in their work, mainly because of their close contact with their medical and other Health Service colleagues, and also because of the amount of responsibility they can take and the initiative they are encouraged to show.

The latest development is for Group Medical Practices to employ nurses and social workers to care for their own patients.

5 Psychiatric Nursing

An increasing number of general hospitals are opening psychiatric units, and whilst the majority of the nursing staff in these wards and departments will have received specialised training, some students and pupils will be allocated for short periods of experience. In any case, many physically sick people suffer some degree of mental upset, and all nurses should be aware of the signs and symptoms which would indicate the beginning of or the increasing mental illness of their patient.

As in other specialised fields of nursing, the environment both physical and emotional is very different from the general ward, and the inexperienced nurse may be concerned by an apparent lack of treatment and a totally different tempo of ward and departmental life. As she becomes more experienced she will realise that not only is the physical and emotional environment part of the treatment for each patient, but that she is too. It is the establishment of good relationships with her patients which will take all her qualities as a person and as a nurse to make and maintain.

The aim of psychiatric nursing is to heal the diseased mind and to return the patient to his family and the community as quickly as possible. Where cure is impossible, the patient may still be able to return home, provided he receives adequate medical and social support. For a few a return to the community is impossible, and they need constant help even to live in an acceptable way within the hospital community.

For many years there has been a separate register for nurses who have completed a three-year course of training in a psychiatric hospital, and now it is possible to become enrolled in this aspect of nursing after a two-year training. Both training periods may be shortened if the nurse is already trained in general nursing.

6 Mental Sub-normality Nursing

This aspect of nursing calls for a tremendous amount of patience and dedication. Whilst it is now recognised that many subnormal people respond to special educational methods and some may even be able to lead a useful life in the community, there are many who are ineducable, and some who will be bed-fast all their lives. It is these patients whom the nurses know will never leave them, and their care calls for the highest devotion. The roll for this speciality has now been opened and again a two-year training is offered to pupil nurses or a shortened period if general training has been completed.

7 Occupational Health Nursing

This branch of nursing was pioneered in Great Britain at the end of the nineteenth century when Phillipa Flowerday was employed by a firm of mustardmakers to look after their employees both at work and at home. Since then many industrial and commercial firms have started health services, usually individually but sometimes in group schemes. Occupational health nursing offers opportunities to enrolled nurses to work as members of a team whose objects are to promote and protect the health of employer and employee.

No special training is available for enrolled nurses, so it is recommended that they should always work with or under the supervision of a registered nurse who may hold the Occupational Health Nursing Certificate of the Royal College of Nursing or of the Birmingham Accident Hospital. Good experience in casualty and out-patient departments and also in district nursing is a sound basis for nursing in industry, as it combines practical nursing with health and safety supervision.

8 Other Specialities

An increasing number of special hospitals, i.e. Ophthalmic, Ear, Nose and Throat, and special units within General Hospitals, i.e. Theatres, Coronary, Kidney and Intensive Care Units are offering In-service Courses to both registered and enrolled nurses. Particulars of these can be obtained from the individual hospitals. To control the standard of these courses, the profession has set up a Joint Board of Clinical Nursing Studies from whom a list of approved Courses will be available.

FURTHER READING

Care of the Colostomy. A pamphlet for patients. St Thomas's Hospital

Home Management of a Colostomy. Pamphlet for patients. Hallam Hospital, West Bromwich.

Advice to a Patient with an Ileostomy. St Charles' Hospital, London

Stroke—A Diary of Recovery by D.Ritchie. Faber & Faber

A Guide to Medical and Surgical Nursing by Bendall and Raybould. H.K.Lewis.

Modern Gynaecology with Obstetrics for Nurses by Hector and Bourne. Heinemann

Other Aspects of Nursing

Illustrated Guide for Theatre Nurses by Matthias Penfold and Fry. Butterworth.

Essentials of Out-patient Nursing by C.Rayner. Almington Books

District Nursing by Merry & Irvin. Ballière, Tindall & Cox

Handbook for Occupational Health Nurses by M.West. Arnold

Psychiatry for Nurses by J.Gibson. Blackwell

Nursing the Mentally Retarded by Gibson & French. Faber & Faber

Home from Hospital. M.Skeet. Dan Mason Research Committee

INDEX

Abbreviations in prescription 169
Abdomen, distension after operation 209
structure 224
and function, in movement 247
See also Stomach, Intestines, etc
Abortion 478
complete 479
incomplete 479
threatened 479
Abortion Act 479
Abscesses, causes formation and treatment 236
cerebral 39
Accident—Emergency Department 405, 493
Accommodation of the eye 408
Acetest 125
Acids, swallowing 350
Activity, observation of patient 252
Adenoids, enlargement 436
Adenoma 217
Administrative service 20
Admission, bathing the patient 101
principles 85
Adoption 477
Adrenal cortex 457
disorders 457
hormones, undersecretion 457
Adrenal medulla, hormones 458
Adrenaline 458
use as treatment 458
Air, humidified 324, 325
inhalation 324
Air-way, mechanical 203
Albumin, in urine 379
Albustix 125
Alcoholism, acute, management 405
Alimentary tract 337
anatomy 337
clinical investigation 347
disease, signs and symptoms 346
in health and illness 343
medical and surgical conditions 349
Alkalies, swallowing 350
Ambulant patient, care 75
Ambulation, ward routine 36
Amenorrhoea 469
Amputations, management 268
Anaemia 285

blood transfusion for 300
cause 286
iron-deficiency 286
pernicious 286, 352
Anaesthetic, recovery from 203
Anorexia 346
Angina pectoris 290, 291
Ante-natal care 471
Antibodies, functions 175
Antiseptics 184
skin 185
Anti-tetanus serum 174
Apnoea 314
Appendicitis, acute, treatment, complications 354
Appetite, loss 346
Arteries 280
Arteriograms 287
Arterioles 280
Arthritis, rheumatoid 256
rehabilitation 256
septic 255
Artificial kidney 385
Ascites, in congestive heart failure 292
Aseptic technique 182
for dressing wounds 185
Asphyxia 435
after operation 208
Aspiration of stomach contents 204
Asthma, bronchial 321
Astigmatism 409
Atheroma 291
Atrial fibrillation 289
Atrophy, muscle 251
Audiogram 423
Auditory area of the brain 420
Augustinian Sisters 5
Auriscope 422
Autoclaves 183
high-pressure 183
low-pressure 184
Autonomic nervous system 392

Baby, care, at birth 473, 475
normal milestones 144
Bacilli, identification 172
Bacillus Calmette Guerin (B.C.G.) 321
Bacillus coli 172
Back, muscles 245
Back-rests 89

Bacteria, classification   172
Bacteriological Service   12
Balance, sense   420
Bandages   213, 417
  breast   216
  care and use   50
  ear   216, 427
  eye   216
  manytail   214, 215
  roller   213, 214
  T-   214
  triangular   214, 215
  tubular   214, 215
  varicose veins   216
Bandaging   213
  patterns   215
  rules for   214
Baptism, emergency   476
Barbituate poisoning, management   404
Bartholin's glands   467
Barrier nursing   191
Basal metabolic rate   368, 459
Basic needs   26
Basil the Great, Bishop of Caesarea   5
Bath, cleaning   102
Bathing, infants   142
  the patient on admission   101
  the patient in the bathroom, proce-
    dure, 101
  the patient in bed   97
    equipment   99
    preparation   99
    privacy   98
    procedure   100
Bed(s), care and use   48
  cradles   89
  linen, infected   179
  making, principles   88
    reasons   92, 93
    simple   91
  nursing care of patient in   59
  pans   118
    care and use   49
  sterilisation   180
  sides   90
  sores   60
    in children   144
    degrees   235
    prevention   114, 131, 232
    in traction patients   275
    treatment   117
  tables   90
Behaviour   394
Bile   342
  function   340
Bladder   375

carcinoma   381
conditions   380
function, after operation   205
  in unconscious patient   133
rupture   380
stones   381
Blankets, care and use   48
Blepharitis   414
Blindness, rehabilitation   417
Blood, circulation   230
    during illness   231
  clinical investigations   284
  components   223
  count   284
  disease, symptoms and signs   284
  groups   284
  physiology   278
  pressure, changes in heart disease
    290
    method of taking in children   139
  sugar urea   285
  transfusion, checking of blood   302
    equipment   301
    observation of apparatus   302
    observations of patient   302
    procedure   301, 302
    reasons   300
    Service   12, 303
  vessels   280
    diseases, clinical investigations   287
      and conditions   287
    grafts or repairs   289
    symptoms and signs   287
Board of Governors   10
Boils, cause, formation and treatment
    236
  ear   423
  nose   433
Bone marrow, see Marrow
Bones, in disease   249, 251
  face   244
  head   243
  in health   248
  lower limb   247
  neck   243
  rigidity, and prolonged bed rest   60
Body, structure   223
    and functions   242, 243
Bottles, changing during infusion   299
  feeding sterilisation   185
  hot-water   90
Bowel action, after operation   205
  function in unconscious patient   133
  large, cancer   356
Brain, anatomy   389
  stem   391

Brain—*cont.*
  tumours 399
Breasts, diseases 489
  enlargement, in newborn 489
  mastectomy 489
  structure 489
  tumours 489
Breathing exercises 309
Bronchial asthma 321
Bronchioles 305
Broncho-pneumonia, prevention 132
  and prolonged bed rest 60
Bronchitis 318
Bronchogram 316
Broncho-pneumonia 318
Bronchoscopy 316
Bronchus 305
Buddhists 70
Burns, first aid management 157

Calcium, in diet 327
  requirement 248
Calorie, requirements 327
  use, in body 327
Cancer, *see* organs and regions of the
  body
Carbohydrates 326
Carbon monoxide poisoning 322
Carbuncles 236
Carcinoma 217 *see also* organs and
  regions of the body
Cardiac arrest 152, 289
  asthma 293
  massage, external method 152
Cardiospasm 349
Cardiovascular system 278
  in disease 283
  in health 283
Care, basic 78
  intensive 79
  progressive 77
Caries, dental 446
Casilan, 331, 335
Cataract 414
Catheterisation, bladder 377
  preparations 386
  procedures 385
Catheters, self-retaining 388
Cells, body, definition 223
  white, in blood, function 175
Central nervous system 391
Cerebellum, anatomy 390
Cerebro-spinal system 391
Cerebro-vascular accident, hemiplegia,
  nursing care 402
Cerebrum, anatomy 389

Cervix, carcinoma 481, 486
  smear 486
Chairs, care and use 48
  making comfortable 74
Chest 223
  aspiration 317
    procedure 317
Chicken-pox 193
Childbirth 472
  emergency, management 474
Children, administering medicines to
  144
  admission 138
  bathing 142
  feeding 140
  normal milestones 144
  nursing 138
  observations and examinations 138
Cholecystectomy 358
Cholecystitis, acute 358
  chronic 358
Chorea 291
Choroid 406
Christian Scientists 69
Chronic sick, special needs 147
Circulation, extracorporeal 300
  portal 281
  pulmonary 280
Circumcision 383
Cirrhosis of the liver 357
Cleanliness, body 66
Cleft palate 254
Clinistix 125
Clinitest 125
Clostridia, identification 172
Clothes, patients, storing 50
Clothing, suitability, patients in bed
  63
Club-foot 254
Coeliac disease 353
Cold, common 318, 433
Colon, physiology 341
  washout 367
Colostomy 356
  management 356
Coma, diabetic 371
Commodes 119
Communicable diseases 192
Communication by patients 67
Complan 330, 335
Conception 470
Concussion 264
Condition, changes in, observation 128
Congenital dislocation of the hip 254
Conjunctivitis 414
Consciousness, levels 265, 395

Constipation 347
  management 345
  after operation 210
  relief 59
Contraception 478
Convalescence 76
Convulsions 250, 295
Cooling, in high temperature 452
Co-ordination, loss 395
Cornea 406
  injury, ulceration 410
Coronary thrombosis, management 291
Cortico-steroids, oversecretion 457
Cortisone 457
Cosmetics, in hospital 233
Cranial surgery 401
Cranium 223
Cretinism 460
Crockery, cleaning and sterilising 53
C.S.S.D. 184
Culdoscopy 482
Curtains, care and use 48
Cushions 90
Cutlery, cleaning and sterilising 53
  observation during 370
Cystocele 483
Cystitis 380
Cystoscopy 378
Cytotoxic drugs 218

Dangerous Drug Cupboard 161
Dangerous Drugs Act 161
Deafness 421, 423
  causes 428
  congenital 428
  degrees 427
  rehabilitation 427
Death, customs surrounding 69
Deborah, the first nurse 4
Defaecation, act 341
  problems during illness 344
Dehydration, after operation 204
Dentures, care 113, 445
Derbyshire neck 460
Dermatitis 238
Dermis, structure 227
Dextran 295
Dextrose 351
Diabetes insipidus 457
Diabetes mellitus 368
  diagnosis 369
  and pregnancy 481
  treatment 369
    observations during, 370
Diabetic Association 371
Diacetic acid in urine 125

Dialysis 385
Diaphragm 246
Diarrhoea 347
  management 345
Dickens, Charles 5
Diet, in diabetes 332
  emergency 372
  factors controlling 328
  fluid 330
  and food, religious considerations 69
  gastric 331
  gluten-free 331
  high-protein 331
  low-fat 331
  low-protein 331
  after operation 204
  requirement for bone 248
  special 330
  weight-reducing 331
  without milk 332
Digestion in small intestine 340
  in the stomach 340
Digitalis administration 293
Dilatation of cervix and curettage of
    uterus 482
Diphtheria 193
Disabled Persons (Employment) Acts
    1944 and 1958 12
Disasters, major 160
Discharge, hospital preparation for 78
  principles 85, 87
  self 88
Discharge from wounds and drainage
    206
  disposal 181
  vaginal 481
Disease, causes 148
  treatment 148
Dislocation, first aid management 156
  management 258
    cervical spine 258
    hip, 259
Disposable equipment, collection and
    disposal 188
  use in hospital 186
Disseminated sclerosis 400
District Nursing 494
Drainage from the chest 207
  postural 326
  tube 207
  under-water in lung surgery 323
  from wounds 206
Dressing, care and use 50
  disposal 181
Dressing station, care and use of equip-
    ment 50

Dressing and undressing a patient in bed 64
Drop foot, prevention 110, 249
Drops, instillation into ear 426
  eye 415
Drugs, administration 163
  during intensive care 81
  by mouth 163
  under tongue 164
  checking 162
  dangerous 162
  eye 417
  habit-forming 162
  inhaled 325
  overdose, management 403
  see also Medicines
Duodenum 340
Dust, removal, to prevent infection 178
Dying, care of 134
Dysmenorrhoea 469
Dysphagia 346, 435
Dyspnoea 314

Ear-ache 422
  bandaging 427
  care during health and illness 421
  conditions 423
  discharges 422
  drops, instillation 426
  examination 422
  inner, diseases 425
  internal, 419
  investigation 422
  middle 419
  nose and throat 418
  nursing techniques 426
  signs and symptoms 421
  structure and function 419
  tenderness 422
Eclampsia 480
Ectopic gestation 480
Education Act 1944
Ego-structure 25
Electric pads 91
Electro-encephalogram 396
Electrolytes, after operation 204
  balance 124, 266
Elevators 89
Embolism, cerebral 288
Embolus 287
  pulmonary 288
Emergencies, in intensive care unit 82
  urgent treatment 152
Endocrine system 389
Endotracheal tubes 59, 265

Enemas 361
  procedures 362, 363, 364
Enrolled nurse 7
Enteric fevers 194
Enteritis 352
Epidermis, structure 227
Epilepsy 399
  first aid management 159
Epistaxis 153, 430
  mild, treatment 432
Epithelium 223
Equipment, ward, care and use 48
Ethics, nursing 22
Etiquette, nursing 21
Eustachian tube 419
Eve's rocking method 152
Excreta, observation on 124
  see also Faeces, Urine, etc
Exercise, after operation 207
  foot 110
  hand 108
  muscle 428
Exophthalmos 410, 460
Expiration 304
External otitis, acute 424
  chronic 424
Eye, accessory organs 408
  anatomy 405
  applying drops 415
  applying ointments 415
  applying steam 416
  bandages 417
  care, during illness 410
  care in health 409
  disease and conditions 413
  disorders, nursing care 411
  drugs 417
  infections 413
  injuries 413
  investigations 412
  irrigation 416
  observations 412
  prevention of infection 410
  prevention of injury 409
  shape, abnormalities 409
  structure 406
  swabbing 416
  symptoms and signs 412

Fabiola 7
Face, bones 244
  expressions, muscles used 245
  injuries, management 262
Factories Acts 1937 13
Faeces, abnormalities 126
  in children 139

Faeces—*cont.*
  collection 127
  disposal 180
    during enteric fever 180
  examination 347
  impacted, management 345
  incontinence 347
  observations of 126
Fallot's tetralogy 294
Family Allowance 12
Family Planning Association 478
Farsightedness 409
Fats, absorption 330
  animal, in diet 327
  in diet 327
  vegetables in diet 327
Feeding, infant 140
    artificial 141
  naso-oesophageal 332
  oral-oesophageal 336
  patients 344
  under-feeding 140
Feet, care 109
  exercises 110
  function 247
Fertility 476
Fever, nursing care 196
Fibroids 485
Fibroma 217
Fire, extinguishers 51
  instructions in case of 56
  precautions 55
First Aid, equipment in factories 13
  object 149
  qualifications 148
Fits 395
  first aid management 159
Flatus, retention after operation 209
  relief 210
Floors, care and use 48
Fluid, administration in heart surgery,
    intravenous 295
  balance charts 123
  measuring 122
  intake 123
  output 123
Food, poisoning 352
  preparation 52
    and prevention of infection 179
  storage 52
Foot board 89
Foreign bodies, first aid management
    159
  nose 431
  in small intestine 355
  swallowed, management 350

  throat 437
Fracture boards 89
Fractures, complications 263
  first aid treatment 155
  jaws 448
  management, 259
  nose 431
  reduction 261
  reduction, by traction 272
    fixed 274
    methods 272
    preparation 273
    sliding 274
  signs and symptoms 260
  treatment 261
    immobilisation 262
  types 259
Fry, Elizabeth 5

Gait 394
Gall-bladder, function 342
  medical and surgical conditions 358
Gangrene 171
  cause 268
Gas gangrene 173
Gases, interchange in lungs and body
    tissues 308
Gastric analysis 347
  aspiration, procedure 359
  juice 339
  suction 359
Gastritis 350
Gastroscopy 348
Gastrostomy 336, 352
General Dental Services 11
General Medical Services 10
General Nursing Council 7, 16
General Practitioner Services 10
Geriatrics, care in 145
  maintenance 146
  psychological help in 146
  rehabilitation 146
  special needs 145
German measles 192
Giddiness 422
Gingivitis 447
Glands, adrenal 457
  endocrine 455
  parathyroid 461
    disorders 461
  parotid 441
  pituitary 456
    posterior lobe, damage 456
  salivary 441
  sebaceous 229
  sweat, structure 229

Glands—*cont.*
 thyroid 459
  clinical investigations 459
  disorders 459
Glaucoma 414
Glucose in urine, test 125
Gluten-free diet 353
Goitre 460
Gonococci 172
Gonorrhea 196
 dangers in pregnancy 481, 485
Grooming, of patients in bed 66
Group Medical Practice 495
Gynaecology, conditions 483
 disorders, nurse's approach 486
 nursing techniques 487
 examinations 482
 signs and symptoms 481

Haematemesis 153, 346, 351
Haematest 126
Haematuria 153, 377
Haemoglobin 284
Haemoptysis 126, 153, 315, 319
Haemorrhage, after amputation operations 268
 after operation 208
 cerebral, and hemiplegia, nursing care 402
 in childbirth 476
 external, management 154
 following dental extraction 447
 management in emergency 153
 severe, management 285
Haemorrhoidectomy 357
Haemorrhoids 357
Haemothorax 319
Hair, patient's care 103, 232
 washing, in bed 104
 lice 105
  treatment 106
 structure, and distribution 227
Halitosis 346
Hallux valgus 254
Hand, exercises 108
 patient's, care 107
 structure and function 247
 washing, to prevent infection 182
Head, bones 243
 injuries, management 263, 264
  treatment and nursing care 264
   diet 266
   fluid and electrotype balance 266
   rehabilitation 266
   restlessness 266

 surgery 265
Headaches 394, 430
Heaf test 321
Health, communal 30
 personal 28
 return to 71
Hearing aids, importance 427
 in hospital 421
Hearing, pitch, intensity and quality 418
Heart, anatomy and physiology 281
 conditions, congenital 294
 diseases 290
  clinical investigations 290
  symptoms and signs 289
 failure 290
  congestive, management, and general nursing care 292
  left-sided 293
  pulmonary 294
 muscle, rate of activity 393
 operations 294
 surgery, preparation, fluid administration, intravenous 295
Heartburn 346
Heat, applied to the skin 239
 body, loss 450
  physiology 449
 dry 184
Heating, methods 40
Hemicolectomy 356
Hemiplegia, nursing care 402
Hepatitis, acute 357
Hernia, inguinal, umbilical, femoral 354
 strangulated 355
Herniorrhaphy 355
Herpes simplex 349
Herpes zoster 193
Hiatus hernia 349
Hindus, religious and dietary problems 69
Hoarseness 435, 461
Holger Neilsen's method 152
Hordeolum 413
Hormones 455, 456
 anterior pituitary, undersecretion 456
 antidiuretic 456
 growth, oversecretion 456
 sex 462
Hospital, departments, function 19
 Management Committees 10
 and specialist services 9
Hydrocephalus 398
Hygiene, communal 30
 personal 29

506 Index

Hygiene—*cont.*
  ward kitchen 51
Hypermetropia 409
Hyperpyrexia 452
Hypertension 291
Hypodermic needle, administering drugs
  164
Hypoglycaemic coma 371
Hypothermia 294, 454
  accidental 455

Ice poultices 257
Ileostomy 356
Immunisation 177, 192–3
Immunity, definition 175
  natural 175
  passive 177
Impetigo 237
Incinerators, ward, care and use 49
Incontinence, equipment 103
  faecal 347
  urine 376
Indigestion 346
Industrial nursing 495
Industrial Relations Act 1971 24
Infant, at birth, care 473, 475
  toilet 142
  See also Babies, Children
Infected bed linen and clothing, man-
  agement 179
Infection, body's defences 174
  droplet 178
  and inflammation 170
  local effects 171
  prevention 177
  regulation 177
  of spread 178
  sources 174
  of wounds 235
Infertility, investigations 477
Inflammation and infection 170
  treatment 171
Influenza, epidemic 195
Infra-red cabinets 184
Infusion, continuous, milk 337
  intravenous 295
    apparatus, taking down 299
    changing bottle 299
    equipment 296
    in infants and children 300
    observation of the patient 298
    preparation of patient 296
    procedure 297
    supervision of patient 297
  rectal 362, 364
    continuous 364

preparation and procedure 365
Inhalations in respiratory procedures
  324
  steam 324
Inhaler, Nelson's 324
Injection, hypodermic, administration of
  drugs 164
  procedure 165
  intramuscular, procedure 166
  intravenous, preparation 167
  subcutaneous, administration of drugs
    164
Injuries caused by articles near bed 67
Injuries, *see also* Head, Multiple etc.
  sources 170
Insomnia, relief 62
Inspiration 304
Instruments, care and use 50
  disinfectant 181
  sterilisation 184
Insulin 369
  production 462
    disorders 462
  protamine 370
  soluble 370
  strengths 370
  zinc suspension 370
Intensive care units, clinical investigations 82
  emergencies 82
  equipment 80, 82
  general environment 81
  nursing of patients 79, 83
  observations and reports 82
  reassurance of relatives 83
International Council of Nurses 18
  Code of Ethics 22
Intestinal juice 340
Intestine, small, absorption of foodstuffs
  340
  digestion 340
  disorders 352
Invalid cookery 53
Iodine, in diet 327
  deficiency 460
  radioactive, uptake 459
Iron, in diet 327
Irradiation, delay in wound healing
  235
Irrigation of eyes 416
Islets of Langerhans 464
  oversecretion 462
Isolation nursing 188
  in general ward 191
  in side ward 189
Izal 170

Jaundice 347
Jaws, fractures, treatment 448
Jehovah's Witnesses 69
Jews, care of, after death 135
 customs and diet 69
Joints
 cartilaginous 243
 disease 251
 fibrous 243
 in disease 249
 in health 248
 synovial 243

Kaolin poultices 239
Keloids, treatment 37–38
Ketosis coma 371
Kidneys, anatomy 373
 artificial 385
 calculi 380
 cancer 380
 functions 375
  after operation 205
 stones, and prolonged bed rest 60
 see also Nephritis, Urinary tract, etc.
Kitchen, food preparation 53
 ward hygiene 51
 storage of food 52
Kosher meat 69

Labour, emergency, management 474
 three stages 472
Labstix 125
Lachrymal apparatus 408
Language difficulties with patients 68
Laryngectomy, communication with patient after 68
Larynx 307
 carcinoma 435
 malignant growth 437
 trachea and bronchi, inflammation 437
Laying out 135
Legal aspects of hospital stay 85
Legal aspects of Nursing 24
Lens 406
Leucorrhoea 481
Leukaemia, acute myeloid 286
 chronic lymphatic 287
 chronic myeloid 287
Lice, body and head 105, 106
 removal 106
Lifting and moving the patient 94
Ligaments 243
Lighting 43
 and health of eyes 410

Limb, lower, bones 247
 shortening in 254
Linen, care and use 47
Lipoma 217
Liquids, measurement 169
Liver, function 342
 medical and surgical condition 357
Local Executive Councils 10
Local Health Authority Services 11
Lockers, care and use 48
Lockjaw 173
Locomotor system, medical and surgical conditions 254
 symptoms and signs 250
Lotions, measurements 170
Low-residue diet 355
Lumbar puncture, procedure 396
Lungs, anatomy 304
 cancer 321
 resection 323
 surgery, preparation of patients 322
 under-water drainage 323
Lymph, contents 303
 definition 303
 nodes 303
Lymphatic system 303
Lymphocytes 303

Malaena 153, 347, 351
Malnutrition 329
Marrow, failure to form blood 286
 puncture 285
Mastectomy 489
 radical 490
Mastitis, acute 489
Mastoid process 420
Mastoiditis, acute 425
Mattresses 88
 care and use 47
 and prevention of infection 180
Meals, ward, times 35
Measles 192
Measurement of liquids 169
Meatus, external auditory, cleaning 426
Medical Social Worker 213
Medicines, administering to children 144
 definitions 161
 state of 6
 storage 163
 see also Drugs
Membranes, serous, mucous and synovial 225
Menière's disease 425
Meninges 391
Meningitis 398
 tuberculous 398

Meningococci 172
Menopause 464
Menorrhagia 469
Menstrual cycle 467
Menstruation 468
  disorders 469
  hygiene 468
Mental apathy and prolonged bed rest
    61
  sub-normality nursing 495
Metabolic rate 368
  basal 368
Metabolism 367
  physiology 367
Metastases 217
Methyltestosterone 462
Metrorrhagia 469
Michel clips 205
Micturition, frequency 376
Milestones, normal, in children 145
Milk infusion, continuous 337
Minerals, deficiencies 329
  in diet 327
Mitral stenosis 294
Mohammedans 70
Moles 238
Monilia 485
Monoplegia 276
Morphine, excess, management 403
Mouth, abscess, aspiration 446
  administration of drugs by 163
  anatomy 337
  carcinoma 447
  care 344
    in health 441
    in illness 442
  cleaning, of ill patient 444
    of mentally confused patient 445
    of unconscious patient 445
  diseases 349
  examination 446
  hygiene in children 144
  investigations 446
  irrigation 443
  to-mouth breathing 312
  observations 445
  structure 438
  and teeth, care, 111, 443, 444
  toilet, after operation 205
Movement, muscle bone and joints 240
  observation of patient 252
  and posture in bed 60
  purposes 248
Moving and lifting the patient 94
Multiple injuries, management 267
Mumps 193

Muscles, in disease 249, 250
  face 245
  in health 248
  involved in movement 240
  neck 245
  tone, loss, and prolonged bed rest 60
Myasthenia gravis 401
Myopia 409
Myxoedema 460

Nails, care 107
  structure 227
Naso-oesophageal feeding 332
  equipment 333
  procedure 333
National Health Service Act 8
  ancillary services 12
  see also individual services
  finance 14
    future developments 14
  nurse's place 15
  structure 8
National Insurance Acts, 1946, 1948
    12
Nearsightedness 409
Neck, bones 243
  traction 274
Needles, sterilisation 184
Neomercasyl 461
Nephrectomy 383
Nephritis, acute and sub-acute 379
Nerves, cranial 391
  motor 391
  sensory 391
  severed 397
  spinal 391
Nervous system 388
  anatomy 389
  functions 392
  medical and surgical conditions 397
  symptoms and signs 394
Neurological examination of patient
    396
Nightingale, Florence 5
Night-time, nursing of patients 62
Nobecutaine 206
Noise, elimination 44
  intense, effect 421
  prevention 45
  source in hospital 45
Noradrenaline 458
  use in treatment 459
Nose, bleeding 430
  boils 433
  care in illness 430
  condition 431

Nose—*cont.*
  discharges 430
  examination 431
  infections 433
  injury 430
  investigations 431
  obstruction 430
  and pharynx, structure 428
  swab 431
  symptoms and signs 430
  throat, and ear 418
    infections 421
Nurse, derivation 3
  ethics 22
  etiquette 21
  and professional relationships 21
Nurses Act 1919 and 1943 7
Nurses and Midwives Whitley Council
    18, 23
Nursing, care of patient, basic 58, 78
    breathing 58
    nutrition 59
  development 3
  isolation 188
  minimum 77
Nutrition 326
  adequate, during intensive care 81
  of patient 59
  provision in unconscious patients 132

Obesity 329
  diet for 331
Observation of patient's response to
    treatment 128, 253
Occupational health nursing 495
Occupational Health Service 13
Occupational therapy 78, 79
  after operation 207
Oedema, in congestive heart failure
    295, 293
Oesophagitis 350
Oesophagoscopy 348
Oesophagus 339
  obstruction 349
  stricture 350
Oestrogens 463
Old people *see* Geriatrics
Operating theatre, techniques 491
Operations, *see* Surgery
Ophthalmic Services, supplementary 11
Opium, excess, management 403
Oral-oesophageal feeding 336
Orbit of the eye 408
Organ, definition 223
Osteo-arthritis 255
Osteoma 217

Osteomyelitis, acute 255
Otitis media, acute 424
Otorhinolaryngology 418
Out-patients' Department 491
Ovaries 465
Overfertility 478
Oxygen administration 310, 293
Oxygen-therapy, precautions 311
  tent 310

Paediatric nursing 138
Pain, in alimentary tract 347
  in bones 251
  following operation 209
  heart 290
  in muscle 250
  in traction patients 276
  urinary tract 376
  in wounds 235
Pancreas, diseases 358
  function 342
  head, carcinoma 358
Pancreatic juice 340
Pancreatitis, acute 358
Papilloma 381
Paralysis 394
  flaccid, muscle 250
  following spinal injury, treatment and
    care 276
  spastic 250
  see also Hemiplegia
Paraplegia, management 276
  nursing care 277
Parasites, intestinal 352
Parasympathetic nerve supply 392
Parathormone 461
Patients, accomplishments during illness
    72
  in bed, movement and posture 60
  in bed, toilet 59
  communication by 67
  convalescent 76
  dangers to 67
  nursing care, basic 58
  property 86
  recreation 70
  sitting, care 73
  toilet 97
Paula 7
Pediculosis, treatment 106
Pelvis, structure 224
Peripheral nervous system 391
Peristalsis 339
Peritonitis 354
  gonococcal 354
Personal development 24

Personality 28
  changes after injuries 395
Petit mal 400
Pertussis 192
Pessaries, insertion 488
Pharmaceutical Services 10
Pharynx 306
  in health and illness 434
  pain 435
  structure 434
  symptoms and signs 435
Phimosis 383
Phrenic nerve 392
Physiotherapy 78, 79
  after operation 207
Pillows, care and use 48
  and prevention of infection 180
Placenta 472, 476
Plasma, administration in heart surgery
    295
Plaster of paris splint, preparation 269
  arm, foot 269
  special care while drying 270
Plastic equipment, sterilisation 184
Plastic surgery 237
Platelets, physiology 279
Pleural effusion 319
Pneumococci 172
Pneumonectomy 323
Pneumonia 318
  acute lobar 318
  broncho- 318
  influenza 319
  staphylococcal 319
Pneumothorax 320
Poisoning, management 403
  first aid 157
Poisons Act 161
Poisons, definition 161
  schedule 161
  removal from stomach 361
Poliomyelitis 194, 399
  respiration in 309
Politics, influence on nursing 6
Pole and chain 89
Polypi, nasal 432
Portal circulation 281
Positions used in nursing 94
Post-operative nursing 203
Posture 309
Potasssium 295
  see also Electrolytes
Poultices, ice 257
  see also Kaolin
Prayers, children 69
  consideration for 69

Pregnancy, complication 478
  and diabetes 481
  ectopic 480
  in patients with general medical con-
      ditions 480
  signs and symptoms 470
  special observations 481
  termination 479
Pre-operative drugs 202
Pressure areas, care 114
  routine treatment 116
Pressure points 154
Presure sores, *see* Bed sores
Prestige 27
Progesterone 463, 466
Prolapse, uterus 483
Property, patient's 86
  management in infection 180
Proctoscopy 348
Prosthesis 268
Prostrate gland, enlargement 381
  treatment 382
Proteins 326
  in urine, test 125
Pruritus 482, 484
Psychiatric nursing 495
Public Health Services 30
Puerperium 473
Pulmonary cardiac failure 294
Pulmonary circulation 280
Pulmonary ventilation 309
Pulse, arterial 209
  method of measuring in children 139
  rate 394
  routine observations and method of
      taking 121
Pupils 406
  unequal 394
Pus 175
Pyelonephritis 380
Pyrexia 121, 394, 451
  and infection 171

Quadriplegia 276
Quakers 5
Queen's Institute for District Nursing
    495
Quinsey 326

Radiation sickness 218
  side-effects 218
Radiography *see* X-rays
Radiotherapy, nursing care 219
Rashes 238
Recreation for patients 70
Rectal washout 366

Rectocele 484
Rectum, administration of fluid into 361
    cancer 356
    drugs given by 364
    examination 348
    physiology 341
Red blood cells, physiology 278
Reflex action 392
Regional Hospital Boards 9
Registers (G.N.C.) 7
Rehabilitation 78
    in blindness 417
    deafness 427
    in geriatrics 146
    after operation 213
Religion, arrangements for 68
    diet and food 69
    influence 3
Renal failure 383
    causes 384
    effects 384
Reports, ward, giving, receiving and
        writing 129
Reproduction 226, 470
    organs, female 465
        male 464
Reproduction system 464
Respiration, act 305
    artificial 311
    causes of difficulty 307
    Cheyne-Stokes 314
    depth 314
    physiology 307
    in sleep 314
    and the respiratory tract 304
    routine observations, and method of
        taking 122
Respiratory arrest 152
Respiratory system, clinical investiga-
        tions 315
    diseases 318
    maintenance in disease 309
    maintenance in health 309
Rest, periods 63
Retention of urine 376
    acute 382
    treatment 382
Retina 406
Rhesus factor and blood transfusion of
        babies 300
Rheumatism, acute 290
Rickets 254
Rohere 5
Roll (G.N.C.) 7
Roman catholics, religious and dietary
        considerations 69

Roughage in diet 327
Rounds, doctors', and ward routine
        36
Routine observations and reports 120
Routine procedures 85
Royal College of Nursing 18
Rubber equipment, sterilisation 185
Rubbish, disposal 51
Rubella 192, 481
    and deafness 428
Rules, hospital 85, 86

St Bartholomew's Hospital 5
St Mary of Bethlehem Hospital 5
St Thomas's Hospital 5
Salicylate poisoning, management 404
Saliva 441, 442
    functions 338
Salmon Report on Senior Nursing Staff
        Structure 16
Salmonellae bacilli 172
Salpingitis 484
Salpingogram 477
Sani-chairs 119
Sarcoma 217
Scabies, treatment 106
Scalds, first aid management 157
Scalp wounds 263
Scar prevention 235
Scarlet fever 194
School Health Service 12
Sciatica 255
Screens, care and use 48
Scrotum 463
Sea-sickness 420
Sedation, before surgery 202
Self discharge 88
Semicircular canals 420
Sensation, loss 394
Sense organs 226
Sepsis, avoidance 182
Septum, deflected 431
Serum, anti-tetanus 174
Shafer's method 152
Sheepskin 116
Shingles 193
Shock, after operation 208
    electric 398
    management 155
Shoulder girdle 246
Sight 405
Sigmoidoscopy 348
Silvester's method 152
Sim's position 482
Sinus, tumours 434
Sinusitis 433

Sitting out of bed, ward routine   36
Sitting patient, care   73
Skeleton   224, 242
Skin   226
    application of medicaments   240
    circulation of blood   230
        during illness   231
    cleanliness   230
        during illness   231
    deformities   237
    during illness   231
    foreign objects, management   237
    functions   229
    general care   230
    heat applied to   239
    infections   236
    nursing procedures   239
    nutrition   230
        during illness   231
    observations   128
        on admission   233
        in children   138
        conditions affecting   234
        while in hospital   233
    plastic surgery   237
    protection   230
        antiseptics   185
        during illness   231
    rashes   238
    structure   227
Skull   223
    structure   243
Sleep, after operation, sedatives   209
    and rest for patient in bed   61
    ward, times   35
Small-pox   193
    vaccination   193
Smell, sense   430
    loss   430
Smith-Petersen nail   262
Smoking, effects   318
Soups   330
Spasms, muscle   250, 394
Specimens, collection   127
    labelling   128
Speculum, aural   422
Speech, impaired communication with
    patients   68
Spermatozoa   463
Spinal column, structure and function
    245
Spleen, rupture   358
Splenectomy   358
Splint, Braun's   271
    metal   271
    plaster of paris, preparation   269

plastic   271
Thomas's   271
wooden   272
Sprains, management   257
    first aid   157
Sputum, collection   127
    examination   315
    observations   126
Squint   415
Staphylococci, identification   172
Starches, in diet   326
Starvation   328
Status   27
Steam, application to eyes   416
    tent   325
Sterilisation   480
    methods, 183
    storage of equipment   187
Sterilisers, care and use   50
Steroids   457
Stilboestrol   463
Streptococci, identification   172
Stress-incontinence   482
Stitches, see Sutures
Stomach, anatomy   339
    cancer   352
    digestion   340
    diseases   350
    removal of poisons   361
    washout, purposes, procedure   360
Strabismus   415
Structure of the human body   223
Strychnine, poisoning, management   403
Styes   413
Sugars, in diet   326
    in urine, test   125
Suppositories, rectal   366
Surgery   199
    complications   208
    cranial   401
    examination and investigations   200
    heart   294
    preparation of patient   200
    routine nursing attention   211
    sedation and pre-operative drugs   202
Surgical equipment, sterilisation   184
Surgical nursing, routine   211
    see also Surgery
Sutures   205
    removal   206
    tension   205
Swab, throat   436
Swabbing eyes   416
Swallowing   339
    difficulty   435
Sweat   450

Sweat—*cont.*
  structure 229
Sympathetic nerve supply 392
Syphilis 195
  and pregnancy 481
Syringe, disinfection 181
  sterilisation 184
Systems, body 225

Talipes 254
Tears 408
Teats, sterilisation 185
Teeth 338, 439
  charts, deciduous and permanent 440
  cleaning 422
  extraction 447
  medical and surgical conditions 446
  and mouth, care 111, 112
  in unconscious patient 113
Temperature, body, maintaining normal
      range 65
    method of taking 120
      regulation 449
    method of taking, in children 139
    subnormal, relief 66
    reduction 65, 451
      nursing treatment 452
    routine observations 120
Tendons 243
Tenesmus 347
Terminal nursing 146
Testes 463, 464
Testosterone 462, 463
Tetanus 173, 250
Tetanus toxoid 174
Thermometers, sterilisation 185
Thiouracil 461
Thorax 223
  movement, muscles and bones 246
Throat, conditioning 436
  examination 435
  foreign object 437
  nose and ear 418
    infections 421
  swab 436
Thrombosis 288
  venous, after operation 210
Thrush 349
  in children 144
Thyroid crisis 461
Thyroidectomy, partial 461
Thyrotoxicosis 460
Thyroxine 368, 459
  undersecretion 459
Tinnitus 422
Tissue, body, definition 223

types 223
  connective 223
  germinal 224
  muscle, types 223
  nerve 223
Toilet, children's 143
  infant 142
  patient's 35
  training 143
Tongue 439
  administration of drugs under 164
  function 439
Tonsillectomy 436
Tonsillitis, acute 436
Tonsils 441
Torticollis 254
Tourniquet 154
Toxaemia, pre-eclamptic 480
Tracheostomy 312
Tracheotomy 437
Transfers, principles 85, 87
Transillumination 431
Traction, fixed 274
  -methods 272
  -nursing care 274
  -preparation 273
  -sliding 274
Treatment, observation of patient's re-
      sponse to 253
Tremor 394
Trichonomas 196, 485
Trigeminal neuralgia 401
Trolleys, care and use 50
Tubercle bacilli 172
Tuberculosis 195, 320
Tuberculous infection of the joints
      225
Tubes, drainage, shortening 207
  Jaques oesophageal 333
  Levin's 333
  nasopharyngeal 204
  Ryle's 333
  tracheostomy 312
Tumours 217
  benign 217
  malignant 217
  treatment 218
  types 217
  See also individual organs and regions
Twitchings, muscle 395
Typhoid fever 353

Ulcer, duodenal, chronic 350
  perforated 351
  gastric 351
  perforated 351

Ulcer—*cont.*
  peptic 350
  skin, mouth 238
Ulcerative colitis 355
  diet in 332
Unconsciousness 395
  first aid management 158
  muscles in 249
Unconscious patient, adequate airway
    131
  adequate nutrition 132
  bowel and bladder function 133
  nursing care 130
  prevention of bed sores 131
  prevention of broncho-pneumonia
    132
  prevention of damage to blood and
    nerves 132
  special observations 133
Uraemia 384
Ureters 375
Urethra 375
  conditions 382
  injuries 382
  stricture 383
Urethritis 382
Urinals 118
  care and use 49
  sterilisation 180
Urinary system 372
  clinical investigations 377
  observations 377
Urinary tract, injury 378
  medical and surgical conditions 378
  organs 372
  symptoms and signs 376
Urination difficulties, relief 60
Urine, collection 127
    in children 140
  diacetic acid in 125
  disposal, during enteric fever 180
  glucose in 125
  incontinence 376
  observations, in children 140
    and indications 124
  protein, test 125
  retention 376
    acute, treatment 382
    after operation 209
  sugar in, test 125
Uterine tube, insufflation 483
Uterus 467
  displacements 483
  prolapse 483
  retroverted 483
  tumours 485

  signs 486

Vagina 567
  bleeding 482
  examination 482
  irrigation 488
  packs 488
Varicose veins, bandaging 216
  treatment 288, 289
Veins, cutting down to in intravenous
    infusions 299
Ventilation, importance 37
  methods 38
Vertebrae 244
Vertigo 420, 422
Viruses, identification 174
Visiting times 36
Visual apparatus 406
Visitors, after operation 211
Vitamin B_{12} 340
  failure to absorb 330
Vitamin D requirements 248
Vitamins, deficiencies 329
  in diet 327
  in infant feeding 141
Voice, loss 435, 461
Voluntary organisation 79
Vomit, collection 127
  observations of 126
Vomiting 394
  indications 346
  management 344
  projectile 346
  and semicircular canals 420
Vulva 467
  cleansing 487
Vulvitis 484

Waking a sleeping patient 62
Ward, equipment, care and use
    48
  kitchen 51
  reports, giving, receiving and
    writing 129
  routine 34
    basic 35
    purpose 34
  side, in isolation nursing 189
Washing in bed 102
Water, in diet 327
Water-pillows 90
Wesley, John and Charles 5
White cells, physiology 278
Whitley Council 18, 23
Whooping cough 192
Women, status 6

Worms, intestinal, tape, thread and
        round 353
Wounds, aseptic technique for dressing
        185
    dangers and problems 234
    delay in healing 234
    haemorrhage 235
    operative, abdominal, break-down
        211
      complications 210
    pain 235
    scar prevention 235
    surgical, management 205
Wryneck 254

X-rays of bones and joints 251
    chest in heart disease 290
    gastro-intestinal tract 348
    head 396
    mass 316
    methods used in 218
    nose 431
    preparation of patient for examination
        252
    respiratory tract 316
    stomach 350
    teeth 446
    urinary tract 378